Universal Clinical Reasoning

Optimising the Approach and Care for Patients

Universal Clinical Reasoning

Optimising the Approach and Care for Patients

SOH Jian Yi

National University Hospital of Singapore
& National University of Singapore

World Scientific

NEW JERSEY · LONDON · SINGAPORE · BEIJING · SHANGHAI · HONG KONG · TAIPEI · CHENNAI · TOKYO

Published by

World Scientific Publishing Co. Pte. Ltd.
5 Toh Tuck Link, Singapore 596224
USA office: 27 Warren Street, Suite 401-402, Hackensack, NJ 07601
UK office: 57 Shelton Street, Covent Garden, London WC2H 9HE

British Library Cataloguing-in-Publication Data
A catalogue record for this book is available from the British Library.

UNIVERSAL CLINICAL REASONING
Optimising the Approach and Care for Patients

ISBN 978-981-126-928-8 (hardcover)
ISBN 978-981-126-941-7 (paperback)
ISBN 978-981-126-929-5 (ebook for institutions)
ISBN 978-981-126-930-1 (ebook for individuals)

For any available supplementary material, please visit
https://www.worldscientific.com/worldscibooks/10.1142/13232#t=suppl

DISCLAIMER

All names of patients in the clinical cases are fictitious. Any matching of a name to a real person is by coincidence.

The cases and examples are a mix of hypothetical and real situations. Where the encounter really took place, all unique identifiers have been removed. Where needed, details have been altered to further safeguard confidentiality. Where feasible, I requested and obtained permission from the real patients for their experiences to be shared in this book.

I am not present in some of the real encounters. Some encounters involve other doctors (not necessarily in Singapore), and the patients of other doctors.

NOTE ON INTELLECTUAL PROPERTY AND PURCHASE

Piracy of intellectual property and books is becoming more rampant in the years leading up to 2023. This is disrespectful to the people who came up with the ideas, and then shared these ideas.

If you have obtained this copy of the book through piracy, I cannot stop you from reading the book. If you find the content useful, please purchase a copy of the book from the official publisher. To indulge in piracy is to indulge in the same disrespect towards other human beings, that permeates poor clinical reasoning and poor clinical care.

CONTENTS

Section 2   Decision Making: Tests

Section 3   Decision-making: Treatment

Section 4   Monitoring

Section 5   Clinical Reasoning, Ignored

Section 6   Wrapping Up

INTRODUCTION

The goal of healthcare and clinical reasoning

Clinical reasoning.

Those two words have seen increasing use as doctors and educators recognise the necessity of reasoning for excellent health care.

Robust clinical reasoning drives the information-gathering and analytical process to get the correct diagnosis for every patient.

Getting the correct diagnosis and relevant differentials (if any) facilitates the making of optimal, rational, resource-efficient decisions for healthcare: tests, treatment, monitoring, disposition, and counselling. Without the correct diagnosis, decisions are often dubious and sometimes dangerous.

Since getting the correct diagnosis enables optimal decision-making, getting the correct diagnosis as early as possible, means optimal decisions are made as early as possible. Optimal decisions maximise the chance of the best possible outcome for that patient.

Getting the correct diagnosis as early as possible suggests that the doctor should strive to deduce this diagnosis through the clinical evaluation alone: asking the patient the best questions as early as possible, performing a relevant physical examination, and then weighing all the answers correctly. Obtaining the diagnosis in this fashion is known as getting the correct *clinical* diagnosis.

The benefits of routine accuracy in clinical diagnosis, followed by optimal management, are enormous:

- The patient is happier, healthier, and more productive.
- The patient's family is happier.
- Tests are ordered when necessary.
- Treatment is on-target to obtain the best outcome, without being wholly irrelevant, inadequate or excessive.
- The doctor is more successful, feels more secure and is genuinely confident of themselves.

The benefits are widely felt when more healthcare workers get it right, clinically:

- There is less strain on healthcare facilities and hospital beds.
- There is higher productivity in the population, because more patients can function and contribute instead of being hamstrung by their undiagnosed and improperly treated illnesses.
- Minimising wastage reduces the carbon footprint, thereby aiding sustainability and slowing the pace of climate change.

Getting these benefits for ourselves and every unique patient, requires clinical reasoning to be well-taught and systematically practised.

Even when several patients have the same diagnosis, each patient is unique and can vary in their presentation. Aiming to be correct all the time will require a patient-centred reasoning process.

Is getting the correct clinical diagnosis 100% of the time, a realistic expectation? Not at all. However, the chance of being correct plummets if you do not try. As with everything else in life, you may not always succeed if you try, but you will fail more often if you do not try.

In situations where the doctor:

- Is going to be wrong, or
- Is wrong, or
- Has no idea what is going on,

robust reasoning allows the doctor to recognise the situation immediately and react optimally. Optimal reactions maximise the chance of 'rescuing' the situation and the patient. Without robust reasoning, it is easy to make mistakes and compound one's initial mistakes with more mistakes.

Missing the correct diagnosis predisposes to poor decisions (such as inappropriate tests and treatments), which:

- Waste resources,
- Lead to unnecessary risks for patients, and
- Cause delays in appropriate care, leading to avoidable harm and deaths.

Just as the benefits are widely felt when more healthcare workers get it right clinically, the adverse consequences are widely felt when more healthcare workers get it wrong clinically:

- There is a greater strain (money, manpower and time) on healthcare facilities and hospital beds.
- There is lower productivity in the population, because more patients suffer and are hamstrung by their undiagnosed and improperly treated illnesses.
- Increased wastage increases the carbon footprint, which is detrimental to sustainability and trying to slow the pace of climate change.

Healthcare and training as of the end of 2022

There is a popular folktale about a race between the tortoise and the hare. The hare lost the race despite having the advantage of speed.

The hare lost the race because it took a nap. The hare took a nap because of its complacency. The hare was complacent because of its poor reasoning: the hare had decided that an advantage guaranteed success. Thus, poor reasoning led to the hare throwing away its advantage. The outcome for the hare was poor.

The lessons from the folktale apply to all humankind. Advantages at the individual (such as intelligence, knowledge, experience, and access to technology) and national level (such as having many doctors, many healthcare facilities, high technology, and abundant resources) are often wasted because of poor reasoning.

Despite extremely high healthcare expenditures and boasting many advantages over other developed countries, in terms of many healthcare outcomes, the United States of America (USA) consistently ranks as one of the worst among its peers. These outcomes include outcomes of care for various chronic diseases, rates of hospitalisation from preventable causes, and avoidable deaths. The poor outcomes were seen again when the COVID-19 pandemic struck. This contrast in outcomes between the USA and its less-wealthy, less-technologically-rich peers suggests systematic and major problems with how American physicians train and practice. One problem is a lack of robust clinical reasoning.

Advantages cannot substitute for the right effort in the right direction.

Wealth, technology, experience, and slick-looking tools (such as tests and guidelines) cannot substitute for robust clinical reasoning.

These lessons go beyond the USA. Worldwide, studies of diagnostic accuracy in experienced doctors (often internists, family physicians and emergency medicine doctors) cite across-the-board ceilings of 55–70%. This means that many doctors, including experienced doctors, get the diagnosis wrong for at least 1 out of every 3 patients. These success rates would drop to 30% or less (sometimes single digits!) for more difficult cases. A 30% success rate at most, translates into the doctor getting the right diagnosis for, at most, 1 out of every 3 patients.

If you are a patient, this knowledge hardly inspires confidence. Many patients do not need to read the literature to have this knowledge.

Patients often notice when, and how often, they do not recover despite the doctor's management and assurances.

I have heard patients and non-patients — some are in healthcare themselves — lament how many healthcare professionals seem only to want to follow a rigid sequence. One layperson likened commonplace healthcare to an 'unthinking factory production line approach to patients, instead of focusing on the unique patient'. These comments are accompanied by sadness and frustration, not malice.

Clearly, conventional training and practice worldwide leave much to be desired.

As of the end of 2022, conventional training has many limitations. Healthcare students strain to absorb a tremendous amount of theoretical knowledge. Teachers focus on imparting this abundance of knowledge. Meanwhile, science continues to advance, increasing the amount of knowledge and thus, the burden on the medical student and the doctor trying to keep up with new knowledge.

The many fixed 'approaches' for different symptoms and scenarios are impossible to memorise and apply. Relying solely on approaches to 'the classic patient in the population' means some, if not many, patients would automatically be misdiagnosed because they are not 'the classic patient'.

Trainees encounter patients and strive to learn from each encounter. Often, these lessons focus on common knowledge, which is fixed and easier to learn than patient-centred skills.

Application of the sum of this knowledge — theory, approaches, clinical experience — can be shown and tested. For the sake of simplicity and standardisation, the tests are often based on 'the classic patient'. This is where exams often fall flat: when knowledge is the focus and the 'classic' patient is used for assessment, is patient-centred clinical reasoning being assessed? Patients are not clones of each other.

Though healthcare teachers readily teach knowledge, reasoning is another matter entirely. Some of these teachers lack robust reasoning, and thus teach their students to make decisions based on poor reasoning.

Knowledge versus reasoning

Knowledge is not reasoning.

Knowledge and reasoning are separate entities. Knowledge includes disease knowledge and unique patient information. Reasoning is the process and skill that allows the optimal, patient-centred usage of that knowledge.

Knowledge of one disease can sometimes be extrapolated in a limited fashion to similar diseases, whereas reasoning is readily transferable across diseases, scenarios, and patients.

The real-world distinction between knowledge and reasoning is evident in many ways. The usual example is the knowledgeable doctor who knows the 'standard patient presentation' for a disease, but struggles when handling patients with different presentations of the same disease.

Knowledge and experience do not automatically facilitate clinical reasoning. Experience provides opportunities to learn a skill such as clinical reasoning, but learning any skill is difficult if one does not know what that skill is and how the skill should be learnt. This is a truism of life.

Is knowledge important? Yes. Since clinical reasoning facilitates the optimal use of knowledge, the professional must have some knowledge. However, knowledge without robust reasoning is often useless, and sometimes dangerous. Using knowledge without possessing robust reasoning, is like using the tools of a carpenter without possessing the understanding needed to use those tools properly.

Knowledge and robust clinical reasoning have synergistic effects when wielded together. The phrase 'clinical acumen' is often applied in admiration to the experts who wield knowledge and clinical reasoning, simultaneously and effectively.

Clinical reasoning versus the (ineffective) descriptors and substitutes for reasoning

Since robust clinical reasoning is crucial for excellent healthcare, inculcating this reasoning throughout training, practice and governance would be globally beneficial. The benefits of routine clinical accuracy could be obtained without requiring vast investment in money or technology. The potential improvements in human health, quality of life, and life expectancy are tremendous. The annual savings would easily number in the billions, if not trillions, of American dollars in every developed country.

Acquiring and developing a universally applicable clinical reasoning and learning process, offers huge benefits to the healthcare worker:

1. The overall learning process is more efficient because the two synergistic elements for excellent healthcare (reasoning and knowledge) are being learnt and applied simultaneously and systematically. This contrasts with commonplace approaches and teaching, which are a hodgepodge of seemingly disparate lessons on knowledge of different diseases.

2. Lessons from a clinical encounter can be extrapolated to other patients and other diseases. This contrasts with commonplace lessons, where knowledge of one patient's situation, approach and decisions cannot be readily extrapolated to other patients.

3. By viewing each teacher's and senior's approach and decisions through the lens of that universal effective process, the learner discerns the strengths and weaknesses in the lessons of their teachers. The learner then knows which elements to copy, discard or challenge.

These benefits accelerate the attainment of competence and increase the level of competence. When tackling assessments and exams, undergraduate and postgraduate healthcare students would enjoy these benefits too.

Why has this universally applicable process of clinical reasoning, never been developed?

The answer: **No one, to my knowledge, has ever described what clinical reasoning is, in full**.

'In full', as in: describe clinical reasoning, each subcomponent, the relationship between all subcomponents, and the predictable outcomes linked to each subcomponent and the entire process.

As of the end of 2022, books, studies, assessments, and other documents describe clinical reasoning in terms of:

- What it might look like, or
- What it can do, or
- What it is not, or
- How opportunities should be provided to learn it.

If you tasked someone with building a ship, car or another device, but they were unfamiliar with the device, that person would have considerable difficulty building a reliable, working product if you described:

- What it might look like, or
- What it can do, or
- What it is not, or
- How opportunities should be created to build it…

…all while failing to tell that person what the device is, in full.

These descriptors of appearance, function, what something is not, and how something can be learnt or built, are external descriptors. External descriptors superficially describe the topic or object of interest, but do not give enough detail for complete understanding, reliable production, or proper use.

Imagine tasking someone who does not know of the existence of cars, with building a car. All you say is: 'It carries people from Point A to Point B, faster than they can run on 2 legs.' What are the chances that you will receive a finished car?

- Adding more 'what it does' or 'what it looks like' descriptions, such as 'it has a compartment for carrying objects' or 'it has lights in the front and back' would not make much difference to the abysmally low chance of getting a functional car.
- Stating the 100 things the car is not, such as 'the car is not an aeroplane, or a bicycle, or a train, or a…' is unhelpful.

- Giving that person more opportunities to build a car, does not help if they were not told how to build the car.

In contrast, providing a complete and detailed blueprint, along with the exact materials and sources in each component of the car, and the exact relationship of each component to every other component, greatly increases the likelihood of getting a complete and functional car.

The car analogy mirrors training in all professions, including healthcare.

The literature is filled with external descriptors of reasoning for the past 40-odd years: script concordance, problem representation, cognitive biases, theories of approach, dual-process theory, predictive brain theory, theories of cognition, reflective structure, management scripts, and so on.

All these external descriptors of clinical reasoning, have one or more major limitations. The limitations include the descriptor:

- Being inherently flawed, akin to insisting the car must have a steering wheel composed only of uncompressed tissue paper. The tissue-paper steering wheel will crumple upon being used.

- Being so vague that the average learner or educator has nothing practical to use.

- Being complicated and sometimes, irrelevant to the task. This is akin to providing all the chemical formulae, geographical details, philosophical speculation and historical importance of each material and component of the car whilst failing to specify the material or component itself.

- Isolating 1 component of the entire clinical encounter, and then failing to accurately describe the relationship of that component to every other component. This is like providing detailed plans for the steering wheel of the car and nothing else about the car, to the would-be manufacturer for the whole car.

Suggesting methods that could encourage learning of reasoning without defining the exact mental steps to be learnt, does not work either.

If a teacher said 'if you see more cases, you can learn to reason', a serious learner can easily reply 'what exactly is the reasoning, step-by-step, that I am supposed to learn?' This question by the reasoning learner, and the puzzled expression of the (poorly reasoning) teacher when faced with this sensible question, simultaneously illustrates the necessity and absence of a complete blueprint.

Many 'approaches' books, guidelines, protocols, and algorithms exist. They are often used as substitutes for clinical reasoning: the user adheres strictly to the suggestions of the document and then ignores the entirety of the patient. Unfortunately, medical schools, teachers and learners often fail to recognise these documents for what they are: poor substitutes for patient-centred reasoning. Some teachers and learners mistakenly think that these substitutes for clinical reasoning are, in fact, clinical reasoning.

The widespread use of these documents as substitutes for robust reasoning, is one reason (pun intended) why poor outcomes have continued for decades, worldwide.

Methods for practising or assessing clinical performance, such as virtual patient platforms and simulations, are often based on external descriptors and substitutes for clinical reasoning. Thus, most conventional patient platforms and simulations possess the same flaws and limitations as these external descriptors and substitutes for reasoning. Medical students and doctors can go through hundreds of cases and vignettes, and pass their exams, but learn nothing of clinical reasoning.

Unsurprisingly, with the prolific use of external descriptors or substitutes for clinical reasoning, it is difficult to find evidence that patient outcomes have improved significantly, unless new technology was directly and appropriately applied to the patient.

A complete blueprint of the car is necessary to consistently produce a complete and reliable car. Likewise, a practical and complete blueprint of universally applicable reasoning is necessary to consistently produce patient-centred doctors and optimal outcomes.

Without defining clinical reasoning and all its components in full, it is impossible to consistently and accurately learn, teach, assess, or correct clinical reasoning. Under these unhappy circumstances, only a minority of students will ever attain competence, with that minority being exceptional because they combined dedication, reasoning, self-teaching and raw talent. Hardly the desirable result when training a cohort of medical students or specialist trainees, agreed?

Clinical reasoning — is there a complete process that can be universally applied?

The best professionals, regardless of setting or speciality, show curiosity over and above their peers, learn more quickly and are more adaptable. They acquire knowledge from both theory and clinical experience, and simultaneously organise this knowledge in a clinical-reasoning-friendly way. They prioritise their questions to centre around the patient. Instead of prioritising knowledge over the entirety of each unique patient, they use their knowledge to complement their assessment of the patient.

These top-tier experts have a systematic, patient-centred method of reasoning, which is complemented by their highly efficient and accurate learning. This method is intuitive to them, but not to everyone else. If you observe these experts' approaches to different patients with different diagnoses and can recognise the self-teaching they often subconsciously reveal during discussions, a consistent pattern emerges. However, the complete, invisible mental process that they use is hard to vocalise or teach directly, because no one has defined its entirety and its components.

Until now.

Long ago, I realised the value of a systematic 'best' thought process. This process was absent from conventional teaching. By trying various approaches (including some of my devising), observing the outcome, and tackling each weakness that emerged, that 'best' process gradually became apparent.

I also sought out and observed the best professionals across settings and specialities, prompting them to describe their thought processes. I distilled their strengths and weaknesses. A consistent and systematic pattern of reasoning became evident. This pattern mirrored the 'best' process I was developing. The top healthcare experts:

- Used the same steps in diagnosis and decision-making. These steps directly contributed to their superior speed and accuracy.

- Usually did not omit any fundamental steps in that systematic thought process.

- Had minor variations in the style and execution of some steps, but the fundamental principles and steps were unchanged.

- On rare occasions, made an unnecessary mistake. This mistake was always directly attributable to omitting at least 1 crucial step in that systematic process.

More years were spent on putting this combined, universal mental process into simple diagrams, and trying different ways of teaching this process. Every concept, every diagram, and every example had to add concrete value to the learner. Every lesson had to be applicable immediately.

I found myself using the same phrases and the same language to teach and correct medical students and postgraduate specialist trainees, both locally and internationally trained. Regardless of their intelligence, experience, knowledge, the patient's final diagnosis, or the setting of healthcare, these learners were making the same mental mistakes at the same time points in clinical scenarios and simulations.

Teaching the correct mental process using the 'language of reasoning' at each time point was the most effective way to correct the mental mistakes, instead of merely telling the learner the correct for-that-case-only step or warning them to avoid that mistake. It is more impactful to teach the learner what to do, instead of teaching the 20 things they should not do.

This teaching did more than just stop the mistake being made for that 1 patient with that diagnosis; it prevented the same mistake at the same mental time point when these learners tackled other patients with other diagnoses.

What about the scenarios where patients have multiple bizarre complaints, or have at least 2 simultaneous diagnoses? Conventional, commonplace teaching and practice have not provided any clear solution. Experienced doctors and specialists struggle with these patients. These scenarios are difficult because of the limitations of conventional teaching and healthcare practice.

As the saying goes: if you do the same thing as everyone else, you can expect to get the same result.

If you have not undertaken the learning journey necessary to develop proficiency in this universally applicable reasoning method, you will often lack the knowledge and clarity to fully recognise and understand 1 disease in your patient. Conventional training and practice usually confer a general recognition of the disease. This general recognition is insufficient; there is a huge difference between having a general recognition of the disease, and a full understanding of the disease. If the full recognition of 1 disease is too much for you, how can you hope to handle the patient with multiple bizarre complaints, or two or more diseases manifesting simultaneously?

If you want to have any chance of handling these scenarios properly, I recommend you start with this book.

Overview of this book's content and format

In this book, I will define and discuss the elements of patient-centred clinical reasoning. This universal process can be applied to any patient you will see in your lifetime. I will describe the concomitant learning journey. Where relevant, I will describe commonplace teaching and conventional healthcare as comparisons to patient-centred reasoning, thereby illustrating the vast difference this method will make to personal, educational, regional, and national-level outcomes.

To keep the content simple and accurate, I will not invoke terminology from other sources unless necessary. I have also provided clinically applicable definitions of loosely used words and phrases in healthcare training and practice. I recommend you stick to these definitions, for mental clarity drives diagnostic and decision-making clarity. These definitions helped my students (in this book, a 'student' of mine is anyone who spends significant time and effort learning clinical reasoning from me. Some of them are specialists.) find clarity in the deluge of textbooks and literature, which used similar words whilst meaning different things for the same word.

This method will teach you to 'see' concepts and truths that healthcare training and practice across the world, for decades, have largely failed to see. If healthcare is to improve dramatically, these concepts and truths must be seen and realised.

This universal reasoning technique has many implications for conventional healthcare training, practice, governance, and research. Thus, leaders of healthcare training, leaders of healthcare institutions, clinical researchers, and government officials responsible for healthcare, have much to gain from reading this book. The mistakes and weaknesses of conventional training, practice, research and governance are discussed in various parts of this book. Section 5 focuses on these flaws at a system-wide and global level, and some of the globally applicable solutions to these flaws.

If you deem yourself an experienced healthcare professional, medical educator, or leader of healthcare, here is a word of caution: you have likely surmised from the introduction that this book will be an eye-opener. Many commonplace practices and guidelines are not best practices once they are compared to the full universal process here. Your mind is probably going to be reeling before you reach the end of this book (your mind may already be reeling by this point). Keep an open mind. I am not asking you to instantly discard your habits and usual practice. All I ask is that you consider the entire process step-by-step, with the explanations and outcomes, and decide for yourself. If you need a month or two to mentally digest the content of this book and come to terms with this method, then take this time to do so.

Patients consult healthcare practitioners for their concerns. Healthcare practitioners include more than just doctors. Nurses, pharmacists, dentists, and allied health practitioners such as speech therapists, occupational therapists, and dietitians also provide healthcare to patients.

Many or all of the principles in this book apply to any healthcare practitioner. Throughout this book, when I use the word 'doctor', it is for the sake of brevity (instead of concomitantly mentioning dentists, nurses, allied health, etc.). If you are a healthcare professional but not a doctor, you should decide if each principle is important for your job.

This book is relevant to:

- All healthcare students and professionals who must figure out a patient's illness, and then make or execute healthcare decisions
- Healthcare teachers and schools as an introduction to teaching reasoning
- Researchers, research regulatory and ethics boards, and reviewers as an introduction to impactful, applicable design and conduct of clinically relevant diagnostic and therapeutic studies
- Administrators, system designers and government officials as an introduction to recognising and incentivising patient-centred healthcare
- Anyone else interested in effective, patient-centred diagnosis and decision-making

In each chapter:

- One or more principles will be discussed.
- Common examples will illustrate the difference that those principles make to outcomes.
- Most will have a capsule summary or Frequently Asked Questions section, or both.
- Content will build on the previous chapters, demonstrating how clinical reasoning permeates the entire process of patient care, and drives each successive step in the patient approach and decision-making.

SECTION 1

The Clinical Approach

This section covers the core tenets of clinical reasoning and the effective approach to the patient.

WHAT IS CLINICAL REASONING?

What is reasoning?

The definition is 'Thinking about something in a logical, sensible way'.

By extension, clinical reasoning would be 'Thinking about your patient and the clinical scenario in a **logical, sensible way**'.

This definition demonstrates that robust clinical reasoning must centre around and adapt to each unique patient, to get that patient what they want.

What would patients want?

To get the best possible outcome.

To get the best possible outcome, patients want optimal decisions to be made with them and for them, as soon as possible. Patients know that optimal and timely decisions maximise the chance of getting the best possible outcome.

Patients consult the doctor when they have concerns relating to their health. Since identifying the root cause of their concerns helps to fix those concerns, getting the correct diagnosis is crucial. The correct diagnosis facilitates optimal decision-making. By extension, making optimal decisions as early as possible requires getting the correct diagnosis as early as possible.

When faced with a patient, there are 3 fundamental jobs for any healthcare practitioner:

1. Make the correct, current diagnosis
2. Gather additional information needed for optimal management of that patient
3. Make optimal healthcare decisions in partnership with the patient

Given these 3 jobs, let us consider 'logical' and 'sensible' as per the definition of Clinical Reasoning.

Logically, the approach to every patient must concentrate on making the correct diagnosis as soon as possible, because logic also demonstrates that the correct diagnosis is central to making optimal decisions afterwards. Likewise, 'sensible' requires the doctor to accept reality: why the patient is there, what each clue from the patient means, and the correct use of these clues. Thus, making the correct, current diagnosis is also known as 'Ruling In' the most likely diagnosis because the doctor must be attentive to all the right clues.

Clinical reasoning is not knowledge (algorithms, population-level statistics, guidelines, and so on) used in isolation. Clinical reasoning recognises that you pay attention to the unique patient in front of you.

Healthcare students are often taught lists of questions to ask patients. They are advised to study hypothetical 'approaches' and algorithms, which make suggestions for handling hypothetical 'classic' patients. None of these lists, approaches or algorithms can analyse or adapt to the entirety of each patient and thus, are poor substitutes for patient-centred clinical reasoning.

The outcome is often poor when the doctor is not paying attention to each unique patient's entirety and the proper use of each clue.

If a patient is unhappy over a poor outcome due to your inattentiveness, citing how the outcome was unexpected because they were not 'the average/classic patient', announces your lack of empathy and reasoning. The patient sees you because they are relying on your expertise to pay attention to them and get it right for them. It is no consolation (and in fact, infuriating) to hear the doctor try to justify a poor outcome through an absence of patient-centredness.

If we break down the 3 fundamental jobs further, the sequential steps are:

1. Recognise the reality behind the patient's presentation, which drives effective questioning and the accurate use of patient information

2. Use each piece of initial information, according to its importance

3. Shape and prioritise the information-gathering to match each clue's importance to our task

4. Organise all the information according to their importance

5. Analyse the information according to their importance

6. Mentally decide the most likely diagnosis and reasonable alternative diagnoses

7. Gather additional information to understand the patient as a whole

8. Combine the additional patient-unique information with general medical knowledge, to make decisions with and for the patient

When I teach a new group of students, I begin with the foundation: the patient's perspective.

Almost always, the reaction from the students is one of shock:

- Using the patient's perspective as the starting point, is novel to them.

- They realise that applying the patient's perspective is not just for building rapport or showing empathy, but also enhances reasoning and diagnostic accuracy.

- They realise this foundation, if taught explicitly and in full at the start of medical school, could have transformed their acquisition of knowledge and approach to patients, thereby reducing the cognitive load, headaches, and frustration they had had for years.

Let us start with the patient's perspective.

The patient's perspective

When patients notice or suspect something concerning their health, they consult a doctor. Much of the time, there will indeed be a disease.

The information proffered by the patients about what they notice or feel about themselves, is known as the symptoms. The possible symptoms are many: tiredness, nausea, fever, vomiting, pain, dizziness, itch, swelling, rashes, and so on.

If the patient has a disease, symptoms occur because of the disease. The disease may:

- Be relatively benign, such as the common viral flu or gastroenteritis that resolves on its own.
- Require simple help for recovery, such as a common bacterial infection requiring antibiotics, or an illness that requires routine surgery.
- Be the beginning of a long-term common illness, such as hypertension or diabetes mellitus.
- Be a rare and potentially-lethal illness, such as a cancer or autoimmune disorder.

Since symptoms are direct manifestations of the current disease, they are direct clues to the current disease.

When a patient has more than 1 symptom, they usually describe the most troublesome symptom first. If the patient has:

- Vomiting and other symptoms, but the vomiting troubles them the most, they will volunteer their history of vomiting up front.
- Severe breathlessness, fainting and an itchy rash, they will complain of the breathlessness and/or fainting up front. They would not mention the rash up front, and then refuse to mention the other 2 symptoms.

The initial symptom(s) the patient volunteers to the doctor is the Presenting Complaint.

Since humans tend to volunteer the most troublesome and severe symptoms in their Presenting Complaint, the symptom(s) in the presenting complaint is (or are) the most important of all the patient's symptoms.

Applying the patient perspective to drive the clinical approach and analytical weightage

Since symptoms are direct clues to the current diagnosis, and the presenting complaint has the most important clues, applied clinical reasoning means:

- At the start of the encounter, listen carefully to the symptom(s) in the presenting complaint.

- When you get the chance to respond, your first reply to the patient must be: 'Tell me more (about the presenting complaint).'

- Weigh the patient's information accordingly. The presenting complaint always carries greater weight than any other symptom in isolation.

- Any other information that ranks below symptoms in importance, should usually be asked later and processed as such in weightage.

These 4 points described the first step in the 8 steps outlined earlier in this chapter. There are still the other 7 steps, which will be discussed in the rest of this book.

Overview of the doctor–patient encounter

The next figure demonstrates the flowchart of a doctor–patient encounter. Each path is the result of a chain reaction.

The Doctor–Patient Encounter

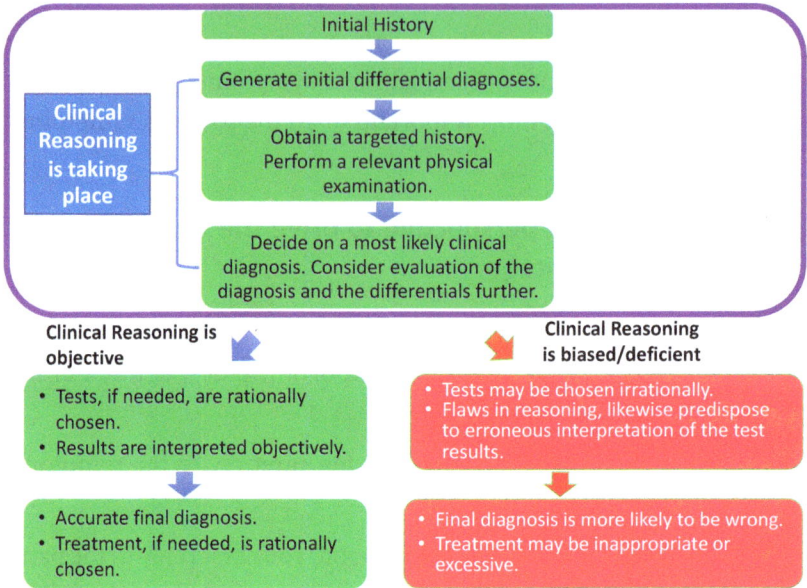

The green boxes encompassed by the purple border, depict the steps necessary to stay on the optimal path:

- Relevant differentials are generated and then explored in a targeted fashion, maximising the chance of reaching the correct clinical diagnosis.

- The green boxes in the lower half of the figure depict the correct diagnosis and optimal decisions.

- Resources are used rationally, efficiently and effectively.

- Outcomes are usually excellent.

- Risks of poor outcomes and side effects are minimised.

This optimal path is shown in the green boxes in the lower half of the figure.

In contrast, failure to follow the initial green boxes leads to a chain reaction of mistakes. This chain reaction increases the likelihood of the wrong diagnosis, which then predisposes to inappropriate decision-making.

The path of poor decision-making and outcomes is shown in the red boxes in the lower half of the figure. At the individual level, consequences include:

- Tests are ordered unnecessarily and the results are misinterpreted, resulting in unnecessary costs (such as money, discomfort, anxiety and wasted time) and risks posed to the patient.

- Unnecessary treatment is provided, resulting in unnecessary costs and risks to the patient.

- Appropriate care is delayed or not provided, which leads to poor outcomes, including prolonged hospital stays, permanent disability and death.

The adverse consequences go beyond the individual doctor and patient, especially if the doctors making these mistakes work in a hospital:

- Given the limited manpower and facilities to perform investigations, a multitude of unnecessary investigations results in delays of urgent, appropriate investigations for other patients in the same hospital.

- Stocks of medication and other treatments may be strained by many inappropriate, wasteful treatment orders.

- Some of the funding for healthcare comes from taxes. Thus, the extra costs are partially borne by the taxpayers. The wasted money is unavailable for other purposes for the country and its people.

- The healthcare resources that were wasted, were generated through processes that produced greenhouse gases, increasing the carbon footprint. Wasted resources must be generated anew for other patients to use. Thus, this wastage accelerates the pace of climate change and global warming, which is in everyone's interest to avoid.

Thus, clinical reasoning sets off a chain reaction during the healthcare encounter. This is like lining up a row of dominoes, and then knocking over the first domino to strike the next — the rest will fall in rapid succession.

There are 2 'chains of dominoes'. One chain represents robust clinical reasoning (all the green boxes in the figure). The other chain represents a lack of robust reasoning (events leading to the red boxes in the figure):

- If the doctor has sufficient skill in clinical reasoning to meet the needs of a patient, the optimal chain of dominoes shows up: making the correct clinical diagnosis, making optimal testing decisions, interpreting test results correctly, and choosing optimal treatment. The outcome is often excellent.

- Conversely, if the doctor's skill in clinical reasoning is insufficient to meet the needs of a patient, the disastrous chain of dominoes shows up: making the wrong (or having no) clinical diagnosis, making poor decisions in testing, frequently erroneous interpretation of test results, and making suboptimal choices in treatment. The outcome is often poor.

The chains of dominoes demonstrate another aspect of patient-centredness: though it is advantageous to be as skilful as possible in reasoning, the adequacy of the doctor's reasoning for each patient depends on the complexity of that patient's diagnosis and care. Robust reasoning is also required to gauge one's adequacy of reasoning relative to the patient's disease.

The robust reasoner would be an accurate and optimal doctor for most patients. When encountering a potentially too-difficult patient for them, this reasoner is aware of the disastrous chain of dominoes. This reasoner hesitates to rush into ordering tests and treatments. They recognise that if their reasoning skill might not be good enough diagnostically for that patient, using the same potentially inadequate reasoning skill to order tests and treatments, is often suboptimal. They would proceed carefully and summon help.

In contrast, a poor reasoner would be more likely to make mistakes with every patient. The more complex the patient, the exponentially higher chance of making mistakes. Since poor reasoning often accompanies inattention and leads to difficulty with correctly interpreting information, poor reasoners are often unable to notice or recognise a mistake in time. Sometimes, poor reasoners recognise their mistakes but lack the reasoning and humility to admit these mistakes, and thus insist on continuing down their mistaken path, whilst hoping for a miracle and refusing to summon help. Thus, initial mistakes are often compounded with yet more mistakes: the disastrous chain of dominoes.

Throughout this book, I will use the labels 'robust reasoner' and 'poor reasoner' to describe the usual behaviours that differ between these 2 groups of doctors. However, the ability to reason lies on a spectrum. The frequency of the behaviours in the individual doctor like you or me depends on our reasoning. Using the earlier doctor–patient encounter flowchart:

- Robust reasoners tend to stay on the optimal green-box path on the left. The stronger their reasoning, the less often they stray from this path and the quicker they 'rescue' themselves from the red-box path if they stray.

- Poor reasoners tend not to follow the green boxes. The weaker their reasoning, the more often they stay on the disastrous red-box path.

- In-between-robust-and-poor reasoners may follow the initial green boxes for 'simple' patients, but often get on the red-box path (even more so when they face surprises or rare diseases) afterwards. Their ability to rescue themselves and get back on the green path is dependent on their reasoning. Stronger reasoners will rescue themselves more often than weaker reasoners.

In conclusion, robust clinical reasoning is central to reaching the correct diagnosis and making excellent decisions.

Capsule summary

- The correct clinical diagnosis is required for all healthcare decisions to be excellent.

- Effective clinical reasoning starts with the reality that drives patient information.

- Symptoms are direct clues to the current diagnosis. Among all the symptoms, the symptom(s) in the presenting complaint is (or are) the most important.

- Robust clinical reasoning drives an optimal chain of dominoes: correct diagnosis and optimal decisions. The outcome is often excellent.

- Poor or no clinical reasoning drives a disastrous chain of dominoes: wrong or no diagnosis, and poor decisions. The outcome is often poor.

THE INITIAL INFORMATION, CATEGORIES OF DIAGNOSTIC INFORMATION, AND ILLNESS SCRIPTS

Patients often volunteer the Presenting Complaint at the start of the patient encounter.

The doctor may have other information about the patient at the start of the encounter:

- The patient demographics: name, age, gender, race, and so on. The demographics can be obtained from the registration data of the patient. Demographics are data that belong to Epidemiology.

- The past medical history may be known from existing healthcare records. The past medical history is data that belongs to Risk Factors.

- Some physical clues may be immediately apparent upon seeing or hearing the patient. For example, the patient may be limping, gasping, have a rash, or have an open wound. These clues are data that belong to Clinical Features.

- In many Emergency Departments, triaging provides the patient's vital signs. The vital signs are data that belong to Clinical Features.

Note the colour coding of the words in blue and green. These are separate categories with separate levels of importance:

1. Green refers to Clinical Features, the most important category of information.

2. Blue refers to Epidemiology/Risk Factors, the less-important category of information.

All direct manifestations of the current diagnosis are classified as Clinical Features, including:

- Symptoms of the current diagnosis.

- Current physical data on the patient. Physical data includes the vital signs, as well as the clues on examining the patient. In medical parlance, these are called Signs.

All other information that may modify (increase or decrease) the likelihood of the current diagnosis, is classified as Epidemiology/Risk Factors. This category includes the patient's demographics, past medical history, travel history, contact history, and so on. Symptoms and signs of other already known co-morbid diseases in the patient, where the co-morbid diseases modify the risk of the current diagnosis or differentials, would also be considered Risk Factors.

Information that is not a direct manifestation of the current diagnosis, is not as important as the information that is a direct manifestation of the current diagnosis. Therefore, Epidemiology/Risk Factors are clues of secondary importance, ranking below Clinical Features in importance.

Since the Clinical Features are direct clues to the current diagnosis:

- The correct diagnosis must explain <u>all</u> the Clinical Features. Not one, two, or half of the Clinical Features, but all of them.

- Most of your diagnosis-seeking questions should focus on Clinical Features.

- To get the correct diagnosis early, you must ask diagnosis-seeking questions focused on the Clinical Features early in the consultation.

Since the category of Epidemiology/Risk Factors comprises clues that may or may not be related to the current diagnosis:

- It is often unnecessary to explain any of the information in this category, with the patient's diagnosis.

- Questions in this category should comprise the minority of your questions.

- Questions in this category should generally be asked (if still necessary) after you have exhausted the questions addressing the patient's Clinical Features.

Consider these examples.

CASE #1: Patient X

Patient X comes in complaining of headache and fever, for 3 days.

--

Clinical reasoning-based mental process: The patient has symptoms of fever and headache lasting 3 days. These are direct clues to the current diagnosis.

Next course of action: You tell the patient, 'Please tell me more (about the headache and fever).'

--

In this example, I did not furnish the patient's name, age, gender, race, or past medical history. These fall under Epidemiology/Risk Factors.

Might you want to know these? Yes.

Do you <u>need</u> to know these to make the diagnosis? Maybe not.

Do you <u>need</u> to pursue the Clinical Features to make the diagnosis? Yes.

Case #1 lacks details. Now, let us add more information to Case #1, which becomes Case #2:

CASE #2: Tina

Tina is a 13-year-old Chinese girl with a past medical history of cystitis (this is a lower urinary tract infection). She consults you with the Presenting Complaint of headache and fever for 3 days.

--

Clinical reasoning-based mental process: The patient has symptoms of fever and headache lasting 3 days. These are direct clues to the current diagnosis.

Next course of action: You tell the patient, 'Please tell me more (about the headache and fever).'

--

In this example, there is the patient's name, age, gender, race, and past medical history. These fall under Epidemiology/Risk Factors.

Though this information is 'nice to have', is it more important than exploring the Clinical Features? No.

Do you <u>need</u> to pursue the Clinical Features to make the diagnosis? Yes.

Would any of these sentences be sensible or logical?

- Tina has a disease because she is female. Her gender caused the illness.

- Tina has a disease because she is a child. Her age caused the illness.

- Tina's current disease must be due to her history of cystitis. The past always predicts the future.

Let us try another example.

CASE #3: Sam

Sam is a 50-year-old Danish man with a past medical history of cystitis, heart disease, diabetes mellitus, alcoholism and a fracture of his right forearm from playing baseball 20 years ago. He consults you with the Presenting Complaint of headache and fever for 3 days.

--

Clinical reasoning-based mental process: The patient has symptoms of fever and headache lasting 3 days. These are direct clues to the current diagnosis.

Next course of action: You tell the patient, 'Please tell me more (about the headache and fever).'

--

In this example, there is the patient's name, age, gender, race, and a much longer past medical history than Tina had. These fall under Epidemiology/Risk Factors.

Though this information is 'nice to have', is it more important than exploring the Clinical Features? No.

Do you <u>need</u> to pursue the Clinical Features to make the diagnosis? Yes.

Would any of these sentences be sensible or logical?

- Sam has a disease because he is male. His gender caused the illness.
- Sam has a disease because he is an adult. His adulthood caused the illness.
- Sam has a disease because he is middle-aged. His age category caused the illness.
- Sam's current disease must be due to cystitis. The past always predicts the future.
- Sam's current disease must be due to something in his medical history. The past always predicts the future.

Across the examples, the clinical reasoning remained unchanged regardless of the Epidemiology/Risk Factors. The optimal path always focused on the Clinical Features.

Notice the nonsensical thought process that prioritises Epidemiology/Risk Factors instead of Clinical Features. A doctor who prioritises Epidemiology/Risk Factors would tend to fixate on information that may not relate to the current diagnosis. When there is the choice to pursue information that is directly relevant to the current diagnosis (Clinical Features) at the start of the consultation, choosing to pursue potentially irrelevant information instead is foolish.

A flawed thought process alters your questioning for the worse. For example, deciding the patient's disease must be due to a history of cystitis, would shift the focus of initial questioning towards diseases linked to cystitis and the details of previous cystitis.

Do medical students and doctors have ample time to pursue potentially unrelated threads?

Would a doctor who cannot prioritise the patient's information, suddenly be able to prioritise the best decisions for that same patient?

Rule #1 of clinical reasoning: Try to explain all clinical features

Sherlock Holmes was a mythical detective able to solve any mystery. He accomplished this by pursuing the details of all relevant clues to the crime. He then put all these clues together to figure out the crime.

Being a skilled doctor is no different from emulating Sherlock Holmes. A skilled doctor is a skilled 'medical detective'. The patient's diagnosis is the 'crime'. Discarding clues directly manifesting from this 'crime' would be foolish.

Clinical features directly manifest from the current diagnosis. Therefore, the robust reasoner does not cherry-pick which clinical features to explain. Instead, this doctor realises that he or she must try to explain all of them. The details of the clinical features must also be explained. If the patient has:

- Severe persistent abdominal pain over the epigastric region for 2 days, the doctor should strive to explain the pain and its details, with their diagnosis.

- Abdominal pain and 3 other symptoms, the doctor should strive to explain all the symptoms and their details, with their diagnosis.

The more of the clinical features and their details that can be explained, the more accurate the diagnosis. The most accurate doctors explain all clinical features in all their patients.

Clinical diagnostic skill is the biggest and most crucial difference between a doctor and a layperson with Internet access. 'Doctor Google' can often tell a layperson the tests and treatments for a particular diagnosis. What Doctor Google cannot do, is get the correct diagnosis consistently.

The correct diagnosis is 'ruled in' by obtaining and then putting all the relevant clues together whilst respecting their relative importance: Clinical Features versus Epidemiology/Risk Factors. This combination of recognising the relative importance of the categories of diagnostic information and Rule #1, is the <u>basic diagnostic reasoning requirement</u> for all patients. This requirement is essential for excellent and safe healthcare, and will be referred to repeatedly in the rest of this book.

Rule #1 — How a top expert shapes their learning over the years

Since everyone starts as a novice, it is unrealistic to expect trainees to be able to explain all clinical features overnight in all their patients.

However, it is important to try. Trainees will not undertake the necessary learning journey if they do not try to master this skill.

In the trying, the trainee is compelled to follow up on their patient to learn the final, correct diagnosis. The trainee is also compelled to read about their patient's clinical features, especially the clinical features and details they cannot explain. These steps facilitate the building of detailed and accurate illness scripts, which are required for expert-level performance.

In this manner, experts rapidly build up illness scripts over the years and simultaneously hone the clinical reasoning to use these scripts effectively. In contrast, doctors who do not obey this rule, can remain novices even after decades of experience. Experience does not automatically confer skill, especially if the skill requires a focused effort to hone.

The illness script is a representation of the knowledge of the ways each disease can manifest, combining clinical features with other information such as risk factors, epidemiological data, and results of testing. Strong clinicians include pathophysiology in their illness scripts. Each disease has an illness script.

To make a diagnosis, doctors mentally reference the information from each patient, against their illness scripts for relevant diseases.

Imagine you are the welcoming driver/official, tasked with identifying and escorting 1 person out of the crowd of people leaving the airport terminal. Though many welcoming drivers and officials hold up signs with their target's name emblazoned in huge letters, you have no sign. You must identify your target with your eyes. All you have is a description of the person.

- Suppose you only have 2 to 4 scant bits of information about the person: Male, Adult, Tall, Wears a shirt. I wish you luck trying to find this person out of the hundreds of people streaming out of the airport.

- Now, suppose you have 15 detailed bits of information about the person: Male, middle-aged adult, looks younger than his age, 1.9 metres tall, wears a blue shirt with an eagle emblazoned across the centre, etc. You are likely to identify this person easily and rapidly.

The job of identifying your target out of the crowd mirrors the doctor's job of identifying the patient's disease out of all the possibilities. The more details you have, the more you can use to do your job well. The more detailed your illness script is for each disease, the more accurate and rapid you will be at identifying that disease.

The steps of obeying and pursuing mastery of Rule #1, one patient at a time, often look like this:

1. These future experts get all the details of the direct clues (Clinical Features) to the diagnosis. They ask themselves: 'Do I know enough about my top diagnosis and differentials to explain all the patient's clinical features?' When the answer is 'No', they consult their textbooks.

2. They soon realise that standard textbooks, and sometimes even subspecialty textbooks, do not suffice to explain all of the patient's clinical features (and details of these features), for the patient's differentials.

3. They then turn to journal articles and content experts for these answers. These answers are not written in many textbooks because of word limits and the perceived lack of interest in details.

4. Sometimes no source explains all the patient's clinical features with a diagnosis.

5. All patients are followed up to obtain the final correct diagnosis. Follow-up is crucial for assigning the patient information (especially the clinical features) to the correct diagnosis, for learning. The keeping of patient logs for this purpose, is explained in the next chapter, 'Targeted evaluation: history'.

6. These doctors apply their new knowledge to subsequent patients.

This is the acquisition of patient knowledge at the **patient-centric** level. The journey to meet this standard requires far more than the commonplace reading of standard disease entries in standard textbooks. The process must match the desired results. Superficial pursuit of knowledge is insufficient for consistently excellent patient care.

Through this dedication and extended effort, the top experts develop the ability to consistently make the correct clinical diagnosis, sometimes needing only the details of the presenting complaint.

The consequences of disobeying Rule #1

Rule #1 maximises the chance of getting the correct diagnosis.

Obeying Rule #1 comes from accepting that all of the patient's symptoms and signs are real, and important for getting the correct diagnosis.

It can be tempting to ignore clinical features that you cannot explain with your diagnosis. The temptation arises from either reluctance to change your diagnosis, or reluctance to read up to explain these clinical features with a diagnosis, or both.

Thus, many doctors disobey Rule #1.

To disobey Rule #1 for the patient in front of you, is *to pretend that some or all the patient's symptoms and signs do not exist*. This pretence increases the chance of mistakes.

Would Sherlock Holmes have been as accurate if he ignored clues, and instead consulted the list of 'the most common or dangerous crimes in this area'?

Beyond the immediate danger to the patient (and your career) posed by unnecessary mistakes, there are 2 major problems:

1. Opportunity cost
2. Habituating the ignoring of inconvenient-to-explain information

Opportunity cost: The first major problem arises from the opportunity cost of not asking yourself: 'Do I know enough about these diseases to explain all of my patient's clinical features?'

By not asking yourself this question, you see no need to read up on the diagnosis and differentials in this patient-centric manner. By never addressing your ignorance, you continue to lack detailed illness scripts, even years and decades later. Experience provides opportunities to learn, but does not automatically confer learning. This is 1 reason why many experienced doctors lack the knowledge required for excellent patient care. They know *something*, but that 'something' is not good enough. Some experienced doctors seem more ignorant than medical students, as if they stopped studying since medical school, forgot what they learnt in medical school, and assumed experience automatically confers knowledge.

Habituating the ignoring of inconvenient-to-explain information: The second major problem comes from disobeying Rule #1 for years.

If you disobey Rule #1, you are not practising the skill of 'explain all clinical features' for every patient you see.

If you never follow Rule #1, you are not practising this skill for *any* patient you see.

To disobey Rule #1 is to practise ignoring the most important clues from the patient.

Ignoring the clues to the crime makes it much harder to figure out the crime.

Ignoring the clues to the diagnosis makes it much harder to figure out the correct diagnosis.

When you practice ignoring the direct clues to the diagnosis, ignoring these clues becomes a habit. It is a dangerous habit. It predisposes you to be dismissive of any patient's symptoms and signs that you do not wish to acknowledge.

Experience matters little if your experience has been used to habituate to ignoring patients.

If you are habitually ignoring the patient, I would hate to be your patient.

Someone who has chosen to ignore Rule #1 (the first major problem) usually wants to carry on doing so (the second major problem). Thus, both major problems usually coexist simultaneously in the same doctor.

Poor reasoners often attempt to compensate for their inattention towards patients, in ineffective ways, such as ruling out a fixed or arbitrary checklist of diseases, batteries of tests, and engaging in polypharmacy. Ineffective attempts fail to prevent mistakes because they do not address the root cause of the disastrous chain of dominoes: habitually ignoring the clinical features that the doctor deemed too troublesome to explain or learn about.

Here is one of the typical conversations I have with students on this topic. As a preface to such conversations, I usually explain the importance of building up illness scripts. This contrast between what should be done, and what is usually done, helps lead the learner to wisdom and self-reflection.

Me: 'What do you usually do after clerking a patient?'

Student: 'I refer to the electronic entry made by the doctor.'

Me: 'And you assume the diagnosis the doctor made is correct?'

Student (uneasily): 'Yes.'

Me: 'Assuming your senior is always right? Oh dear, that is a problem. Anyway, assuming your senior is correct, what do you do if their diagnosis disagrees with your clinical diagnosis?'

Student: 'I look at the tests and treatment they ordered. I assume those are correct too.'

Me: 'And if your diagnosis agrees with their diagnosis?'

Student: 'I still look at the tests they ordered, and the treatment. I assume those are correct too.'

Me: 'The decisions made for the patient would depend on the accuracy of the clinical diagnosis. Do you review your clerking notes on the patient's clinical features? And then check your mental banks — your illness scripts for that disease — and see if you can explain all of that patient's clinical features with the presumed diagnosis?'

Student (often with a mixture of dawning realisation and horror in their expression): 'No.'

Me: 'If you are not trying to explain all clinical features, then you are ignoring the inconvenient clinical features you cannot explain in your patient. This will become a habit. Without trying to explain all clinical features, how are you going to build up detailed illness scripts? And therefore, how are you ever going to master this crucial skill if you are not checking and refining it?'

Student: 'Uh oh.'

Me: 'Let us review the issue of assuming your senior is always right. Reality is the best check for the final diagnosis. You need to follow up on your patient after that encounter. Follow up to the time of discharge or, better yet, at the subsequent clinic review. If you have rotated out of the posting, there are ways of following up. For example, you can identify the doctor reviewing the patient, and then ask that doctor for permission to ask them about the patient's outcome after they have reviewed the patient.'

'Most diagnoses, if missed, will become more obvious within 2 weeks. If the assumed diagnosis was wrong, more clues will emerge at that point to the correct diagnosis. The patient often returns because they do not recover or seem to recover very slowly. Some patients get readmitted for the diagnosis that was missed, or a complication of that diagnosis. You must learn the final correct diagnosis if you are to place the information you gathered, in the illness script of the correct diagnosis.'

Student: 'Yes.'

Me: 'If you assume your seniors are always correct, you are gambling your clinical learning on them. I do not know anyone who is 100% accurate, myself included. If your seniors are not 100% accurate but you assume their diagnosis is correct, you will assign the information of some patients to the wrong disease, which makes it difficult for you to learn how to differentiate between diseases.'

'Suppose you have clerked 10 patients whom your seniors labelled as having "viral gastroenteritis". You assume all 10 of them have viral gastroenteritis because you assume your seniors are always correct. This is a mistaken assumption. Therefore, some patients did not have viral gastroenteritis. Following up may reveal that some had acute appendicitis, some had bacterial gastroenteritis, and perhaps one or two might have had a rarer disease like diverticulitis and inflammatory bowel disease.'

'If you never followed up and therefore never learnt the true diagnosis for each patient, "viral gastroenteritis" based on your seniors' diagnosis seems to have many different presentations that mimic other diseases. Some of the patients labelled as having "viral gastroenteritis" had those other diseases instead, but you never followed up to discover the truth. You will have great difficulty differentiating clinically between viral gastroenteritis and those diseases. If the patient had tests performed, you will also mistakenly assume all the test results belonged to "viral gastroenteritis". So you cannot differentiate between viral gastroenteritis and those other diseases clinically and on testing.'

'This inability to differentiate between diseases clinically and on testing because you never followed up to verify the exact disease in each patient, is true for all diseases in all the patients you have ever seen and will ever see.'

The degree of horror on the face of the student correlates with the number of years they have spent assuming their senior was always right.

Student: 'Uh oh.'

Me: 'When you have the final correct diagnosis and can then retrospectively review your clerking notes, you can learn if you were right or wrong. You can assign the patient's information to the correct diagnosis, filling your illness script with accurate information about that disease. Furthermore, you also learn the true accuracy of your seniors, as I did long ago.'

The student often goes silent at this point. They must now weigh the unpleasant truth, which compels extra work to follow up on patients, against the temptation to stick to their beliefs; the beliefs that encourage them to carry on doing what they were doing, stay inside their 'comfort zone', and not follow up on the patients.

Me: 'The quality of your seniors will vary greatly. I noticed long ago that age, intelligence, knowledge, and title matter little when it comes to clinical accuracy. Why do you think some of your seniors are often inaccurate?'

There is a long pause, followed by the light of understanding appearing in the eyes of the student: 'They did the same thing as I did. They assumed their seniors were correct. They did not deliberately follow up on the patients. So, they copied the mistakes of their seniors. They never learnt to differentiate between the diseases clinically and on testing. If they continued like this as doctors, they would never improve.'

Me: 'Correct. If you do the same thing as someone else, you can expect the same result that person got.'

Student: 'No one has ever taught us this!'

Me: 'Should you expect others to teach you everything you need? I thought about this and taught myself. All of you have excellent brains. Do not shortchange yourselves. You should observe, think, teach yourself, and learn to question. Asking the right question gives you half the answer.'

--

After the above conversation, some students protest: 'Many teachers tell us to "see more patients". What you are suggesting is that we invest the time properly in one or a few patients and their diseases, to fully recognise and understand one or a few diseases every day instead of seeing many patients every day!'

The unspoken statement by the student is: Why should I believe you? No one has ever said this to us before. You seem to be alone in your view.

This is the fallacy of quantity over quality: believing that the quantity of people holding one view is more important than the quality and accuracy of that view.

Me: 'Is the quantity of friends you have, more important than the quality of your friends?'

Student: 'No. Unless I am egotistical.'

Me: 'If you were training to be a cook, is rushing through the cooking of a dish many times, more important than slowly and carefully cooking the dish to get it right and learn how to do it properly?'

Student: 'No.'

Me: 'Is quantity more important than quality?'

Student: 'No.'

Me: 'Is quality more important than quantity? In friendship, in training, and everything else too?'

Student: 'Yes. I see.'

Me: 'Anyone who understands true friendship and is a true friend knows the answer. Any master cook knows the answer. Any master *professional* knows the answer. You do need some quantity to have a chance to learn quality, but quantity matters little if you never bothered to ensure the quality of your learning. Furthermore, the phrase "See more patients" is misleading. Like the equally popular and misleading "Experience is important".'

Student (horrified): '*What?!?*'

Many students have heard the soundbites 'see more patients' and 'experience is important' from many teachers and doctors. Thus, their horror is understandable.

I sigh. 'Any phrase quoted without the full context can be misleading. The full sentence for "See more patients" is "See more patients *after you have ensured your learning from each patient is excellent and patient-centric.*" Likewise, the full sentence for "Experience is important" is "Experience is important *as an opportunity to learn, provided you recognise what you must learn and how it should be learnt.*"'

'Consider the remaining 80% of each of those sentences. Your reaction reveals that you have never heard the full sentence. The full sentence transforms the implied meaning of those three-word phrases. The full sentence demonstrates that quantity and experience are important *after* you have addressed a more crucial priority: realising what you must learn and how to learn that properly during your experience. If your seniors believed that quantity mattered more than quality, would they be tempted to see a patient, assume their seniors' conclusions are correct, and then rush on to the next patient?'

Student: 'Yes.'

Me: 'If you believed quantity mattered more than quality, would you likewise be tempted to do the same thing as these seniors?'

Student: 'Yes.'

Me: 'So, can you see why misleading phrases and misconceptions, passed through word-of-mouth with the accompanying assumption "my seniors are always correct", can harm successive generations? Teachers do not want to harm their students intentionally, but they can harm their students *unintentionally* because they never checked their assumptions or words. It is unlikely that the people who uttered those soundbites to you ever knew the full sentence. If they had known, it is unlikely they would have given you the misleading soundbite alone.'

Student: 'Yes.'

Me: 'Being encouraged to rush from patient to patient and failing to prioritise quality over quantity, is common. However, seeing more patients is unhelpful if you cannot differentiate between the diseases clinically and on testing. Instead, I recommend that you pick one or a few patients and their diseases, then learn accurately and fully about them every day.'

--

Many humans dislike having to think about the information they receive. Simplifying concepts and resorting to sound bites like 'experience is important' helps to make information appealing to the masses. Simplification drives the lucrative mass market, such as the sale of books.

However, simplification can become distortion. Failure to present the full context of a message, is often misleading. Research is no exception, especially if an author presents part of a study's conclusions whilst omitting the rest of the crucial context. Such presentations become half-truths or half-myths; they contain some grains of truth, but the absence of the full context often means that their conclusion is far from the whole truth and can readily mislead readers.

One half-myth is the '10,000-hour rule'. This half-myth suggests that the time and experience spent on training, with emphasis on a cut-off of 10,000 hours, is crucial to mastery of a skill. To rephrase this half-myth in another way: 'Experience is important'.

The original paper 'The Role of Deliberate Practice in the Acquisition of Expert Performance' acknowledged that though the time spent on practice seemed to contribute to expert performance, there was far more to expertise than just the time spent. The authors concluded that 'Contemporary elite performers have overcome several constraints. They have obtained early access to instructors, maintained high levels of deliberate practice throughout development, received continued parental and environmental support, and avoided disease and injury.'

One author of that paper, Professor Anders Ericsson, was displeased when others misrepresented this information to invent the '10,000-hour rule'. In 2012, he wrote another article, titled 'The Danger of Delegating Education to Journalists', wherein he expressed his displeasure at the invention of the 10,000-hour rule. To quote him, 'Our research found that the best violinists reported having spent a remarkably large number of hours engaged in solitary practice when, in fact, 10,000 hours was the *average* of the best group; indeed most of the best musicians had accumulated substantially fewer hours of practice at age 20.'

If we want to teach our students properly, we must teach the full context of the lessons and messages. We must avoid the use of misleading soundbites. We must teach them to recognise and pay attention to mistakes: our mistakes and others' mistakes. Not to shame or blame ourselves or others, but to accept that we make mistakes. And then teach them what to learn and how to learn from those mistakes.

Experienced, intelligent and knowledgeable doctors of all ranks make mistakes. To pretend those mistakes never occurred and say nothing to our learners, is to deliberately neglect to teach our learners how to avoid those mistakes. If we neglect this teaching, our learners are likely to repeat those mistakes, thereby harming more patients. This is a disservice to our learners and their patients.

Thus, throughout this book, I do not avoid the truths the world needs to accept.

Let us go back to the building up of one's illness scripts.

The effort needed to excel may not seem worthwhile. Furthermore, humans often like to 'fit in' with the crowd:

- Most medical students and doctors do not undertake such dedicated follow-up and systematically accurate learning. (If they did, I would not need to write this book.) If you lack compassion or reasoning, it becomes easy to think: 'Why should I bother? The other doctors seem to get by just fine.'

- Doctors living in wealthy societies often see their peers ordering batteries of tests and treatments. Therefore, it is easy to think: 'Why not copy my peers, and try lots of tests and treatments instead of learning how to get it right from the beginning? Many guidelines and protocols suggest approaches, so why bother to think when I can just follow those?'

Under these circumstances, the question about the quality of healthcare is often ignored.

The only consistent way to get it right for each unique patient is to have detailed illness scripts and robust clinical reasoning. No other option comes close.

However, when students and teachers are oblivious to the dual requirements of detailed illness scripts and robust clinical reasoning, this is the setup for routine disaster in every crop of medical graduates. These graduates often have few or no detailed illness scripts, cannot think straight, and unnecessarily harm the patients and themselves.

When these graduates remain oblivious to the dual requirements, they continue to lack detailed illness scripts and reasoning, to the continued detriment of their patients and themselves.

Illness scripts, illustrated

Consider the earlier example of Case #1: the patient with a headache and fever for 3 days.

Suppose 3 different doctors are handling this patient. All 3 doctors are thinking of bacterial meningitis. Here are their illness scripts:

Bacterial meningitis: Illness script

Novice, freshly graduated from medical school, and did not obey Rule #1	Novice, spent 5 years working and trying to memorise defensive guidelines, and did not obey Rule #1	Expert-to-be, spent 2 years asking patients in detail about clinical features and building expert-level illness scripts to obey Rule #1
• High fever	• Fever of at least 38 degrees Celsius	• Rapidly progressive illness
• Looks very sick	• Looks very sick	• Fever is universal, usually at least 38 degrees Celsius
• Headache	• Headache, severe	• Headache (?universal), unremitting (?secondary specific), severe
• Seizures	• Seizures	
• Vomiting, nausea	• Decreased consciousness	• Appearing toxic, may take up to 3 days
• Neck stiffness and hyperreflexia are always present	• Vomiting, nausea	• Vomiting, nausea
	• Neck stiffness always	• Seizures uncommon
	• Hyperreflexia often	• Decreased consciousness
• Kernig's sign positive	• Kernig's sign may be positive	• Neck stiffness often
		• Hyperreflexia sometimes
	• Brudzinski's sign may be positive	• Kernig's sign may be positive
• Demographics: any		• Brudzinski's sign may be positive
		• Tachypnea uncommon
		• Perfusion may be compromised
• CSF cell counts are high	• The elderly are at higher risk	• Babies and the elderly are at higher risk
• CSF cultures positive		• Immunocompromised (uncontrolled diabetes mellitus, HIV, spleen removed) at higher risk of meningitis and universal features may be delayed
	• CSF may look turbid	
• Pathophysiology: some memory of infections and immune response	• CSF cell counts are high	
	• CSF chemistry abnormal	• CSF may look turbid
	• Gold standard: CSF cultures positive	• CSF cell counts are high, not always neutrophilic
		• CSF chemistry abnormal
		• Gold standard: CSF cultures positive
	• Pathophysiology: forgotten virtually everything	• Pathophysiology: understands infections, immune response, neuroscience

Notice the width of the rightmost column and the sheer detail of that script, in contrast to the other 2 columns.

The exact content and composition of these illness scripts may vary among these doctors' peers. When considering like-minded peers, their illness scripts, the subsequent history taken, and the likely outcome of the clinical evaluation, can look like this:

	Novice, freshly graduated from medical school, and did not obey Rule #1	Novice, spent 5 years working and trying to memorise defensive guidelines, and did not obey Rule #1	Expert-to-be, spent 2 years asking patients in detail about clinical features and building expert-level illness scripts to obey Rule #1
Length of illness scripts	Up to 10 bits of information for each common disease with headache alone or fever alone, some diseases may cause both fever and headache	Up to 12 bits of information for each common disease with headache alone or fever alone, some diseases may cause both fever and headache 15 to 20 bits of information for the 'dangerous diagnoses not to miss' listed in defensive guidelines Up to 5 bits of information for rare diseases with similar presentation	30+ bits of information for each common or dangerous disease with headache alone, fever alone, and both headache and fever simultaneously 8 to 10 bits of information for each rare disease with headache alone, fever alone, and both headache and fever simultaneously
Composition of illness scripts and their details	60–70% clinical features. 10–20% risk factors and epidemiology. Pathophysiology <5%, and the remainder are test results	50–60% clinical features. 10–20% risk factors and epidemiology. Pathophysiology <1%, and the remainder are test results	80–85% clinical features. 5% risk factors and epidemiology. Pathophysiology 5 to 10%, and the remainder are test results

(Continued)

(*Continued*)

	Novice, freshly graduated from medical school, and did not obey Rule #1	Novice, spent 5 years working and trying to memorise defensive guidelines, and did not obey Rule #1	Expert-to-be, spent 2 years asking patients in detail about clinical features and building expert-level illness scripts to obey Rule #1
Number of differential diagnoses being immediately considered	0 to 3, some of which will not explain the presenting complaint	Up to 5, mostly based on 'dangerous diagnoses not to miss'. Some or all will not explain the presenting complaint	3 or more, all of which will explain the presenting complaint completely (or almost completely)
Pattern of questioning on Clinical Features	Asks about presenting symptoms and other symptoms, then launches into a list of significant negatives	May ask about presenting symptoms and other symptoms briefly, then rapidly launches into questions to rule out dangerous diagnoses. Goes through a long list of significant negatives	Focuses on presenting complaint, exploring details and using targeted questions that check for details in detailed illness scripts. Asks about other symptoms broadly and in a targeted manner without pause
The usual proportion of enquiry on risk factors	10–40%	20–50%	5–20%
Accuracy of clinical diagnosis	Variable	Poor. Excluding the dangerous diagnoses does not reveal the patient's current diagnosis	Good
Chance of missing a dangerous diagnosis	Moderate	Moderate to High, because of multiple mistakes that have become automatic bad habits over the years	Almost zero

The previous 2 tables illustrate the consequences of obeying Rule #1 versus not obeying Rule #1, over time.

A defensively obsessed, experienced doctor often has more knowledge than a fresh medical school graduate. Despite that slight advantage, this defensive-minded doctor's outcomes will often be the same or worse than the fresh graduate's outcomes.

Ironically, this experienced novice who follows arbitrary checklists of dangerous diseases 'to rule out' in the belief this will make them safe, is as likely (or even more likely!) to miss a dangerous diagnosis as the inexperienced graduate:

- The inexperienced graduate may pay attention to 'weird' clinical features and test results.

- The defensive-minded novice has cemented many dangerous habits, such as the habit of ignoring 'weird' clinical features and inconvenient test results.

When the experienced-but-defensively-obsessed doctor (middle column) is compared to a less-experienced peer who prioritised clinical reasoning in their learning and approach (rightmost column), the difference in accuracy, detail of illness scripts, and subsequent performance is dramatic.

If you assumed the expert-to-be in the rightmost column must be a doctor who has worked for 2 years, you would be wrong. Look at the heading of that column. I never mentioned 'working'. I mentioned the time spent on this dedicated learning journey. Thus, a diligent medical student who undertakes this learning journey from the start of medical school, can demonstrate the detailed illness scripts, questioning style and outcomes of the expert-to-be, by the time they graduate.

Illness scripts can include the pathophysiology of that disease. Skilled clinicians often understand the pathophysiology of diseases well, which is useful in puzzling circumstances. The chapter 'Pathophysiology in reasoning' explains the importance of pathophysiology in greater detail.

Capsule summary

- Patient information can be split into 2 categories: Clinical Features, and Epidemiology/Risk Factors.

- Clinical Features are the most important clues for the current diagnosis. These include all symptoms and physical data, such as Signs.

- Epidemiology/Risk Factors are not a direct manifestation of the current diagnosis. Thus, this information ranks below Clinical Features in importance.

- Since Clinical Features are direct manifestations of the correct diagnosis, you should try to explain all of the patient's clinical features with your diagnosis. (Rule #1)

- Following Rule #1 drives a patient-centred approach and effective learning.

- The combination of the priorities of the 2 categories of diagnostic information and Rule #1 of clinical reasoning, is the requirement of 'basic diagnostic reasoning'.

Frequently asked questions

Q: If there is more than 1 symptom in the presenting complaint, can't we just cherry-pick 1 symptom and get the details of that? Then focus less on (or ignore) the other symptoms?

A: You cannot cherry-pick a symptom in the presenting complaint, and then pay less attention to other symptoms in the complaint. All symptoms are the most direct clues to the correct diagnosis.

This cherry-picking of one or two symptoms and subsequent inattention to other symptoms in the presenting complaint, is a common mistake that impedes diagnostic accuracy. This mistake impedes learning too; when you have less clinical information about the patient's disease, you have less information to use to learn about that disease.

Q: What if the patient comes in requesting a test or treatment, without volunteering symptoms?

A: This is a common scenario. Examples include:

- An allergy test
- A blood test for (insert disease the patient suspects)
- A specific treatment, such as injections, for (insert problem).

Instead of giving in to the request or refusing the request right away, ask the patient for the symptoms that led to the request. Ask for their concerns. Sometimes, they have no symptoms but have a perception of needing the test/treatment. A concern is not always a symptom.

If the patient has symptoms, you need to know those symptoms because they are the direct clues to the correct diagnosis. Getting the correct diagnosis is more useful for the patient's health than performing a test or treatment that may be irrelevant to the underlying disease.

Q: Is the terminology in this book, directly synonymous with terminology from other sources such as journal articles?

A: No. If readers are to have mental clarity as they read this book, definitions must be specific and clear.

For example, I described how Risk Factors are second-line information that may change the likelihood of the patient having a disease. In the literature, the term 'Risk Factors' has been used to suggest factors that increase the risk of various things: outcomes of the disease, the presence of the disease, and non-compliance.

Some words have been so carelessly used that the basic meaning of the word and the implications of that meaning, have become muddled. When learners can comb through journal articles and supposedly reputable online resources and then encounter the same word being used haphazardly across different sources, confusion often sets in.

This confusing, careless use of words includes words like 'Diagnosis' (the next chapter) and 'Complication' (covered later in this book). Being clear and using these words correctly, gives mental clarity to the doctor. Clarity drives effective patient approach, decision-making and learning.

Think of the terminology, definitions and steps in this book as 'the language of universal clinical reasoning'.

The Glossary near the end of the book defines several important terms and their significance in clinical care.

Q: How are detailed illness scripts crucial to handling patients with more than 1 simultaneous diagnosis/disease?

A: Patients with more than 1 simultaneous diagnosis are far less common than those with just 1 diagnosis.

If you lack detailed illness scripts, from the perspective of Rule #1, you are ignorant. You would not know if the patient has one or two diseases because you do not know enough to 'explain all the patient's clinical features' with 1 disease. If you are too ignorant to fulfil the basic diagnostic reasoning requirement for a patient with 1 disease, how can you expect to promptly recognise the patient with more than 1 disease?

Inability to fulfil the basic diagnostic reasoning requirement in the early stages of your learning journey will usually mean your illness script is lacking, or your diagnosis is wrong. Sometimes, it is both: you lack detailed illness scripts *and* your diagnosis is wrong.

Lacking both detailed illness scripts and an understanding of the basic diagnostic reasoning requirement will also predispose you to make the same mistake in reverse: diagnosing 2 diseases simultaneously when there is only 1 disease. This mistake occurs because you struggle to prioritise, and do not know enough about any of the diseases to explain the patient's presentation and test results. Thus, you are more likely to suggest multiple simultaneous diagnoses as you go through each piece of patient information.

Conversely, having detailed illness scripts for each disease will warn you when a patient with two or more active diseases shows up. There will be some clinical features you cannot explain if you only used the illness script for 1 disease. This inability to fulfil Rule #1 has different implications because you have detailed illness scripts for most diseases; thus, the 'ignorance' reason is gone. By elimination, the remaining possibilities are:

1. You insist the patient has only 1 disease. Your inability to explain all the patient's clinical features with that disease, means that you are probably wrong.

2. The patient has more than 1 disease.

Further elaboration on the answer to this question is provided in the FAQ section of the chapter 'Putting it all together: the most likely diagnosis'.

Q: Since Rule #1 is to 'explain all clinical features', after hearing the patient's presenting complaint, would it be better to immediately request that they tell you about any and all symptoms they have, instead of focusing on the Presenting Complaint?

A: This request is not ideal, for 3 reasons. The first reason is disregard of the higher priority of symptom(s) in the Presenting Complaint, over all other symptoms. Focusing on the highest-yield symptom(s) initially to guide the flow of the consultation and adapt your evaluation, is more efficient.

The second reason is the signal you will be sending your patients. They have just told you their biggest concern in the Presenting Complaint. If you respond in any way other than showing direct interest in their biggest concern, some will get the impression that you are not listening or prioritising properly.

The third reason is the cost of getting all of that information, before moving on mentally. If the patient has many symptoms and details to describe, you can be potentially overwhelmed getting all this information without apparent prioritisation. If you are listening to all that information without generating relevant differentials, you may run out of time for a proper, targeted clinical evaluation.

Q: If the patient is 'faking', or has a psychosomatisation disorder or Munchausen syndrome, does this make 'explain all clinical features' futile?

A: Not at all. Rule #1 of clinical reasoning and the simultaneous pursuit of knowledge to obtain detailed illness scripts, gives you the awareness that you cannot explain these patients' clinical features with organic diseases.

You will have to study these patients like all other patients, to obtain a detailed illness script for these situations: faking, psychosomatisation and Munchausen syndrome.

WHAT IS A DIAGNOSIS?

If you had to purchase a bicycle, vehicle, or other manufactured product, how important is it that the manufacturer knows the materials and components for a reliable product?

I ask this question routinely. Virtually every medical student and doctor replies, 'Very!'

I continue: 'Good. if a manufacturer does not know what is needed to manufacture the product, would you trust the quality of their product?'

The reply is always 'No.'

I then say, 'Good. If the correct diagnosis is required for excellent decisions for patient care, would you trust a doctor who does not know what a diagnosis is?'

The reply is always 'No.'

I go on. 'By extension, should any patient trust us if we do not know what a diagnosis is?'

At this point, most students and doctors are puzzled by the simple-sounding questions and statements. Some start looking a bit wary because I am obviously not a fool.

Their concerns are justified when I proceed to state, 'You have been a medical student/doctor for some time now. You have seen many patients in many settings, and they all need the correct diagnosis. So, tell me the *universal* elements of the correct diagnosis.'

Almost everyone fails this question, and needs a lot of prompting to get to the answer. The components required to obtain the correct Diagnosis have never been taught to them, nor have they ever asked themselves this question (and thus, never learnt the answer).

--

Getting the correct diagnosis is central to making optimal decisions.

All practical, correct Diagnoses must have 3 universal elements. The correct diagnosis should:

1. Explain all the patient's Clinical Features…(if 'all' is not possible, at least 'most'…while you learn more to try to explain 'all')

2. …with a Disease/Illness…

3. …and include your impression of the Severity of the illness.

The following table demonstrates the short-term and long-term importance of using all 3 elements.

Element	Importance for the immediate patient	The consequence for your learning, short-term and long-term
Explain all clinical features	You maximise your chance of being right about the Disease and its Severity.	If you cannot explain all clinical features, you are either wrong about the Disease, or you guessed the right disease but are ignorant of some of its clinical features. Or you are both wrong and ignorant. Adhering to this element prompts you to fix your weaknesses.
Disease	The Disease decides all potentially reasonable decisions. This element helps you to focus on these decisions, instead of wildly thinking of 'everything I can do'.	Follow up on this patient. If you were right, affirming the correct diagnosis and seeing the response to your management reinforces your mental processes. If you were wrong, committing to a Disease gives you the chance to identify the personal weaknesses that led to this mistake.
Severity	Among the potentially reasonable options for all decisions (including tests and treatment), you select the best options: those that match the severity of your patient's illness. Estimating the correct severity, avoids excessive healthcare and inadequate healthcare.	You learn to clinically estimate the urgency and intensity of care that each patient needs. When you follow up with the patient, you then discover if your skill at assessing severity is accurate. If you were inaccurate, having previously committed to a severity level, you now get the chance to reflect and re-calibrate your assessment skill.

In comparison, if you ignore any of the 3 elements, the short-term and long-term consequences are:

Element ignored	Importance for the immediate patient	The consequence for your learning, short-term and long-term
Explain all clinical features	Your chance of making the wrong diagnosis, increases. Having no diagnosis or the wrong diagnosis, predisposes you to poor decisions and outcomes.	You do not learn how to explain all the clues that point directly to the diagnosis. Thus, you do not improve in diagnostic skill. You do not pursue the additional knowledge to build up the detailed illness scripts required for diagnostic skill.
Disease	You make decisions that are unfocused or irrelevant because you do not commit to the Disease.	You would not improve on your mental processing or learn your weaknesses, because you did not attempt this step.
Severity	Your decisions for the patient ignore the illness' severity. Therefore, the healthcare you provide is often excessive or inadequate.	You would not learn to instantly match your management plan to each unique patient's illness severity.

What is a disease?

A Disease is a specific, often pathologically definable condition arising from one or more derangements in the normal development, structure and/or function of the human body.

Therefore, Disease is *not* any of the following non-specific descriptions:

- A category of disease, e.g. infection, inflammation, cancer
- A vague organ-level description of the patient's information, e.g. nephrotic syndrome, nephritic syndrome, congestive cardiac failure
- A label of any single symptom, sign, or test abnormality, e.g. sepsis, pyrexia of unknown origin, prolonged headache for investigation,

altered mental state, anaemia, hyponatremia, '(insert symptom/sign/test abnormality) for investigation'

- A mix of categories or labels, such as 'secondary bacterial infection' or 'neonatal pyrexia'.

Medical students and doctors who do not practice making up their minds about specifics, do not learn to be specific. Their subsequent documentation and healthcare decisions often mirror the same lack of focus. Labelling a patient with a non-specific descriptor, is often followed by an unfocused battery of tests and treatments. The outcomes are often poor.

Does this mean that medical students and doctors should never learn these non-specific descriptors? Not at all. During medical training, future doctors are taught these descriptors and their general importance. For example, 'nephrotic syndrome' versus 'congestive cardiac failure' implies possible decisions for the patient.

These non-specific descriptors can be used as stepping stones towards the final correct diagnosis.

They are stepping stones along the way, *not the end that the doctor must reach.*

The end the doctor must reach for each patient, is the fulfilment of all 3 elements of the correct diagnosis. One element requires committing to a specific disease.

By obeying Rule #1 and following up on the patient as described in the previous chapter, medical students and doctors learn if they were right or wrong, and strive to attain the patient-centric standard of knowledge necessary to obey Rule #1. This is a cycle of ownership of one's outcomes and learning. By asserting ownership of themselves and their actions, this positive feedback cycle compels the learner to use the outcomes of their decisions to improve the quality of their learning and clinical practice.

The underlying disease ultimately dictates the optimal decisions. Let us use the descriptors of 'nephrotic syndrome' and 'congestive cardiac failure' to illustrate the contribution of knowing the underlying disease:

- There are important differences in treating nephrotic syndrome due to diabetes mellitus, versus nephrotic syndrome due to systemic lupus erythematosus.
- There are important differences in treating congestive cardiac failure due to uncontrolled primary hypertension, versus congestive cardiac failure due to viral myocarditis.

However, many commonplace teachings stop at vague descriptors, and then suggest an unfocused battery of tests and treatments. Doctors who stop at vague descriptors and then make decisions, often put themselves into a vicious cycle of failure.

Imagine that you are a doctor who has decided not to commit to specifics.

In failing to commit, it is harder to decide if you were right or wrong. By making it harder to conclude if you were right or wrong, following up on the patients can seem unnecessary. Without following up, patient-centred learning does not occur. This mess is compounded by pushing responsibility for the patient's outcome to the tools of our profession, such as tests, treatments and guidelines. Pretending that the doctor who (mis-)used those tools has little or no responsibility for the outcomes, enables denial of personal responsibility for poor outcomes. Since poor outcomes can be blamed on the tools, and the doctor is not responsible for the outcomes, why even bother to learn what the outcomes are? In this manner, the doctor can spend years seeing patients while not improving themselves at all.

This cycle of failure to commit, failure to see any need to learn, failure to learn, and pushing blame, to justify a continued lack of committing and learning, is a self-created vicious cycle. This cycle is the opposite of asserting ownership: it is a denial of ownership of one's actions and responsibility towards the patient.

Going back to the title of this chapter, a diagnosis (without needing to be correct) comprises the 2nd and 3rd elements: a specific disease and its severity level. Hence the need for the 1st element: Rule #1 of clinical reasoning. Without the 1st element, it is difficult to be consistently accurate and learn over time to become more accurate.

Though the 3 elements do not require explaining all risk factors or patient demographics, this category of information — the Epidemiology/ Risk Factors — does play a role in some situations. The situational use of Epidemiology/Risk Factors will be covered in the chapter 'Epidemiology and Risk Factors'.

Capsule summary

- The correct diagnosis will fulfil 3 elements: explain all clinical features, by committing to a specific disease, and estimate the level of severity of the illness.

- Striving to make complete diagnoses in all patients with these 3 elements, maximises your chance of getting it right and simultaneously increases the number of learning opportunities you have with every patient.

Frequently asked questions

Q: Can we make diagnoses by prioritising something else instead of Rule #1?

A: Yes, if you wanted to make mistakes. To any expert diagnostician, the answer to that question is always 'No'.

Making other diagnoses by prioritising something else, often occurs because of biases. The doctor can choose to diagnose:

1. The disease they or someone close to them has
2. The disease they have recently read about in the textbook
3. The disease that must be in their speciality
4. The dangerous disease they are most afraid of missing
5. The disease that they see most often in everyone else

The disease the doctor or someone close to the doctor has, has no relationship to the patient's disease. The same is true for the most recent disease they learnt in the textbook.

To think that all patients see a specialist for diseases that must fall within that specialist's expertise, is a fallacy. If you choose to look at everyone through rose-tinted glasses, they all look red to you. A specialist who cannot diagnose the patient's illness should refer the patient to the appropriate colleague.

The dangerous disease the doctor is most afraid of missing, focuses on the doctor's fears instead of the patient. Since patients come to the doctor for the disease they have, not the disease the doctor fears, prioritising the doctor's fears will defeat the purpose of the consultation.

The disease that the doctor sees most often in everyone else, is a manifestation of 'common things happen commonly'. Insisting that the most common diagnosis in everyone else must therefore be the most *likely* diagnosis in everyone regardless of their presentation, is a mistake. Each unique patient wants the doctor to get it right for them all the time instead of being right only when they have a common disease.

The only viable solution to 'how to teach doctors to make the correct diagnosis' is to teach the steps to the correct diagnosis, instead of trying to teach what not to do. That is why I have not listed the many (over 30) biases described in the literature.

Q: Are diagnostic tests crucial for the diagnosis?

A: No. It is no accident that top diagnosticians 'go clinically'.

When you do not have the diagnostic tests available, or the time to wait for the results of these tests (such as in rural areas, primary care clinics, and some emergencies), you must make the correct clinical diagnosis.

If you develop robust reasoning, diagnostic tests are valuable in a minority of patients.

In all professions, the accuracy and usefulness of the tool are entirely dependent on the skill of the professional. Tools can help to get the job done if they are used properly.

- If you are a novice tennis player, does using the world champion's tennis racket significantly increase your chance of victory in any match? No.

- If you are a novice cook, does having a high-technology oven significantly increase the chance of you producing a tasty meal? No.

- If a player has the world champion's technologically advanced tennis racket, who makes the best use of the racket: the novice, or the world champion? The answer is the world champion. The champion has the skill to wring every bit of performance from the racket. The novice does not.

- If a cook is given a high-technology oven they have never used before, who benefits most from the oven: the novice cook, or the master cook? The answer is the master cook. The master understands the nuances of every cooking option better than the novice.

Every tool requires skill to be used well. In the hands of the unskilled, tools can be useless or even harmful.

Tests are tools. Therefore, giving a poor reasoner plenty of testing options is often unhelpful and might be harmful to the patient. Those with poor reasoning often argue that tests can substitute for poor clinical competence. Merely making that argument proves the arguer has poor reasoning and is oblivious to reality, too. The universal truth about all tools and all professions is obvious to any half-attentive human.

If you have robust clinical reasoning, you rarely need diagnostic tests. When you do need diagnostic tests:

- You choose the relevant tests. Robust reasoners sometimes choose tests that surprise almost everyone else, who lack the reasoning to make or understand that choice.

- You correctly interpret the results of these tests. When a robust reasoner chooses a seemingly bizarre test, everyone else receives a double shock when the test result comes back supporting the clinical diagnosis the robust reasoner made. This occurs virtually every time the robust reasoner makes this seemingly bizarre choice.

- Even when the test results are false negative or false positive, you are not fooled.

If you have poor reasoning, you tend to rely on diagnostic tests in hopes they can substitute for your lack of reasoning. Since tests are tools and are dependent on your reasoning to choose and use properly, your hope is often futile. You tend to choose the wrong tests. Even when you choose the right tests by accident (you 'get lucky' by ordering the correct test among a battery of mostly irrelevant tests), you tend to see what you want to see, thereby misinterpreting the test results:

- You are falsely reassured by the plethora of normal-looking test results.

- When there are several abnormal results, you jump onto the wrong abnormality instead of recognising another genuinely disastrous abnormality for what it is.

- If a test is false-positive or false-negative, you would not realise it until it is too late.

- Being habitually inattentive, it is easy to ignore any inconvenient test result you cannot interpret.

In the hands of the unskilled, any tool is often useless and sometimes harmful.

Some doctors abandon clinical reasoning entirely. They consistently make wrong diagnoses based only on batteries of test results whilst ignoring the patient's clinical information. The diagnosis is cherry-picked from the textbook list of 'causes of that test result'. For example:

- A low white cell count is 'possible congenital immunodeficiency', in a middle-aged adult who has lived for decades without any history suggesting immunodeficiency.

- One positive test result on an 'allergy panel' of dozens of allergens is labelled as 'the patient has this allergy' even though the patient has been exposed to the purported allergen hundreds of times, with no symptoms.

Textbooks and other references can list several possible causes of each abnormality in the test results. The patient's clinical context narrows down the possibilities on any list to 1 cause or a few relevant causes for that patient.

I have had to counsel worried, totally asymptomatic patients who are given 5 or 6 such misdiagnoses simultaneously, based on over a hundred or more tests performed with apparently no valid reason. Performing a proper clinical evaluation each time revealed the truth (most had no disease) and enabled me to reassure them.

Decades of gross medical negligence, lawsuits, and mistakes in healthcare worldwide demonstrate the immutable truth: tests are often unhelpful and sometimes harmful in the hands of poor reasoners. An abundance of tests often fails to stop a major mistake, tragedy or lawsuit.

Instead of preventing disasters, an abundance of tests is likely to predispose to such disasters, because poor reasoners can complacently think the tests will make them safe, and thus see no need to be attentive towards patients or improve themselves.

Before you assume I am decrying all tests, notice I was referring to diagnostic tests. In some specialities and diseases, tests are frequently necessary for adjusting treatment after the diagnosis is known. Tests for these purposes are not diagnostic tests.

Q: You had said that non-specific descriptors of illness are 'stepping stones along the way' instead of stopping there. However, some labels can suggest there is no need to try to make the diagnosis clinically, such as 'pyrexia of unknown origin' (PUO). Why do you disagree?

A: Some labels are misleading because they ignore the doctor's job. Consider PUO. This is often defined as a prolonged fever of an unknown source after 3 weeks or longer, including at least 3 days of hospital evaluation or 3 outpatient visits.

This definition omits 1 crucial element: the doctors' inability to figure out the diagnosis. The source of the fever is unknown for at least that long because the doctors were unable to figure out the diagnosis and thus, cure the disease that was causing the fever. This element can imply that the doctors are not competent enough to figure out the diagnosis within that time frame, for that patient. This implication can offend some doctors.

This implication is the truth. The doctor seeing the patient is supposed to make the diagnosis. The number of days of hospitalisation and the number of outpatient encounters is not the deciding factor for the diagnosis.

If I cannot figure out the diagnosis before a patient meets the definition of PUO, I am not competent enough to figure out the diagnosis. Accepting this truth encourages me to do 2 things:

1. Getting help to make the correct diagnosis as soon as possible, instead of waiting until the definition of PUO is fulfilled

2. Be self-honest, which then prompts self-reflection and self-improvement

If I am not competent enough, I should get help. My duty is to the patient, not to my ego.

By extension, if I was not competent enough to get the correct diagnosis for the patient, my clinical reasoning was insufficient for that patient.

A lack of reasoning explains why some patients eventually, but unnecessarily, become labelled as PUOs.

Poor reasoners often fail to undertake a proper clinical evaluation and get the correct diagnosis. The patient can be labelled as 'Fever for investigation' day after day, visit after visit. Wild guesses at tests and treatments are often attempted. The source of the fever continues to be unknown. If the disease causing the fever does not self-resolve or respond to common treatments (such as courses of antibiotics), the patient eventually meets the definition of PUO.

Getting help in clinical reasoning for these patients, could have avoided the patient suffering until they fulfil the definition of PUO.

By the time the patient fulfils the definition of PUO, their prolonged suffering makes it even more important that the correct diagnosis is made. If a proper clinical evaluation and careful reasoning were never undertaken, this should be remedied immediately. If the diagnosis is still unclear after this evaluation and reasoning, the doctor should get help in terms of reasoning. Though some of these patients eventually need several tests, treatment and referrals, there is a huge difference between making decisions without trying to reason properly, and reasoning properly to avoid inappropriate decisions and delays in treatment.

Robust reasoning allows appropriate and focused management in at least some if not most of the patients labelled as PUO, thereby avoiding batteries of unnecessary tests, treatments and poor outcomes.

Poor reasoning explains why patients continue to be mismanaged even after they are labelled as PUOs.

When a poor reasoner sees a patient who fulfils the definition of PUO, the common reaction is to label the patient as PUO, fail to undertake a proper clinical evaluation or reason, and then do any or all of the following:

1. Resort to batteries of tests

2. Make referrals to specialities such as Infectious Diseases, Oncology and Rheumatology

3. Attempt trials of antibiotic treatment, broadening the coverage if previous antibiotics had failed

Batteries of tests, treatments, and referrals to multiple specialists, do not always lead to the correct diagnosis and optimal management. Sometimes, it is clinical reasoning that provides the solution instead. The importance of clinical reasoning is starkly illustrated by this example: a patient has undergone multiple tests and treatments, with results from many biochemical tests, repeated septic workups, and imaging modalities with no answer. The patient has languished in the hospital with the label of PUO for weeks. Multiple trials of treatment have failed. Many specialists have been consulted, each offering diagnoses and plans that are proven inaccurate. Finally, a diagnostic expert is summoned. The expert seems uninterested in the results of the tests and opinions of the many specialists who had seen the patient, and performs an independent clinical evaluation. After an exploration and understanding of the patient's presenting complaint, this expert suggests the correct clinical diagnosis that no one else thought of.

Some patients labelled with PUO have infections that common broad-spectrum antibiotics would fail to treat. Using ineffective antibiotics provide no benefit to the patient, waste time and increase the chance of complications.

Some patients labelled with PUO have autoimmune or malignant diseases. Antibiotics do not treat these diseases. Waiting in vain for the antibiotics to work only prolongs suffering and can increase the chance of complications, permanent harm and death.

In my experience, which has been echoed by my students, a proper clinical evaluation and obedience to Rule #1 are crucial in patients labelled with PUO:

- This evaluation and reasoning often reveal the correct clinical diagnosis, thereby avoiding the batteries of unnecessary tests, treatments and referrals.

- In many patients, a review of the history or documentation recorded at previous visits before the patient suffered long enough to fulfil the definition of PUO, already pointed to the correct clinical diagnosis. If robust reasoning had been applied to this information during the previous visits, the doctor could have diagnosed and treated them properly, thereby saving them from suffering until they meet the definition of PUO.

If a poor reasoner is not compelled to make the correct clinical diagnosis to avoid the patient suffering long enough to be labelled as PUO, and is also not compelled to make the correct diagnosis after the patient has been labelled as PUO, then this poor reasoner will not improve.

GENERATING EARLY DIFFERENTIAL DIAGNOSES: THE 3-MINUTE HABIT

You have just heard the presenting complaint. About 20 to 60 seconds have passed since the patient began talking.

You ask for more details of all the symptoms in the presenting complaint.

As you ask for more details, you may customise your history-taking to ask high-yield questions. These high-yield questions target specific details that can help you nail the correct diagnosis instantly. Expert diagnosticians do this automatically.

This customisation to ask the highest-yield questions occurs because you have the most relevant differential diagnoses in your head.

Thus, differential diagnoses should be generated early.

Differential diagnoses are all the relevant diseases the doctor must consider, for the patient before them.

The initial questions, such as 'tell me more about (insert symptom)', are open-ended.

When pursuing specific differentials, questions usually become close-ended. Expert diagnosticians can often be seen switching to these high-yield, close-ended questions within 3 minutes of the start of the consultation.

However, the speed at which open-ended questions are replaced by close-ended questions is not a reliable indicator of accuracy or competence. Many defensiveness-obsessed doctors rapidly switch to close-ended questions, because they focus on ruling out their arbitrary list of dangerous diagnoses.

Robust reasoners who are not getting useful information with close-ended questions may switch back to open-ended questions. Their questions flow with the differentials they are considering.

Why you must generate likely possibilities to pursue, early

When generating differential diagnoses, generate at least 2 differentials. The sooner you generate the relevant differentials, the sooner you can customise your evaluation to focus on these differentials. The ability to generate differential diagnoses and evaluate each of them is based on the richness of your illness scripts for multiple diseases.

If your illness scripts are non-existent or scant, it is difficult to generate relevant differentials. This is common at the start of medical school. If medical students and doctors do not dedicate the effort necessary to build up accurate and rich illness scripts, the inability to generate and evaluate for relevant differentials can persist for decades.

The doctor with no differential diagnosis can use the rigid list of questions that is often seen in 'approaches' books. Questions about potential symptoms can be asked in a head-to-toe fashion, without any apparent relationship to the presenting complaint and without relevant differentials. There are 3 problems with this approach:

1. Asking questions in a rigid sequence without adapting to the patient's information, demonstrates a lack of focus on the patient. The questions are 'fishing expeditions'. Failure to prioritise questions often accompanies failure to understand the significance of the answers to those questions. This lack of understanding explains how some medical students and doctors can ask a long list

of questions and get some of the crucial answers (buried among the many answers to their many questions) that point to the patient's diagnosis, and then proceed to completely miss the diagnosis.

2. Checklists of standard questions are very long. If the questioner intends to complete the entire checklist, they will need a long time. This time is often not available in medical exams and real-world consultations. Therefore, to finish within the time limit, the questioner must randomly abandon some questions because they do not know the importance of each question and its answer. They must also randomly abandon steps in the physical examination.

3. Students and doctors tend to miss diagnoses that they never considered. In a tutorial or exam, when the teacher asks the student for the diagnosis and relevant differentials, the student often cannot come up with relevant differentials. When asked, 'Did you enquire about this bit of information / examine the patient for this sign?' — the teacher is often suggesting information that would have pointed to the relevant differentials, but the student often says 'No'. To handle those tasks properly, the student would have needed to think of the relevant disease, then think of the illness script for that disease, and then think of that piece of information to evaluate before time ran out!

This is where the previous chapter comes in. Recall the first 2 elements of the correct diagnosis:

1. Explain all the patient's Clinical Features…(if 'all' is not possible, at least 'most'…while you learn more to try to explain 'all')

2. …with a Disease/Illness…

Generate the relevant diseases that fulfil both elements with whatever information you have, early in the consultation.

From a timed perspective, I suggest the 3-minute mark. This means trying to generate at least 2 to 3 relevant diseases that fulfil the first 2 elements of the correct diagnosis, by the 3rd minute after the patient begins mentioning their symptoms. This is called the 3-minute habit.

Why 3 minutes?

- Three minutes is enough time to get a fair amount of detail of the presenting complaint, sometimes allowing the doctor to ask for any other symptoms too.

- The 3-minute mark gives many doctors enough time to use illness script information to customise their history to their satisfaction.

- As many exam scenarios and consultations allow 10 minutes or more, this buys the candidate at least 7 minutes to evaluate for the relevant differentials, secure the correct diagnosis and gather information to customise the patient's management.

Consider using a stopwatch, phone timer or any other device to systematically train yourself to develop this time sensitivity.

If you obey Rule #1 of clinical reasoning, your illness scripts will grow in tandem with your learning and experience. You will be able to generate the relevant differentials, earlier and earlier. An expert diagnostician can consistently generate these as early as the 1-minute mark, and can sometimes nail the correct diagnosis in less than a minute. By following the basic diagnostic reasoning requirement, your close-ended questions will be accurate because they will identify the correct diagnosis early on.

How to generate relevant initial differential diagnoses

Relevant differentials fulfil the first element of the correct diagnosis: they 'fit' the entirety (or at least most) of the patient's clinical features. Thus, this element is called 'Clinical Fit'.

The following diagrams demonstrate how you use the patient's Clinical Features to generate differential diagnoses.

Clinical Fit: Start Here

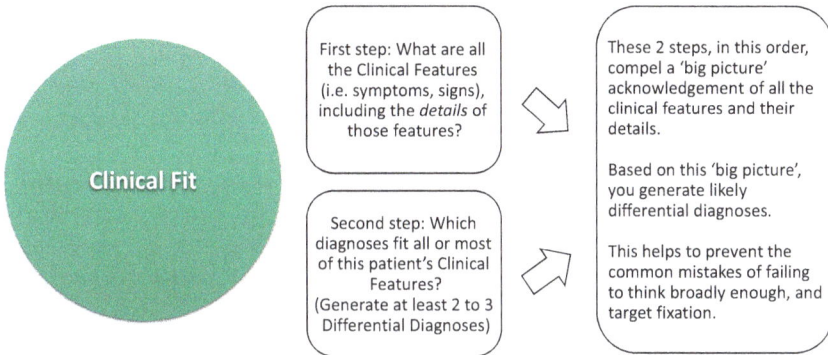

Clinical Fit

First step: What are all the Clinical Features (i.e. symptoms, signs), including the *details* of those features?

Second step: Which diagnoses fit all or most of this patient's Clinical Features? (Generate at least 2 to 3 Differential Diagnoses)

These 2 steps, in this order, compel a 'big picture' acknowledgement of all the clinical features and their details.

Based on this 'big picture', you generate likely differential diagnoses.

This helps to prevent the common mistakes of failing to think broadly enough, and target fixation.

'Explain all clinical features' to choose relevant differential diagnoses, can be shown as a Venn diagram.

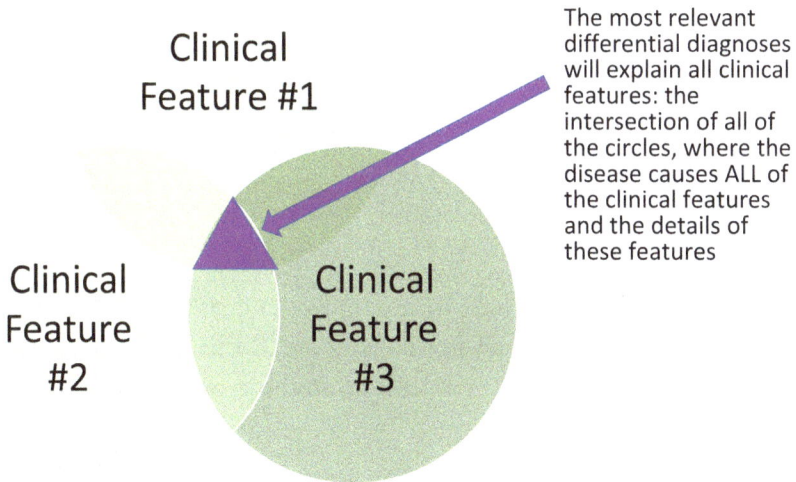

Clinical Feature #1

Clinical Feature #2

Clinical Feature #3

The most relevant differential diagnoses will explain all clinical features: the intersection of all of the circles, where the disease causes ALL of the clinical features and the details of these features

Afterwards, think quickly through the patient demographics and known risk factors (Epidemiology/Risk Factors category). This category is shown as a blue circle, which is not part of the Venn diagram.

... now look at the Blue Circle

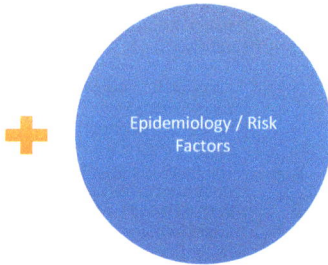

- Epidemiology / Risk Factors information helps you to weigh and prioritise your differentials, sometimes suggesting new differentials.
- Consider the patient's demographics (age/race/gender/etc.)
- For each of the differential diagnoses you generated using the Clinical Features, think of the epidemiology and risk factors. Match the Epidemiology/Risk Factors of those differentials, to your patient.
- If there are new differentials that are suggested by the patient's demographics and risk factors, which also clinically fit the patient, add these to your existing differentials.

Consider whether the initial differentials should be re-ranked based on Epidemiology/Risk Factors. This re-ranking targets the differentials that seem equal in Clinical Fit.

Re-ranking the differentials that are unequal in clinical fit is usually unnecessary; any diagnosis that has less clinical fit to the patient is automatically less likely than the diagnoses with superior clinical fit.

A diagnosis that fits all of the patient's Clinical Features better than the rest, is automatically the most likely diagnosis. The most likely diagnosis should not be re-ranked unless you have overwhelming proof that this diagnosis is impossible.

Sometimes, the patient's demographics and risk factors may suggest new differentials you had not considered. To be relevant, these new differentials must totally (or at least mostly) explain the patient's clinical features:

- For example, a young man presents with 1 day of severe, unremitting right iliac fossa pain. On examination, he has tenderness over the right iliac fossa, and abdominal guarding. Acute appendicitis is the most likely diagnosis. In the absence of any chronic co-morbidities or prior surgery, there are few relevant differentials for his clinical presentation.

- If a woman with the same profile (except for gender) and presentation as the man appears, some doctors might not think of the relevant differentials involving the ovaries until they think of her gender (a demographic), as ovarian diseases are relevant differentials only in females.

Let us illustrate this by using Tina's example.

CASE #2: Tina

Tina is a 13-year-old Chinese girl with a past medical history of cystitis (this is a lower urinary tract infection). She consults you with the Presenting Complaint of headache and fever for 3 days.

--

Clinical reasoning-based mental process: The patient has symptoms of fever and headache lasting 3 days. These are direct clues to the current diagnosis.

Next course of action: You tell the patient, 'Please tell me more (about the headache and fever).'

If you have just begun medical school and thus have little to no knowledge of diseases, the generation of differential diagnoses may be based on single symptoms and non-specific.

For Tina's 3 days of fever, you might think of:

1. Any infection
2. Inflammatory diseases

For Tina's 3 days of headache, you might think of:

1. Primary headaches such as migraine
2. Meningitis (viral, bacterial)

3. Infections outside the brain with the symptom of fever, as a headache can be caused by fever

4. Intracranial haemorrhage

There are 2 suggestions under 'fever' and 4 suggestions under 'headache'.

The next step is the Clinical Fit: which diseases cause both fever and headache for 3 days?

Two possibilities seem the most likely: meningitis, as well as non-brain infections with fever.

The mental Venn diagram looks like this:

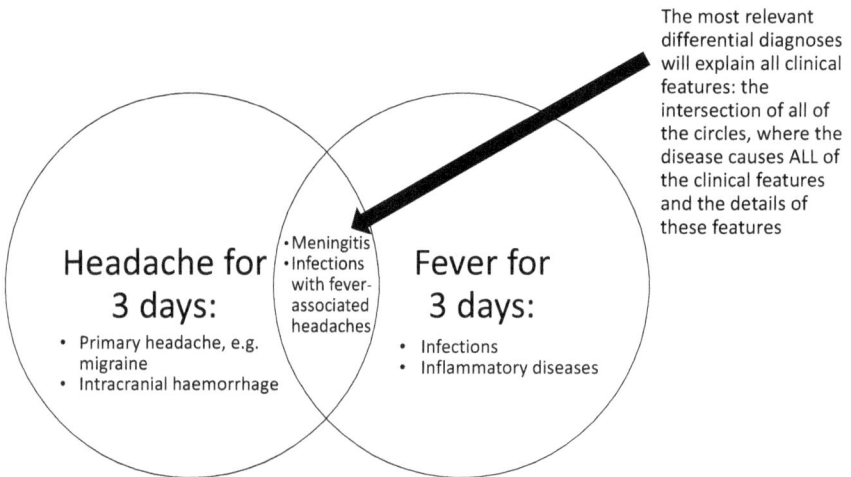

The most relevant differential diagnoses will explain all clinical features: the intersection of all of the circles, where the disease causes ALL of the clinical features and the details of these features

Headache for 3 days:

• Meningitis
• Infections with fever-associated headaches

• Primary headache, e.g. migraine
• Intracranial haemorrhage

Fever for 3 days:

• Infections
• Inflammatory diseases

Then consider Tina's demographics and risk factors: none of these has any bearing on the differentials. Both meningitis and non-brain infections are common in teenage girls with cystitis.

Imagine that a medical student has generated these differentials for Tina, and is discussing the differentials with a teacher.

If the student suggested 'cystitis' because the patient has the Risk Factor of cystitis, the teacher can point out that the patient has the Clinical Features of headache and fever. Cystitis does not cause either symptom.

The student could suggest that the patient has pyelonephritis, an infection of the kidneys because of the risk factor of cystitis. The student could argue that since patients with pyelonephritis often have a fever, they might also have a headache, which was caused by the fever too.

The teacher could agree that even if a patient with pyelonephritis happened to also have a headache, these patients would be very unlikely to have a Presenting Complaint of headache and fever. Kidney infections tend to produce other more troublesome symptoms such as severe flank pain, which the patient would have immediately volunteered instead!

These examples reinforce the importance of the presenting complaint. The presenting complaint alters the top differentials for the patient.

If you have 2 patients, each with identical symptoms #1 to #5, the most likely diagnosis and top differentials can be vastly different between both patients if the presenting complaint of the 2 patients is different. Suppose the first patient's presenting complaint is symptoms #1 and #2, whilst the second patient's presenting complaint is only symptom #5. Even before exploring the details of the presenting complaint, the difference in 1 detail of the Clinical Features is apparent: the presenting complaint is different between the 2 patients.

The next chapter will demonstrate how targeted history-taking is altered by these early differential diagnoses.

Capsule summary

- Generating relevant differential diagnoses requires the first 2 elements for the correct diagnosis.

- Generating relevant differential diagnoses early gives you enough time to target your subsequent evaluation, make the correct diagnosis, and gather information for management.

- Differential diagnoses are generated based on Clinical Fit. Afterwards, any patient demographics and known risk factors are usually used to re-rank differentials of equal likelihood. Sometimes, these demographics and risk factors can suggest new differentials.

Frequently asked questions

Q: Why can't you generate differential diagnoses based on all known information (Clinical Fit, known Risk Factors and patient demographics) simultaneously?

A: Attempting to process all of that information simultaneously has 2 major disadvantages compared to the stepwise approach.

The first disadvantage stems from cognitive load: the more information you use simultaneously when trying to generate early differentials, the slower you are.

The second disadvantage comes from ignoring the relative importance of each piece of information. If you want to be accurate, less-important information cannot be assigned the same importance as more-important information.

Try this exercise. Pick a patient. Generate the initial differentials in 3 ways:

1. Patient demographics and risk factors
2. Patient demographics and risk factors and all clinical features (Clinical Fit)
3. Clinical Fit

Consider Way #1. When you use patient demographics and risk factors whilst ignoring Clinical Fit, you will often be overwhelmed. If the patient is a male teenager living in the city, would you want to think of all the diseases that can occur in males, teenagers or city dwellers? Is the patient's gender, age or place of residence, the cause of the disease?

Since attempting to generate differentials using all of this lower-priority information is overwhelming, poor reasoners usually cherry-pick 1 piece of information in this category, ignore all the other information in this category, and then ignore the clinical features they are unable to explain. This is 1 reason why poor reasoners often seem unable to suggest any relevant diagnosis.

Consider Way #2. When you use all the patient's information as if it is all equally important, you move very slowly and your accuracy is compromised. Recall Tina's example, earlier in this chapter. If you tried thinking of 'causes of 3 days of fever and headache, with a history of cystitis and 13 years old and Chinese and female', it would take you longer to think of all the relevant differentials while trying to remember all that information. Once you compare Way #2 to Way #3, the difference in speed and accuracy becomes obvious. Way #3 requires you only to think of 'causes of 3 days of fever and headache', which generates the relevant differentials shown in the Venn diagrams in this chapter.

When you use clinical fit first (Way #3), you are often faster and more accurate than the other 2 ways.

There are some situations where you need to ask about the Epidemiology/Risk Factors early on, to think of the correct diagnosis early on. Those rare situations are discussed in the chapter 'Epidemiology and Risk Factors'.

Q: Patient demographics and risk factors are not the mainstays of generating differentials. Does this mean you ignore this information completely if there is only 1 clinical diagnosis?

A: No, you do not ignore patient information.

If you are left with only 1 diagnosis that seems unlikely based on the patient's demographics and risk factors, this does not mean that diagnosis must be automatically correct or automatically impossible. You must evaluate both angles: check your existing knowledge of that diagnosis (is it really impossible?), and ask yourself one more time if there are other relevant differentials upon consideration of the patient's demographics and risk factors.

Q: When is it necessary to interrupt a patient soon after the start of the consultation?

A: Doctors must guide the course of the consultation. Thus, interruption of the patient can become necessary in 2 situations:

1. The emergency where the patient is likely to die unless the diagnosis is obtained within the next few minutes, but the patient/ accompanying person providing the information is wasting time by rambling about less-crucial topics (example: 'Why did not I realise he was going to be sick before this? Oh! I should have! This is all my fault! I really should come home and pay attention to my family more closely! However, sometimes I do not see him when I come home from work. Why, just the other day, when I got home…')

2. The non-emergency where the patient provides a rambling and seemingly irrelevant discourse for a few minutes, and there is an unspoken limit as to how much time can be spent in the encounter. Other patients are waiting to be seen.

Situation #1 is rare. Most of the time, when the patient is near death, they cannot ramble and the people accompanying them do not ramble. If you do encounter situation #1, step in and take charge politely.

Situation #2 is common. The patient is giving disorganised and/or irrelevant information soon after the encounter begins. Even if this situation crops up, sit quietly and pay close attention for at least 1 minute. Gathering information is not just about the actual words being said. The mood of the patient and the nature of the information provided give the doctor insight into the patient's emotional state and priorities, which can be used to shape the subsequent handling of the patient.

The usual Situation #2 in my Paediatric Allergy clinic is a child brought by their parents with pages of test results spanning months to years. These results can be tests related to allergy, invalid tests purporting to relate to allergy, and sometimes other common laboratory tests such as a full blood count, blood chemistry, and so on.

The parents will usually provide the test-based diagnosis the previous doctor allegedly mentioned, along with prior advice and management plans. There is no mention of the symptoms or signs.

After the initial minute, I gently interrupt with, 'I am sorry that I must interrupt you. I hear what you are saying and I see these results. The most important information is the problem you initially noticed, which led you to bring your child to see the doctor in the first place. Without information on that problem, it is hard to accurately figure out what is going on and interpret these test results. Can we start with that problem?'

Q: 'Common things happen commonly'. Based on this saying, many teachers tell their students that 'you should always think of common diseases first'. However, 'Common' is disease epidemiology, which you rate as low in importance. How do you explain this?

A: It is true that common things happen commonly. However, you must focus on the patient's Clinical Features first.

Let us go back to Tina, the patient with 3 days of headache and fever.

Let us try using 'you should always think of common diseases first', as the first step in generating possibilities to pursue. The most common diseases would be 'infections in general' and 'primary headaches'. Meningitis and infections with fever-associated headaches would be less common than the 'most common diseases causing headaches'. If you further expanded on infections in general, the most common would be a viral upper respiratory tract infection.

Imagine trying to argue along these lines: the most likely diagnosis for this patient with 3 days of fever and headache is a:

- Viral upper respiratory tract infection because it is the most common infection in everyone else on Earth. A decent reasoner would counter, 'Do you expect someone with a viral upper respiratory tract infection, to routinely present without any mention of cough or nasal symptoms? Yes, it is possible, but we are not talking about whether "anything on Earth is possible". We are talking about *this patient*, not everyone else on Earth.'

- Primary headache such as migraine, because it is a common primary headache in the population. A decent reasoner would counter, 'The patient has a fever, too. Primary headaches do not cause fever. Are you ignoring the fever? Or are you saying the patient has 2 diseases simultaneously, which should never be the first proposal unless there is truly no single disease that explains every clinical feature?'

'Common things happen commonly' is true. Over hundreds to thousands of patients, the common diseases will be the most common diseases you encounter. If you rely solely upon 'common things happen commonly', you will naturally be right in many patients.

However, if you use 'common things happen commonly' to ignore inconvenient-to-explain clinical features from patients, you dramatically increase the chance of being wrong in patients who do not have the most common diseases.

Someone who wants to be making excellent decisions all the time, would not want to be correct only in patients with common diseases. They would want to be correct all the time.

If you decide 'common things happen commonly' is your primary focus, ask yourself: are you now deciding 'common things happen always'?

Is it a mistake to teach 'you should always think of common diseases first'? Yes. However, most of your teachers were not intentionally trying to mislead you. They are not aware of their thought process.

Upon hearing a student mention rare diseases and nothing else, the teacher may have admonished them with 'you should always think of common diseases first'. However, clinically competent teachers who say this, often do not follow their own advice and fail to recognise that their teaching does not match their thought process. Thinking of common diseases was the 3rd or 4th step in their thought process. The first step was listening to the patient and generating the possibilities based on the clinical features; the second was generating the mental Venn diagram earlier in this chapter. Since the teacher did not describe their first 2 steps, their students may mistakenly think the teacher did always think of common diseases first.

The full and accurate statement that applies to 'common things happen commonly' is: You should think of common diseases that *explain all of the clinical features of the patient*, before thinking of rare diseases that can also fit this patient.

This full statement reflects Rule #1 and the stepwise method described in this chapter.

TARGETED EVALUATION: HISTORY

Clinching the correct diagnosis clinically in the first doctor-patient encounter, is often feasible.

Generating the relevant differential diagnoses is necessary for a targeted clinical evaluation that is relevant to the patient. Calling upon one's illness scripts for those differentials enables a thorough exploration of each relevant differential. When learners struggle with this exploration because they lack detailed illness scripts, obeying Rule #1 of clinical reasoning compels these learners to expand their illness scripts.

In contrast, generating irrelevant differential diagnoses, using labels that do not fit the definition of 'Disease', or having nothing in mind, results in an unfocused a-little-bit-of-everything evaluation that is insufficient to get the correct diagnosis clinically.

The targeted evaluation usually starts with the targeted history.

Targeted history: Clinical Features first, then Risk Factors

Based on the relevant differential diagnoses, mentally recall and compare the illness scripts of the differentials.

Questions that focus on the most likely disease the doctor already suspects, usually have a higher yield than questions that focus on unlikely diseases.

The most rudimentary questions target information within each illness script in isolation. The doctor's questions to the patient, probe for this information. The doctor goes through each script one at a time, gathering information on each disease without regard to the other differentials in that patient.

Higher-yield questions are more useful than rudimentary questions. These higher-yield questions require the doctor to have detailed illness scripts for all the relevant differentials. One example is the high-yield question that targets information exclusive only to 1 illness script among the illness scripts of all the relevant differentials for the patient. Such questions come from Rule #3 of clinical reasoning, which is discussed later in this chapter.

Clinical Features and their details are direct clues to the correct diagnosis and thus should be pursued first. Risk Factors can be asked after the enquiry for Clinical Features is complete. Sometimes, it is unnecessary to pursue any Risk Factors.

After completing the questioning for your top suspect in the differentials, move on to the next most likely disease.

Rudimentary targeted questioning

CASE #4: Joe

Joe is a 20-year-old man with the Presenting Complaint of severe pain in the right lower abdomen for 2 days. The pain is so severe that he is unable to walk properly. You saw him limping into your consultation room. He also has fever of up to 38 degrees Celsius, nausea, and vomiting once over the last 2 days.

--

(Continued)

Generation of relevant differentials, order of descending likelihood:

1. Acute appendicitis

2. Septic arthritis of the right hip

3. Acute viral gastroenteritis

4. Intestinal obstruction (exact Disease causing this is unclear)

Let us illustrate the use of rudimentary questions, with Case #4.

Acute appendicitis would be the most likely diagnosis. It explains all the Clinical Features. The other diagnosis that appears to fit this initial information on the clinical features, is an infection in the region of the right hip, such as septic arthritis of that hip. If we contend that septic arthritis does not tend to present with lower abdominal pain whereas acute appendicitis does, then acute appendicitis becomes more likely than septic arthritis of the right hip. Even after considering Epidemiology/Risk Factors, there is no re-ranking based on Epidemiology/Risk Factors, because such re-ranking only applies to differentials of equal Clinical Fit.

Suppose we decide that septic arthritis and acute appendicitis are equal in Clinical Fit. We move on to the Epidemiology/Risk Factors category. Based on the information in the Epidemiology/Risk Factors category, we would re-rank acute appendicitis and septic arthritis because we had decided they had equal Clinical Fit. Acute appendicitis is far more common than septic arthritis in the general population and young adult men. Thus, acute appendicitis moves above septic arthritis in the initial likelihood.

Acute viral gastroenteritis is less likely than the top 2 possibilities because it has less Clinical Fit: the patient has crippling pain in the right lower abdomen and did not mention diarrhoea. Diarrhoea is expected in acute viral gastroenteritis, and the primary concern is usually not the pain, but marked vomiting and/or diarrhoea. We move on to the Epidemiology/Risk Factors category. Though acute viral gastroenteritis is more common than both acute appendicitis and septic arthritis of the right hip in the general population, re-ranking based on Epidemiology/Risk Factors only applies to differentials of equal Clinical Fit.

Intestinal obstruction (the cause of this is currently unclear) may come up as another differential. However, most diseases causing intestinal obstruction do not cause fever. In addition, by the end of the second day of intestinal obstruction, it is unusual to have such severe pain whilst vomiting only *once*. Therefore, using Clinical Fit, intestinal obstruction is the lowest of the 4 possibilities. Epidemiology/Risk Factors will not change the ranking of intestinal obstruction.

Now, the targeted questioning begins. Start with the most likely diagnosis: acute appendicitis.

You recall your illness script for acute appendicitis. A sample question in each category of diagnostic information would be:

- Clinical Features: 'Did the pain begin elsewhere, then move to the part you are pointing to now?' — because the pain in acute appendicitis may begin in the upper-to-middle abdomen, then migrate to the right lower abdomen.

- Risk Factors: 'Have you previously had your appendix removed?' — because the previous removal of the appendix is a strong risk factor against having acute appendicitis now.

After completing your questioning about acute appendicitis, your subsequent steps would depend on the likelihood of the patient having this diagnosis.

If you were almost 100% certain the patient has acute appendicitis, you might briefly ask a few questions about the other differentials. Or you might not; when a single diagnosis is already almost 100% certain, it is debatable if asking more diagnostic questions will add any value to the consultation. Whether you ask about other differentials or not, you should hasten to the physical examination to look for signs that affirm or refute your suspicions. If you are certain this is acute appendicitis, call the surgeon immediately. Prompt treatment of acute appendicitis leads to improved outcomes.

If you were not at least 90% convinced the patient has acute appendicitis, you would move on, and then spend a fair amount of effort and time on the next differential diagnosis, septic arthritis. A sample question in each category of diagnostic information would be:

- Clinical Features: 'Is the pain markedly worse when you move your right leg?' — if the answer was yes, septic arthritis would be a strong suspect. Though the answer to this question can also be 'yes' in acute appendicitis, you have already evaluated for acute appendicitis and formed a general opinion about the likelihood of acute appendicitis.

- Risk Factors: 'Have you had any recent cuts in your skin?' — because open cuts that enable bacteria to enter the body, can be a risk factor for septic arthritis.

Your subsequent steps would depend on the likelihood of the patient having septic arthritis. If you suspected septic arthritis with near-total certainty, you would hasten on to the physical examination, and then make the appropriate healthcare decisions.

If you were not certain the patient has septic arthritis, you would then move on to the next-lower differential diagnosis, acute gastroenteritis. A sample question in each category of diagnostic information would be:

- Clinical Features: 'Do you have diarrhoea? If so, how many episodes?' — because diarrhoea is a cardinal feature of gastroenteritis. Though you could argue that acute appendicitis can also explain an absence of diarrhoea or a few episodes of diarrhoea, you have already evaluated for acute appendicitis, and deemed acute appendicitis unlikely.

- Risk Factors: 'Is anyone else in your family having vomiting or diarrhoea?' — because a positive contact history in the family, if recent, is a risk factor for having gastroenteritis.

Your subsequent steps would depend on the likelihood of the patient having acute gastroenteritis. If you were sure the patient had gastroenteritis, you could either examine the patient or complete the rest of your history, and then manage accordingly.

If you were unconvinced the patient had gastroenteritis, you would move on to intestinal obstruction. A sample question in each category of diagnostic information would be:

- Clinical Features: 'Do you have any swelling of your tummy?' — because the presence of abdominal distension would make intestinal obstruction a strong suspicion.
- Risk Factors: 'Have you had surgery before? If so, tell me more.' — because intestinal obstruction is unlikely in a young man without risk factors such as previous intra-abdominal surgery.

Your subsequent steps would depend on the likelihood of the patient having intestinal obstruction. If you were certain this was intestinal obstruction, you would examine the patient, and then try to discern the disease causing the clinical picture of intestinal obstruction. Subsequent decisions can involve testing and requesting assistance to manage this patient.

--

The sequence of 4 differentials being evaluated, assumes that no other diagnosis-changing information was revealed during the pursuit of those differentials. If this patient suddenly blurts out, 'Oh! I forgot to tell you that I am not walking properly because I heard that walking makes any pain worse. The pain radiates to the right side of my back and is slightly higher up. Also, my urine is cloudy.' This new information, added to the previous information from the patient, would prompt you to think of acute pyelonephritis instead as the most likely diagnosis.

Let us move on to higher-yield questions. Higher-yield questions call upon Rules #2 and #3 of clinical reasoning.

Illness scripts: Universal Clinical Features (Rule #2 of clinical reasoning)

Many diseases have one or more Universal Clinical Features. These are symptoms or signs that are present in virtually everyone who has that disease. Thus, the absence of that symptom or sign will usually exclude that disease.

This is Rule #2 of clinical reasoning: **The absence of Universal Clinical Features for a disease, makes that disease almost impossible in your patient.**

To use this Rule, you must know that Clinical Feature was a Universal feature for that disease *and* when that clinical feature appears during the course of the disease. Some Universal Clinical Features may appear later in the course of the disease.

As of the end of 2022, there does not seem to be any reference that explicitly names Universal Clinical Features and fully describes them for different diseases. To learn the Universal Clinical Features, keep a patient log listing all patients whom you have evaluated clinically. To safeguard patient confidentiality, anonymise the log by removing all unique patient identifiers such as full name, date of birth, identification card number, and so on.

Since accurately assigning these patients, and by extension their information, to each disease in the log requires maximum certainty that they have that disease, follow up on these patients. Do not assume that your colleague or senior is automatically correct in their initial diagnosis. Reality is the final arbiter and asserts itself through the patient's progress over time. The chapter 'Follow-up' in Section 4 explains the follow-up in greater detail.

Each page of the log should be devoted to 1 disease. The patients with that disease are listed on that page. Thus, if you discovered 10 patients had Disease A and 20 patients had Disease B, the patients with Disease A are listed on one or more pages, without including patients who did not have Disease A, on those pages. The patients with Disease B are listed on one or more pages, without including patients who did not have Disease B, on those pages.

After assembling at least 5 (preferably 20 or more) patients for 1 disease, scrutinise the clinical features you recorded across all the patients for that disease. A feature or detail that is present in every patient, is a Universal Clinical Feature. See the following examples.

The first picture is a sample of a basic log template.

Case log for: (insert disease)

Patient initials	Clinical features	Risk Factors for / against this diagnosis	My differential diagnoses	Did I make this diagnosis initially, Y/N. If N, why?

The next figure illustrates a brief and basic log for 5 cases. The clinical feature that is present in all of the patients, is circled in red.

Case log for: acute appendicitis

Patient initials	Clinical features	Risk Factors for / against this diagnosis	My differential diagnoses	Did I make this diagnosis initially, Y/N. If N, why?
AAL	Abd pain 1 day, diarrhoea once, nausea	No previous appendectomy	Viral gastroenteritis	N, patient had diarrhoea so I thought it was gastroenteritis
BCT	Abd pain 2 days, cannot walk, vomiting 2 days	No previous appendectomy	Brain tumour	N, patient had vomiting so I decided to rule out brain tumour first
MYZ	Fever and vomiting 2 days, abd pain 1 day	No previous appendectomy	Viral illness with vomiting, intestinal obstruction of unknown cause	Y
HJY	Fever 1 day, diarrhoea once, abd pain 1 day	No previous appendectomy	Viral gastroenteritis	Y
DRX	Abd pain 1 day, nausea 1 day, vomiting 2 days	No previous appendectomy	Viral illness with vomiting, intestinal obstruction of unknown cause	Y

In statistical terms, Universal Clinical Features of a disease have a strong negative likelihood ratio. If a Universal Clinical Feature is absent in your patient when this feature should have been present by that day of the patient's disease, that disease is virtually impossible in your patient. Thus, Universal Clinical Features are useful for ruling out that disease.

Illness scripts: Secondary Specific Clinical Features (Rule #3 of clinical reasoning)

Secondary Clinical Features appear with varying frequency; not everyone who has that disease has that clinical feature. For example, urticaria is a secondary clinical feature of an allergic reaction. Some patients with allergic reactions do not have urticaria.

Some secondary features are common in multiple diseases; some are specific only to one or two diseases.

A clinical feature that is specific to only 1 disease, if present in the patient, strongly suggests the patient has that disease. Recall the analogy of your waiting at the airport to identify and escort 1 traveller out of the crowd. This clinical feature which is specific to only 1 disease, is identical to having a clue that is specific only to the target you are trying to identify at the airport. That clue identifies your target from the rest of the crowd.

This is Rule #3 of clinical reasoning: **Secondary specific clinical features of a disease, if present in your patient, strongly suggest that disease in your patient.**

Another analogy: imagine you are in a waiting room full of other people, all waiting to see the doctor. The doctor opens the door and calls out, 'Can the person with 2 arms and 2 legs come in, please?'

In most clinics, this statement is unhelpful — everyone will be wondering who the doctor wants to identify! Conversely, if the doctor calls out the full name of their target, this specificity often identifies their target immediately.

An example of a secondary specific clinical feature is tophi. Tophi are specific to gout; almost no other disease has tophi as a clinical feature.

Therefore, the presence of tophi in your patient instantly and strongly suggests the correct diagnosis is gout.

In statistical terms, highly specific clinical features have strong positive likelihood ratios. Thus, they rule in the correct diagnosis.

Secondary specific clinical features can be fixed (specific, regardless of the other differentials in virtually all patients) or non-fixed (may not be specific, depending on the differentials in that unique patient).

Tophi are an example of a fixed secondary specific clinical feature; they are specific for gout in virtually all patients regardless of the relevant differentials.

Non-fixed secondary specific clinical features vary from patient to patient, because the specificity of these features for 1 differential in that patient, depend on the exact differentials in that patient. If you have 3 differentials for a patient, knowing the 1–2 clinical features that are exclusive to only 1 disease's illness script out of all the differentials' illness scripts, allows you to use that secondary specific clinical feature to clinch the diagnosis instantly. Thus, detailed illness scripts are crucial to identifying these non-fixed secondary specific clinical features.

For example, a patient has diseases A, C and Y as the relevant differentials. These differentials mostly or totally explain the patient's clinical features. You recall the illness script for disease A, disease C and disease Y, and then mentally check them:

- Which clinical feature is found only on the script for disease A, but not C and Y?

- Likewise, which clinical feature is found only on the script for disease C, but not A and Y?

- Likewise, which clinical feature is found only on the script for disease Y, but not A and C?

The clinical feature(s) specific only to one of the differentials, is a secondary specific clinical feature for the disease in this patient. Even if that clinical feature on the script for disease A is also found in diseases B and D, diseases B and D are not relevant differentials for this patient because these 2 diseases do not explain the entirety of the patient's clinical features.

As of the end of 2022, there does not seem to be any reference that explicitly names secondary specific clinical features and fully describes their use, across multiple diseases. Again, I recommend keeping an anonymised patient log listing all patients whom you have evaluated clinically and followed up on. Each page is devoted to 1 disease; more than 1 page can be devoted to the same disease. List the relevant differential diagnoses you were considering for each patient.

After assembling at least 5 (preferably 20 or more) patients for 1 disease, scrutinise the clinical features you recorded across all the patients, for that disease. Check these clinical features against the clinical features of all the differential diagnoses you had listed for that disease. Pick out the clinical features that occurred in some of the patients, but do not exist in any of the differential diagnoses mentioned in the 'differential diagnosis' column for that disease.

Clinical features that are absent in the relevant differentials of most of the patients, but present in the relevant differentials of a minority of patients with that disease, are non-fixed secondary specific clinical features.

Clinical features that are absent in all the relevant differentials for all the patients with that disease, are fixed secondary specific clinical features.

The next figure shows an example of a brief and basic log for learning secondary specific clinical features. The clinical feature, tophi, does not appear in any of the differentials and is circled in red.

Case log for: gout

Tophi (circled in the Clinical Features column) are not seen in any of these differentials

Patient initials	Clinical Features	Risk Factors for / against this diagnosis	My differential diagnoses	Did I make this diagnosis initially, Y/N. If N, why?
KDG	Pain over right ankle 2 days with warmth, redness	Nil	Septic arthritis	N, patient had erythema so I assumed it was septic arthritis
UTH	Pain over both ankles 2 days with tenderness, decreased range of motion, swelling. Tophi seen	Known history of gout, overweight	Osteoarthritis, rheumatoid arthritis	N, I thought decreased range of motion was not seen in gout and suited osteoarthritis. Ignored tophi
RVM	Pain over left knee 4 days, swollen knee	Known history of gout, chronic kidney disease	Septic arthritis, rheumatoid arthritis	Y
QWE	Pain over thumbs and index fingers for 2 weeks with swelling. Tophus seen	Drank beer daily for 12 years	Rheumatoid arthritis	Y
ZER	Pain over right wrist for 4 days, worse on playing badminton. Tophus seen	Nil	De Quervain's tenosynovitis, wrist sprain	N, patient types a lot and is right-handed. I fixated on this risk factor

These are examples of basic, very brief logs. A comprehensive log has far more information, such as virtually every detail of the patient's presenting complaint (pattern, location, progression, day of onset, etc.). The amount of information in a comprehensive log is at least quadruple the amount shown in these brief examples. Detailed records allow you to learn more. Conversely, if you skimp on the history and examination, you have little information to put into and use in your patient logs. The less clinical information you have, the less you can learn.

In my experience, the usual clinical clues that point to the most likely clinical diagnosis are found among the details of the presenting complaint.

The potency of combining all 3 rules of clinical reasoning

The next 2 cases demonstrate the potency of applying all 3 rules of clinical reasoning, to the initial information alone.

CASE #5: Ash

Ash is an 8-month-old boy with the Presenting Complaint of fever once every 3 days, for the past 9 days. There are no other symptoms. The baby is happy and has a normal appetite.

--

Differential diagnoses of doctors (both junior and senior) who had seen the child, and performed a complete clinical evaluation:

1. Viral fever, source unknown

2. Occult bacterial infection, likely mild, source unknown, because 'the child looks well'

Plans: Order urine microscopy, urine culture and full blood count. These returned with normal results. Therefore, continue monitoring. Consider X-rays, blood cultures, inflammatory markers, and other workup for potential 'pyrexia of unknown origin' if the fever does not resolve spontaneously.

--

(Continued)

(Continued)

Doctor X possesses an expert-level illness script and uses all 3 Rules of Clinical Reasoning, on the initial information alone. The relevant differentials, in order of descending likelihood are:

1. Deep-seated abscess in a location free of pain fibres and most types of sensory nerve fibres, likely within the trunk: middle of the vertebral bodies, liver or spleen. The exact bacterial pathogen is not certain

2. Non-typhoid Salmonella infection, possibly group C

3. Malaria

Doctor X asks one more question: 'Was the fever truly once every 3 days?' (Doctor X is checking the secondary specific clinical feature for the top diagnosis.)

Subsequent steps: Check the child to confirm the absence of localising symptoms and signs, and signs of the relevant differentials. After such confirmation, an urgent Magnetic Resonance Imaging (MRI) scan is ordered to address the top differential. Additional tests are needed to titrate antibiotic duration. Whilst awaiting the MRI scan, commence high-dose intravenous Ceftriaxone, given the likely pathogens and location of the abscess. (Doctor X is aware that delay in the correct treatment leads to potential disaster and increased morbidity.)

The other doctors argued: 'Why order an MRI scan? There are no red flags! The baby looks clinically well!'

--

Outcome: The child turned out to have microabscesses of the liver, revealed on the immediate MRI scan ordered by the expert diagnostician.

The child's parents were happy the diagnosis was immediately made and treated. All test results and the outcome affirmed the expert's clinical acumen. This is the positive chain of dominoes.

CASE #6: Veera

Veera is an 11-year-old girl with the Presenting Complaint of unremitting headache over the whole head for 4 days, fever for 4 days, nausea and vomiting twice over the past 4 days.

--

Differential diagnoses of doctors (both junior and senior) who had seen the child and ascertained there were no 'red flags' of raised intracranial pressure, nuchal rigidity, Kernig's or Brudzinski's signs:

1. Viral fever, source unknown

2. COVID-19 infection

3. Occult bacterial infection, likely mild, source unknown, because 'the child looks well'

Plans: Order urine microscopy, full blood count, and COVID-19 PCR test. These returned with normal results. Administer Acetaminophen, Ibuprofen and Ondansetron. Wait for the child to get better. Consider blood cultures if the child does not recover spontaneously.

--

Doctor X possesses an expert-level illness script and uses all 3 Rules of Clinical Reasoning, on the initial information alone. The relevant differentials, in order of descending likelihood are:

1. Meningitis, likely viral

2. Viral infection, non-localising virus, with status migrainosus

Doctor X asks one more question: 'Tell me the details of the unremitting headache.' (Doctor X is checking for the secondary specific clinical features for the top diagnosis.)

Subsequent steps: Check the patient for symptoms and signs of viral meningitis, and relevant differentials. Immediate lumbar puncture. Prescribe analgesia for meningitis-severity headaches. If there is no

(Continued)

(Continued)

evidence of bacterial meningitis, chickenpox or herpes simplex virus, hold off all antimicrobial drugs.

The other doctors argued: 'Why order a lumbar puncture? There were no red flags! No alteration in mental state! No nuchal rigidity! No Kernig's or Brudzinski's signs! This cannot be meningitis!'

--

Outcome: The child turned out to have viral meningitis. Immediate analgesia was instituted, with significant improvement. The expert's decisions, subsequent test results and outcome demonstrated the positive chain of dominoes.

Case #5 described a rare disease. Case #6 described a common disease.

In both cases, the expert wielded all 3 rules of clinical reasoning to generate relevant differential diagnoses. The expert used their detailed illness scripts to identify and then check for the crucial piece(s) of information that pointed to the correct clinical diagnosis. The crucial information was the secondary specific clinical features of the top diagnosis, which the expert already strongly suspected from the initial clinical information alone.

The check for the secondary specific clinical feature(s) manifested as the expert's single high-yield question in each case. This crucial question focused on a particular aspect of the presenting complaint. The subsequent clinical evaluation the expert undertook, which checked for clinical features to rule in or rule out their differentials, was based on the 3 Rules of Clinical Reasoning and detailed illness scripts.

Even if the other doctors in these cases could answer the single crucial question that the expert (Doctor X) asked the patient, they did not have enough detail in their illness scripts to recognise the significance of either the question or the answer.

Cases #5 and #6 also demonstrate a common misconception that commonplace teaching gives to learners: in the absence of 'red flags', the dangerous disease cannot be deduced or present.

Red flags, such as nuchal rigidity, Kernig's and Brudzinski's signs for meningitis, are <u>secondary clinical features</u>. Therefore, a robust reasoner knows that the absence of these red flags does not exclude the dangerous disease associated with those red flags. The absence of red flags for meningitis does not exclude meningitis. The absence of 'looking sick' does not exclude a dangerous sickness. If you meet a robust reasoner, ask them to teach you how to diagnose dangerous diseases before the red flags appear. See the discussion on 'Secondary Clinical Features: common mistakes in their use', later in this chapter.

Doctor X's subsequent assessment and plan went straight for the most likely diagnosis. This is logical: if your reasoning is correct, the highest yield will always come from targeting the most likely diagnosis. The subsequent test results and the patient's outcome will prove the robustness of your clinical reasoning. Conversely, if your reasoning is wrong, it may not matter what you target because your decisions are usually inappropriate.

Notice the precision of the differential diagnoses that Doctor X generated based on initial information alone. This comes from constant dedication to think and commit specifically, until specific thinking and the generation of specific differential diagnoses, are habitual.

One could argue that Doctor X might not have been skilled at clinical reasoning. Perhaps their performance was due to an advantage over the other doctors: in intelligence, age, experience, or speciality training (was Doctor X an infectious diseases specialist, gastroenterologist, or neurologist?). The answer: Doctor X had none of those advantages.

One could argue that perhaps Doctor X got these 2 diagnoses correctly as a fluke, but is often wrong in most cases. There are indeed doctors who 'spot the exciting disease' but are often wrong. Given that no other information was given to you about Doctor X's outcomes in other patients, the concern about Doctor X possibly being this kind of doctor, may be valid. Do not worry; Doctor X does not 'spot'. These 2 cases demonstrate the typical performance of Doctor X across all patients: the performance of a reasoning expert.

Every expert-tier diagnostician (discussed in the chapter 'Tiers of performance') I have seen, gets the correct clinical diagnosis in the first consult in at least 90% of common cases, and over 50% of the conventional 'diagnostic dilemmas'.

Such outcomes far exceed the upper limits reported in the literature: the usual ceiling being 55–70% for common cases, and 30% or less for more difficult cases. The combination of robust clinical reasoning and detailed illness scripts, allows the doctor to break through the ceiling of conventional performance.

In summary, Rules #2 and #3 confer additional speed and accuracy above and beyond the use of Rule #1 alone. Additional effort to build up illness scripts and proficiency in clinical reasoning, is required to employ these 2 Rules effectively.

Universal Clinical Features: common mistakes in their use

Universal Clinical Features of a disease are necessary for a patient to have that disease. Thus, the absence of these clinical features when they should have been present in the patient because enough time has elapsed, makes that disease virtually impossible.

Some doctors have an awareness of universal clinical features but do not realise that these features may appear later on during the course of the disease. When these doctors also lack detailed illness scripts, they cannot recognise the disease until the universal feature appears.

For example, Henoch–Schonlein purpura is a vasculitic disorder where the classic universal feature is palpable purpura, which often appears early in the course of illness. However, in a minority of patients, the palpable purpura appears only weeks later. Instead, these patients can present initially with a bizarre pattern of severe abdominal pain, sometimes with other symptoms. Since many doctors rely on the presence of the classic purpura to make this diagnosis and cannot recognise this disease otherwise, such patients suffer severe pain for weeks because the correct treatment was never administered.

Consider this conversation.

Conversation #1

Doctor T walks up to her senior colleague, Doctor Y. Doctor T wants to 'test' Doctor Y's diagnostic skill.

Doctor T: 'I have a difficult case for you! A 9-year-old girl was seen with vomiting, diarrhoea and abdominal pain. The abdominal pain began on the first day of illness and was the main complaint. It was severe. The diarrhoea also began on the first day, with 4 episodes of watery stools every day. The vomiting began on the 3rd day of the illness. She was admitted and treated for gut sepsis...'

Doctor Y: 'Stop. Was the pain unremitting, as per my definition? Non-stop pain with no pain-free periods, since it began?'

Doctor T: 'Yes. Why?'

Doctor Y: 'I thought so. This is not gut sepsis — which is not a proper diagnosis, by the way — and not gastroenteritis. The pattern of pain and the sequence of symptoms do not fit those. I presume she was able to walk and had no tenderness or guarding of the abdomen?'

Doctor T: '...Yes.'

Doctor Y: 'Then that leaves only 2 differential diagnoses in this child. One is more common than the other. How long did the purpura take to appear?'

Doctor T gapes. 'How did you? ...uh, 3 weeks.'

Doctor Y: 'Blood cultures were probably ordered and the child was prescribed antibiotics. She would have undergone irrelevant tests, such as imaging of her abdomen, whilst she was in severe pain for 3 weeks. All of this was unnecessary when the clinical picture at the first presentation already pointed to the diagnosis of Henoch–Schonlein purpura. We could have treated the patient properly and immediately. Notice that I asked you the question about purpura as "when", not "if". Right?'

Doctor T: 'Right.'

--

Being unable to recognise the clinical picture when the purpura is absent, doctors often label patients with Henoch–Schonlein purpura who present with abdominal pain as having 'sepsis', 'gastroenteritis', or 'appendicitis' even though the doctors know the patient has none of those diseases. The doctors then order batteries of tests and trials of antibiotics, to no avail. The purpura appears days to weeks later. Meanwhile, the patient is often left writhing or screaming in pain for weeks in the hospital bed.

This unhappy scenario applies to many patients with various inflammatory disorders. This occurs partly because of fallacies like 'Common things happen commonly, therefore we must always diagnose infection first regardless of the patient' and partly because of insisting that the patient must fulfil enough diagnostic criteria before making the diagnosis.

Obedience to fallacies and sole reliance on diagnostic criteria occur because of an absence of reasoning and detailed illness scripts. Diagnostic criteria are discussed in the chapter 'Theoretical disease approaches'.

Conversely, a robust reasoner with detailed illness scripts can use the secondary specific clinical features of Henoch–Schonlein purpura to make the correct clinical diagnosis in these patients immediately.

If a doctor finds themselves struggling to make the diagnosis for any patient based on the entirety of the patient's clinical features, the first action should be to seek help from a superior reasoner. Thereafter, the doctor should follow up on that patient, build up their illness scripts and improve their reasoning.

Secondary Clinical Features: common mistakes in their use

Secondary Clinical Features appear in some patients with that disease. Since secondary clinical features are not required for the disease to be present, arguing that the absence of these clinical features makes the disease unlikely, is a mistake.

For example, myalgia is a secondary clinical feature of patients with influenza infection. Many patients with influenza do not have myalgia. If you saw a patient who could have influenza upper respiratory tract infection but the patient did not have myalgia, and you then argued that the absence of myalgia makes the diagnosis of influenza upper respiratory tract infection unlikely, you would be wrong.

Sometimes, doctors contend that the absence of the secondary clinical features which are often present in patients with that disease, is an argument against the patient having that disease. Though this argument superficially seems to have merit, most of its weight comes from 1 assumption: the absence of that feature has the same implications for all patients regardless of the unique patient's clinical presentation, as if all patients are clones of each other.

Patients are not clones of each other.

For example, 90% of patients with anaphylaxis (a potentially fatal-allergic reaction that requires immediate treatment) have urticaria. Approximately 10% of all patients with anaphylaxis, do not have urticaria.

If you said that 90% of patients with anaphylaxis have urticaria and 10% do not, you would be correct because you were talking about the patient cohort in general terms, without paying attention to the individual patient's clinical presentation.

If you saw a patient who has clinical features that suggest anaphylaxis, but this patient had no urticaria, and you then thought 'the absence of urticaria makes the possibility of anaphylaxis 10% at most in this patient', you would be wrong. The presentation of each unique patient dictates their probability of having the disease, not the absence of a single secondary clinical feature.

This patient's presentation points to anaphylaxis; the absence of urticaria makes no difference to the probability of anaphylaxis for that patient.

If you thought that the absence of urticaria makes anaphylaxis very unlikely in individual patients, you are likely to miss the 10% of all patients with anaphylaxis who do not have urticaria. Patients can die because you refused to focus on the unique patient first.

The only cohort-level percentages that can be applied directly to all patients, are 0% and 100%. To apply any other cohort-level percentage to a patient directly, the entire cohort must be composed of clones with identical presentations. A clinical feature with 100% prevalence is a universal clinical feature, not a secondary clinical feature.

History by proxy

In some situations, the history cannot be obtained from the patient. This can be:

- Temporary (the patient is delirious or unconscious) or
- For the entire doctor–patient encounter (the patient is uncommunicative due to a major injury or chronic disease).

The history is then obtained from someone else: a proxy. This proxy should have directly witnessed the events relevant to the history. The main caregiver is often the best proxy. This caregiver should be deliberately sought out, especially for young children and adults with severely impaired communication and/or cognition.

If the patient subsequently becomes able to provide a history, such as an unconscious patient who regains consciousness, the history should be obtained from the patient directly. Patients sometimes have symptoms that are unnoticed by the proxy.

Conflicts in corroboration between the history from the patient and the history from a proxy, suggest potential inaccuracies in one or more of the histories. These conflicts point to the need to evaluate the patient and the situation more carefully, as well as react to the implications of the inaccuracy. Though inconsistencies are most alarming when abuse is suspected, these inconsistencies may also point to inattention, tensions or problems with communication between the patient and their proxies. All these require appropriate, corrective action.

A corroborative history is important when school-age children are brought by their parents to consult the doctor. Children who can provide a history may choose not to tell their parents about their symptoms; this occurs in various diseases and cases of suspected abuse. In these situations, I recommend interviewing the children first. Children aged 5 years and above can provide answers to many important questions. If the adult caregiver is also listening in at the same time and agrees with the child's history, there is often no need to repeat the same questions to the adult.

A common mistake is to obtain a history only from the adult, often because it is assumed that the adult always knows everything about the child (this is not true) and will always provide an unbiased perspective (also not true).

Capsule summary

- Generating relevant differential diagnoses enables efficient, relevant clinical evaluation.
- Rules #2 and #3 significantly improve the doctor's speed and accuracy, but require considerable effort to acquire the necessary illness scripts and proficiency. A detailed log is recommended.
- Rule #2 of Clinical Reasoning: The absence of Universal Clinical Features for a disease, makes that disease almost impossible in your patient.
- Rule #3 of Clinical Reasoning: Secondary specific clinical features of a disease, if present in your patient, strongly suggest that disease in your patient.
- Corroborative history is necessary for some patients, but should not be considered an adequate substitute for interviewing the patient directly.

Frequently asked questions

Q: It is often said that with experience, doctors develop pattern recognition and can instantly recognise common illnesses. Thus, when patients seem to present with common illnesses, does clinical reasoning matter?

A: You will indeed see common diseases again and again, to the point you recognise the general pattern within the first few minutes of the consultation.

Pattern recognition cannot replace the basic diagnostic reasoning requirement. A minority of patients who 'fit the general pattern somewhat' do not have the common illness tied to that pattern. These patients will have other subtle symptoms or signs that point to their disease.

If you do not follow Rule #1, it is easy to complacently assume that this minority of patients has the same disease as the majority, ignore the subtle symptoms and signs, and miss the correct diagnosis. This predisposes to missing some dangerous diseases, with tragic consequences.

The classic example is acute myocarditis. Patients with myocarditis can present with seemingly trivial symptoms resembling the common cold or viral gastroenteritis. In addition to presenting with clinical features that resemble the general pattern of a common cold or viral gastroenteritis, the patient has additional, subtle symptoms or signs that cannot be explained by the common cold or viral gastroenteritis. However, it is easy to slip into the mindset of 'oh, yet another flu/gastroenteritis', fail to look for (or ignore) other clinical features that cannot be explained by the common illness, misdiagnose the patient with the common illness, and then mismanage them. Some of these patients then collapse at home or in the hospital ward.

Common, general pattern recognition ascribed to experienced doctors is inferior to patient-centred pattern recognition. Patient-centred pattern recognition combines detailed illness scripts with Rule #1 of clinical reasoning, enabling recognition of the minority with dangerous-but-subtle diseases.

Q: Can we just use Rule #1, and skip the extra work necessary to become proficient in Rules #2 and #3?

A: Yes. Rule #1 is the most important rule of clinical reasoning. Following the requirements for basic diagnostic reasoning (Rule #1 plus the priorities of information categories) would make you a safe doctor.

However, the advantages conferred by proficient use of Rules #2 and #3, are considerable. Whether you face life-or-death emergencies where even a 5-minute delay may mean the patient's death, or want to get the correct diagnosis for all the patients you must see in a busy clinic, the advantages of vastly superior speed and accuracy make a huge difference to the doctor's life and comfort. The extra work is worth the benefits. Upon attaining proficiency in these Rules, the doctor can reap the benefits for the rest of their career.

Without dedicated effort, doctors may develop a vague sense of Rules #2 and #3 for the most common diseases after several years. This hope-we-learn-this-during-daily-work approach is a hope: the learning may not happen. Even if the learning does happen, it is much slower and far less accurate than keeping and analysing the patient logs.

TARGETED EVALUATION: PHYSICAL EXAMINATION

The targeted physical examination should aim to identify the presence or absence of signs that differentiate between the relevant differential diagnoses.

There are 2 steps:

1. Obtain relevant vital signs
2. Execute steps to detect the presence or absence of relevant signs for differentiating between the differential diagnoses

Proficiency in the patient-centred physical examination: the journey

If you need to put in significant effort to do something well, your brain can consciously focus on only 1 task at a time. I have assigned each task to a Level.

Train yourself to master each level, one at a time, starting from Level 1. Mastery means you perform the steps at that level reflexively and excellently.

Once a level is mastered, you can consciously focus on the actions in the next-higher level of proficiency for every patient.

There are 4 levels of proficiency.

Perfect, targeted physical examination is attainable at Level 3.

Level of proficiency	What your brain is doing during the examination	Mastery of this level means habitual, near-effortless execution of:
1	What is the next step in the proper examination sequence?	All the proper steps of examining a single system, without spending any energy to remember them.
2	For every step, can I automatically discern between Normal and Abnormal?	Distinguishing Normal versus Abnormal, instantly and perfectly.
3	How does each Normal/Abnormal finding tie up with everything else I have found so far? What is the most likely diagnosis?	Organising and adding your findings to existing information, whilst analysing the information to decide the most likely and differential diagnoses.
4	What extra steps can I execute regarding this diagnosis or its associations?	Getting the most likely diagnosis almost instantaneously, so you can spend the rest of the time looking for disease associations and complications.

Physical examination proficiency: Level 1 — what is the next step?

At the start of medical training, students are taught (or read from textbooks) the execution of a complete examination of 1 body system and its associated signs. These are usually:

- Cardiovascular
- Respiratory
- Abdominal

- Neurological
- Joints
- Others

Completion of a thorough examination of each system usually takes at least 5 minutes. In medical exams, stations that assess the examination of 1 system are often called the 'short case' or 'focused task'.

The Neurological system's subcomponents include cranial nerves and limbs, each subcomponent requiring at least 4 minutes to examine fully and systematically.

Perform the steps for each system again and again, until the execution of all steps becomes automatic.

Mastery of this level enables the automatic execution of the entire sequence of steps for each system. Virtually no mental energy is needed to recall and execute each step flawlessly.

Forgetting steps of the physical examination arises from failure to master this lowest level of proficiency.

Physical examination proficiency: Level 2 — is my finding normal, or abnormal?

It is crucial to accurately distinguish normal (no sign of disease) from abnormal (a sign of the disease is present).

'Normal' is not just the absence of signs of disease. Some findings, such as the presence of tendon reflexes within the normal range and the anatomical boundaries of certain findings in physical examination, define Normal.

Mastery of this level is rare because it is often not taught in routine medical training, and not learnt by performing routine work.

During training, doctors focus on the body systems affected by the patient's disease. This focus only confers a rough idea of what can be abnormal.

Conversely, mastery of Level 2 proficiency is the Mastery of Normal: the range of normal across all body systems.

To know what is abnormal, you must first learn what is normal.

By extension, to readily detect everything abnormal, you must master normal.

Once you master Normal:

- You know the boundary between Normal and Abnormal. Everything outside Normal is automatically abnormal: the sign of the disease is present! The alternative, which is trying to master everything abnormal, is probably impossible in the human lifetime.

- Your examination technique has become perfect. Before this, if you are examining a 'normal' patient with no signs, failure to detect Normal warns you that your technique was imperfect. You then readjust and improve your technique. Eventually, every time you examine someone without disease, your technique always identifies Normal at the first pass. Perfect examination technique will remove any worry about missing or imagining signs because of imperfect technique.

At undergraduate and postgraduate examinations, candidates who are unsure about Normal will face difficulty upon encountering a patient with a subtle sign. They will guess whether the patient has a sign because they are unsure if the subtle finding is within the range of Normal. They simultaneously worry that their examination technique is so imperfect that they are imagining the sign. Facing uncertainty, some keep repeating a particular step, thereby running out of time to complete that exam station.

If you wish to be able to reliably hear the 1/6 cardiac murmur upon placing your stethoscope on the patient's chest, or palpate the soft-consistency 1-cm-below-right-costal-margin liver with your first touch of the abdomen, you must master Normal. For example, to readily hear the soft cardiac murmur, requires knowing 0/6 (no cardiac murmur) so intimately that any sound above 0/6 warns you that there is probably a murmur.

You need to perform these steps in many people and consciously teach yourself every time that the 'normal examination findings' are Normal, thereby learning the range of Normal for each step. For each step, teach yourself Normal by examining at least a few hundred people who have 'normal' findings in that step.

Such learning does not come automatically with experience.

To illustrate the absence of mastery of Normal despite having experience, ask yourself this: have you, and all your peers, seen thousands of normal people walking? This is the normal gait.

The answer would often be 'yes'.

Now ask yourself: have you mastered the entire range of normal walking gaits?

The honest answer for most students and doctors would be 'no'.

Traditional teaching often focuses on physical examination for disease. Furthermore, learners often pay attention only to the body systems that are diseased in patients. The notion of examining body parts and organ systems in hundreds of normal people to master Normal, is novel to most learners.

Some examples of the silent self-teaching of Normal, are:

- This is the look and feel of a Normal neck without a goitre.
- This is the look of a Normal conjunctiva without pallor.
- These are the findings on examining a Normal pair of lungs.
- These are the findings of Normal first and second heart sounds, without murmurs.
- This is the look of a Normal brisk reflex. (Yes, there are normal brisk reflexes and pathological brisk reflexes. A fine line separates the two.)

Masters of Normal can glance at the patient, and instantly spot 5 or more subtle signs across multiple body systems in that glance. Everything abnormal 'jumps out' at them instantly because they know exactly where the boundary between Normal and Abnormal lies. This is a hallmark of expert diagnosticians: they miss nothing.

Everyone else who has not mastered Normal, often cannot see the subtle signs without help. Sometimes, even with help, they still cannot see the subtle signs, because they have not truly understood the range of Normal. Thus, they do not know where the boundary between Normal and Abnormal lies.

In Singapore and many moderately busy settings, I estimate the time taken to master Normal across human body systems whilst going about your routine training and work, takes 6 to 12 months.

Here is 1 example of the usefulness of Mastery of Normal.

In 2008, the Department of Paediatrics at the National University Hospital of Singapore began holding mock exams to simulate the Membership of the Royal College of Paediatrics and Child Health (MRCPCH) exams. These are the postgraduate exams that trainees must pass, to get beyond the halfway mark of Paediatrics speciality training in Singapore.

The first mock exam comprised several stations, each dedicated to 1 aspect of the exam.

The Neurology station focused on the physical examination of 1 aspect of Neurology. This station took place in a small room with 1 examiner. The patient was a teenage girl.

The task given to each trainee was: 'Watch this girl walk. Then tell me what you see.'

The girl would walk to the end of the room, and then return.

Every trainee who had not mastered Level 2 said that the girl's gait was normal. They failed the station instantly. The signs were so subtle that relying on previously seen signs in patients, videos and textbooks was insufficient.

I had 1 huge advantage over the other trainees: I had been intently examining all the patients in the clinics and the wards to master Normal. I had been paying attention to the normal gait of adults and children.

Mastering normal gait requires looking at hundreds of normal people walking, and observing minutiae such as how and when they lift and plant their feet, shift their weight, swing their hands, and so on. You must then teach yourself 'this is normal' in person after person after person, until you know the range of normal gaits.

I came to the Neurology station.

The girl walked to the end of the room and then returned. I frowned.

I had 2 reference points in my head: all the 'abnormal' signs in my experience, and the mental boundary created by Mastery of Normal.

If I was going by previously seen abnormalities in my experience, it would be tempting to declare the gait was 'normal' because it was not as abnormal as the gait of any of the previous patients with neurological or joint diseases, that I had seen.

However, going by the mental boundary that separated Normal from Abnormal, there was something subtly abnormal about her gait. This abnormality was so subtle that I could not describe it clearly with one 'walk'.

It was as if the abnormality sat immediately outside the boundary of normal; it was so close to Normal, that I had difficulty saying exactly what it was.

I asked her to walk to the wall and back, one more time. This time, I discarded my 'abnormal gaits from experience' reference point, as it was a useless distraction. Instead, I recalled the normal gait I had observed in hundreds of people, and then compared that gait to her gait as she walked.

By her third step away from me, I noticed the first clue: she was lifting her left foot about 0.2 seconds slower than her right foot.

You may say: that difference in time between the lifting of the left and right feet, is impossible to detect!

Such a difference is impossible to detect *if you have never mastered Normal.*

Even so, I was worried. What if I was imagining that subtle abnormality? I scrutinised her left leg carefully, searching for a second sign to back up my suspicions.

Before she took another 2 steps, I noticed the second sign: her left foot was about 5% smaller than the right foot. Again, this is virtually impossible to detect if you have not scrutinised the normal foot sizes of hundreds of people.

When she returned, I turned to the examiner and said, 'This girl has left hemiparesis.'

The examiner, Professor Yap Hui Kim, smiled.

I completed the rest of the examination, provided my diagnosis, and passed the station. However, my final diagnosis was not entirely correct. I eventually discovered that the child had suffered a previous stroke.

Physical examination proficiency: Level 3 — what is the correct diagnosis?

At Level 3, you are constantly analysing the patient's information to decide the correct diagnosis. Mastery of Levels 1 and 2 is a pre-requisite. You cannot generate, consider or re-prioritise differentials accurately if you are missing steps, missing signs or imagining signs.

Proficiency in this level allows the instant generation and ongoing evaluation of the relevant differential diagnoses, with every step of the physical examination. This proficiency also allows you to customise your steps to target the relevant differential diagnoses in any patient.

Let us go back to Case #3:

CASE #3: Sam

Sam is a 50-year-old Danish man with a past medical history of cystitis, heart disease, diabetes mellitus, alcoholism and a fracture of his right forearm from playing baseball 20 years ago. He consults you with the Presenting Complaint of headache and fever for 3 days.

--

By the end of the history, you have decided the differential diagnoses are:

1. Acute bacterial sinusitis

2. Viral meningitis

3. Common viral infection with fever-associated headache, specific virus unknown

When deciding the first steps in the physical examination to complement the history, remember to think of the vital signs.

'Vital signs' refer to numerical information about the function of vital body systems, such as:

- Heart rate (beats per minute)
- Blood pressure (mmHg)
- Respiratory rate (breaths per minute)
- Body temperature (degrees Celsius)
- Pulse oximetry reading (%)

Given the differential diagnoses suggested earlier, you want to know the patient's temperature. Fever is present in both bacterial sinusitis and viral meningitis.

The heart rate and blood pressure can be important: a patient in marked pain may temporarily have a high heart rate and high blood pressure. Bacterial sinusitis may lead to the complication of an intracranial abscess. If the intracranial abscess is present and large enough, the intracranial pressure can increase to the point of seeing a Cushing reflex. Derangements in the vital signs due to the Cushing reflex include bradycardia and hypertension.

Thus, you would:

- Check the temperature, heart rate and blood pressure
- Inspect for the irregular breathing of a Cushing reflex, which would suggest bacterial sinusitis complicated by a massive intracranial abscess
- Inspect for facial and periorbital swelling, which can be seen in acute sinusitis
- Percuss over the facial sinuses for tenderness. The presence of tenderness would point to acute sinusitis

- Then perform a neurological examination focused on eliciting nuchal rigidity, hypertonia, hyperreflexia, and Kernig's and Brudzinski's signs.

Here is an example of Level 3 proficiency.

Several months after I took the first version of the Department's mock exams, I took the next iteration. In the Cardiovascular station, the task was to 'examine the child's cardiovascular system'.

I glanced at the teenage boy's face. I then inspected his chest, axillae and upper back, noting an old left lateral thoracotomy scar. I felt both of his radial pulses.

I then turned to the examiner and said, 'This boy had an aortic coarctation for which he underwent a subclavian flap repair, as evidenced by being acyanotic on room air, the left lateral thoracotomy scar and the absence of the left radial pulse. I am now going to examine the status and associations of the coarctation.'

I then went on to complete the station.

Physical examination proficiency: Level 4 — I am done, early. What else is there to do?

Mastery of the 3 preceding levels opens the door to this final level of proficiency. You instantly detect and assemble all clues to decide the most likely diagnosis. Sometimes, you can get the diagnosis just by glancing at the patient.

If you need to perform any steps of physical examination after your inspection, you think of the high-yield steps instantly and execute them. Thus, the steps of your physical examination may be unconventional. Your mastery of Normal helps you to interpret the outcome of that high-yield step accurately, and your mastery of Level 3 points you to the correct diagnosis instantly.

In a medical exam, this level often grants you the freedom to spend most of the allotted time looking for 'bonus signs', associated diseases and complications.

However, if you are in a medical exam, be cautious in how you proceed. There are standard steps that are expected for examining each body system with marks assigned for each step. Deviation from those steps can cause you to fail the station, even if you deduce the diagnosis instantly.

Thus, strike a balance between following the standard steps and using your mastery of patient-centred physical examination to score extra marks.

Here is an example.

In 2009, I took the MRCPCH exam for Paediatrics. A British examiner oversaw the Neurology station. I entered the small room and was introduced to the 6-year-old boy sitting on the chair. The examiner said: 'Examine this child's lower limbs.'

The boy's calves were slightly larger than those of the usual 6-year-old. There were no other abnormalities on inspection.

I asked the child to walk across the room and then return.

He had a mild waddling gait. Given all the information thus far, including the absence of signs of relevant differentials (evident from my initial inspection and his ability to cooperate with my instructions), I concluded this was Duchenne Muscular Dystrophy.

Once he returned, I instructed him on the steps that would reveal the Gower sign. He demonstrated the Gower sign.

About 1 minute had passed since the station began.

I asked the child to face the wall and showed him the position I wanted him to adopt: arms extended in front of him, wrists extended with the palms facing, and resting against, the wall. I then told him to take up that position, and then press against the wall with his palms.

The examiner said, 'Stop!'

Puzzled, he continued: 'What are you doing?'

I replied: 'The boy has Duchenne Muscular Dystrophy, as evidenced by mild bilateral calf hypertrophy and a positive Gower sign. There are no other abnormalities on inspection to suggest otherwise. I am demonstrating the winging of the scapula, which is a sign of...'

The examiner said: 'Okay, good. Correct. Can you please perform the usual testing of reflexes and so on in his legs, just like the other candidates?'

I went on to finish the motor component of the neurological examination.

Fortunately, despite initially deviating from the standard steps, I scored full marks for the station.

Capsule summary

- The learning journey for patient-centred physical examination has 4 levels.

- Master each level so that you can focus on the next-higher level fully in every patient.

Frequently asked questions

Q: Must the physical examination always occur after completing the history?

A: No. In life-or-death emergencies, you may not have time to take any history. The greater your mastery of physical examination, the more accurate and rapid your detection of all abnormalities (subtle or otherwise), which can make the difference between the patient dying or surviving.

Even in non-emergency situations, there will be patients whose top differential diagnosis prompts you to examine them after asking a few questions. The signs clinch the correct diagnosis. Examples include certain diseases with rashes and many primary joint diseases.

A robust reasoner targets the highest-yield information as soon as possible, whilst simultaneously being mindful of the patient's comfort.

This reasoner may ask the highest-yield questions, then go for the highest-yield physical examination steps for their differentials, and then go back to the history to complete the first fundamental job: getting the most likely clinical diagnosis.

The second fundamental job of all consultations is to gather the information necessary to optimise management for that patient. Since the appropriateness of the management plan depends on the accuracy of the clinical diagnosis, the robust reasoner does whatever it takes to get the correct clinical diagnosis first.

With that diagnosis in mind, the robust reasoner now focuses the rest of the history on patient-centred questions that decide the feasibility of the management plan. This focus is described further in the chapter 'Gathering additional information to manage patients'.

It is illogical for a doctor to insist on performing the physical examination only after completing all the history-taking, regardless of the patient's presentation. You cannot ask relevant patient-centred management-type questions if you do not know the correct diagnosis.

The notion of completing all history-taking before performing any physical examination is perpetuated by some who insist that 'this process looks smooth: finish all history, then finish all physical examination'. This insistence is based on flawed reasoning. The appearance of the process is not the top priority of the encounter. The top priority is the outcome and ultimate goal of the process: getting it right for the patient without wasting time, needing to backtrack unnecessarily or missing important information along the way.

Q: When following up on patients with chronic disease, is there a different focus in the physical examination?

A: Yes. The pattern of history-taking also differs in that situation. However, adequate follow-up of a chronic disease requires understanding the principles covered in Sections 1 through 3. Thus, this follow-up is covered in Section 4, in the chapter 'Tackling the chronic disease'.

EPIDEMIOLOGY AND RISK FACTORS

The patient's clinical features of their current diagnosis, have primacy of place for their diagnosis.

The category of Epidemiology/Risk factors refers to all other information, including:

- Demographics: age, race, gender
- Personal history of other diseases, such as chronic diseases and prior surgery
- Family history of chronic diseases and unexplained deaths
- Travel history and activity history: when, where, and what the patient did exactly
- Contact history of family, friends and colleagues having symptoms of illness
- Sexual history
- Menstrual history
- Birth history
- Vaccination history

- Developmental history
- Treatment history
- Lifestyle and social setup

Demographics: Some diseases are more common or possible only in certain groups in the population. For example, diseases exclusively affecting the female reproductive tract are virtually impossible in males. As another example, femoral neck fractures are more common in people with osteoporosis, and thus tend to be more common in elderly people and females.

Personal history of other diseases: Many diseases exist in association with others, due to similar pathophysiological processes or the consequences of treating the original disease. For example, the cluster of atopic disorders includes asthma, allergic rhinitis, and eczema. A patient with 1 disease in the cluster is more likely to have the other diseases in the cluster.

In some specialities, especially oncological and surgical specialities, some diseases occur after certain treatments. For example, the diagnosis of chemotherapy-induced cardiomyopathy or post-operative wound infection, might not occur to the doctor unless they had thought of asking for the exact name and date of treatment. Thus, enquiry about the personal history of other diseases must include enquiry about treatments of those diseases.

Patients with concomitant other diseases may have symptoms and signs of these diseases. For the current-but-unknown diagnosis you are striving to figure out, the clinical features of the patient's known co-morbid conditions are classified as Risk Factors, instead of Clinical Features.

Family history of chronic diseases and unexplained deaths: Some diseases are more common in patients who have family members with the same disease, compared to patients who have no family members with that disease. This increased risk can be due to similar genes, similar lifestyles or similar environments. Families tend to have similar lifestyles and stay in the same locale. For example, a lady whose mother had breast cancer is at higher risk of developing breast cancer than another identical lady whose mother did not have breast cancer.

Some diseases can cause unexplained deaths. These are deaths in the family members of the patient, where the family could not know or did not want to know the underlying disease that led to the demise. Therefore, questions about family history should also enquire about unexplained deaths, especially if the disease you are suspecting in the patient has a significant chance of causing death.

Travel history and activity history: Upon being told of the patient's clinical features, doctors often need no extra help to think of infectious diseases that are common in their locale. However, doctors are often unfamiliar with infectious diseases that are rare or unheard of in their geographical region. Thus, when an infectious disease is suspected in the patient, the travel history may be important.

Merely naming the country the patient travelled to, is insufficient. The dates are important because each infectious disease has a known incubation period, which points to the window of dates of exposure before developing symptoms and signs of the disease.

Determine the exact activities the patient undertook; some diseases are zoonoses (infections transmitted from non-human animals to humans) or acquired under specific circumstances. For example, leptospirosis is rare in Singapore. However, if a patient presents with symptoms and signs of leptospirosis, the savvy Singapore-based doctor would enquire about travel and activity. This doctor might discover the patient travelled to India and went to play in a waterfall 2 weeks before the start of the symptoms.

Contact history of family, friends and colleagues having symptoms of illness: Infectious diseases can be transmitted between close contacts. When an infectious disease is suspected, enquire about the contacts having symptoms of the suspected disease. The infected contact may not have the same symptoms as the patient. For example, scabies causes an itchy rash. A patient with suspected scabies should be asked about household members with an itchy rash in any part of the body, not just in the same areas the patient shows the doctor.

Sexual history: Sexually transmitted diseases are transmitted mainly through unprotected intercourse. Some of these diseases may present with confusing symptoms, which are explained upon discovering the relevant risk factor in the sexual history. Obtaining this history is also important for the potentially infected contact, for contact tracing and treatment purposes. Examples include trachoma and gonococcal infection.

Menstrual history: Some diseases in women are more likely if they manifest disturbances in the pattern and severity of blood loss during the menstrual period. For example, symptomatic iron deficiency anaemia is more likely in women with menorrhagia.

Birth history: This covers information from the pregnancy where the patient's mother was carrying the patient inside her, until the first few days after the patient's birth. Relevant information can include illnesses in the patient's mother during her pregnancy, anomalies discovered on antenatal scans and tests, the patient's condition at birth, and problems that occurred within the first few days after birth.

The birth history is important when the patient is suspected to have a disease that has its origins, symptoms, signs, or other abnormalities detected during the antenatal and perinatal periods. The exact questions depend on the suspected disease. For example, in the child presenting with severe constipation, the doctor may suspect short-segment Hirschsprung's disease, and then ask the child's parent: 'Did your child pass stools within the first 24 hours of life?'

Vaccination history: This refers to the vaccinations the patient has received. Questions in this area are posed for 2 purposes. The first purpose is to discern the chance of an infectious disease which is difficult to acquire unless the vaccination is missed, such as measles. The second purpose is for anticipatory care in people who should receive vaccinations, such as children, the elderly, and other people whose chronic illnesses put them at higher risk of major harm or death if they catch an infectious disease. The answers to these questions facilitate appropriate and timely vaccinations, thereby protecting the patient and contributing to herd immunity.

Developmental history: This refers to the demonstrated capabilities of the child (called 'milestones') during their pre-school years, covering areas such as comprehension, speech, and motor skills. Some diseases involving the brain are more likely in children with delays or regression in developmental milestones. For example, if a child presents with a seizure and fever, and the doctor is trying to decide if the child had a simple febrile seizure or an epileptic seizure, the presence of delayed developmental milestones significantly increases the suspicion of epilepsy. The developmental history is also part of anticipatory health-maintenance questioning in children, as delayed developmental milestones may require intervention to minimise subsequent handicaps in life.

Treatment history: This refers to any medication the patient recently took or is taking, and any recent procedures. Recent and current medication intakes are risk factors for adverse drug reactions. Recent procedures can be risk factors for subsequent post-procedure problems. This information is also important when trying to distinguish disease severity from disease activity (this distinction is discussed in the chapter 'Diagnosis: disease, severity and treatment').

Lifestyle and social setup: This refers to information related to the patient's occupation, home environment, members of the household, degree of support in relationships (friends, family), and so on. Some diseases are associated with certain occupations or environmental exposures. Some diseases, especially certain psychiatric disorders, are more likely when there are strained relationships or poor social support. For example, depression is more common in estranged patients who feel that they have no friends, family, support or hope. Aside from diagnosis, this information can be useful for adjustment of treatment (this is discussed in the chapter 'Gathering additional information to manage patients').

Do I usually need to know the patient's risk factors to think of the diagnosis?

For most diseases, you should not need to ask for the risk factors to think of the diagnosis. With adequate medical training, common diseases are taught and readily recognisable through their clinical features. By the end of 1 year of work, the doctor can usually diagnose patients with common diseases by using the clinical features alone.

The generation of relevant diagnoses should occur before knowledge of Epidemiology/Risk Factors in the patient. Difficulty in this generation of differentials suggests major weaknesses in information-gathering, knowledge and/or clinical reasoning in the medical student/doctor.

Risk factors can change the doctor's suspicion of the cause of the patient's disease, which can then affect the management plan.

For example, in a patient presenting with vomiting and diarrhoea of 1–3 days' duration, with an unremarkable physical examination, most doctors would think of acute viral gastroenteritis. The age and gender of the patient would not change this.

In this patient, the presence of some risk factors may matter:

- If half the family or all the attendees of a banquet developed similar symptoms simultaneously, suspicion would fall upon the food that was consumed. Food poisoning would be suspected. Though the management of the patient would be similar whether or not their diagnosis is gastroenteritis or food poisoning, the suspicion of food poisoning can have implications for public health. Tracing the source of the contaminated food, and checking the hygiene of the preparers of the food, become important.

- Consumption of certain foods, such as oysters, raw fish or fried rice hours to days before the symptoms, might point to specific pathogens, some of which would require specific treatment.

The absence of these risk factors does not reduce the likelihood of the diagnosis of gastroenteritis.

Uncommon situations when early knowledge of the risk factors may be crucial for making the correct clinical diagnosis

Risk factors can be important for thinking of the uncommon disease that the patient has.

In these situations, the Safety Net questions are asked early on in the consultation. Just as a physical safety net is a useful backup in certain situations to catch someone falling before any major harm or death can occur, Safety Net questions are situationally used risk factor questions that can stop you from missing the correct diagnosis by the end of the first consultation, before any major harm can occur. Asking these questions early enough, under circumstances that suggest a significant possibility of an uncommon disease, buys you enough time to ask more questions that target the uncommon disease.

These questions should be posed after you have obtained the details of the presenting complaint, or after asking the patient for any other symptoms in addition to the presenting complaint.

The main Safety Net questions are:

- Personal history of any chronic problems, major illnesses, recent treatment for these chronic problems or illnesses, and any surgery in the last 1 month
- Contact history of any illness in close contacts (family members, colleagues, classmates) in the last 1 month
- Significant travel history in the last 1 month
- Family history of any chronic illness.

The Safety Net questions can be modified according to your initial suspicions.

The 3 situations where the Safety Net should be used in the initial consultation, are:

1. The patient has a bizarre primary complaint or associated symptoms, such that you struggle to come up with reasonable differentials by the 3rd minute of the consultation (3-minute habit)

2. The patient has skin symptoms, and other symptoms that suggest other organ systems are involved

3. Your top 2–3 differential diagnoses include a 'surgical speciality-related diagnosis'

Safety Net questions tend to be open-ended. However, if you have a specific diagnosis in mind, you may alter your Safety Net question to target the Risk Factor relevant to that diagnosis.

You may wonder: why can it be important to ask specific questions, instead of just relying on open-ended questions all the time?

There are 2 potential problems with open-ended questions. The first problem is that vague, open-ended questions can invite vague, non-specific answers. For example, you ask for 'any family history of illness'. The patient then spends the next 5 minutes telling you about the multiple problems across the 3 generations of the family.

The second problem is that the failure to ask a specific question may lead to the patient failing to tell you the specific answer. Assume you were thinking of lethal cardiac arrhythmias, and you only asked for 'any family history of illness'. The patient had a close relative who had a sudden, unexplained collapse and death at the age of 22 years, but did not tell you about this death because you did not ask for 'sudden, unexplained collapses and deaths in the family'.

The sheer number of Risk Factors that can be mentioned, requires a focus on the specific Risk Factors of interest.

Thus, Safety Net questions do not replace targeted questions on the Risk Factors that are relevant to your differentials.

The next figure depicts the use of the Safety Net, in tandem with the 3-minute habit.

The 3-Minute Habit: how the 'Safety Net' is situationally used

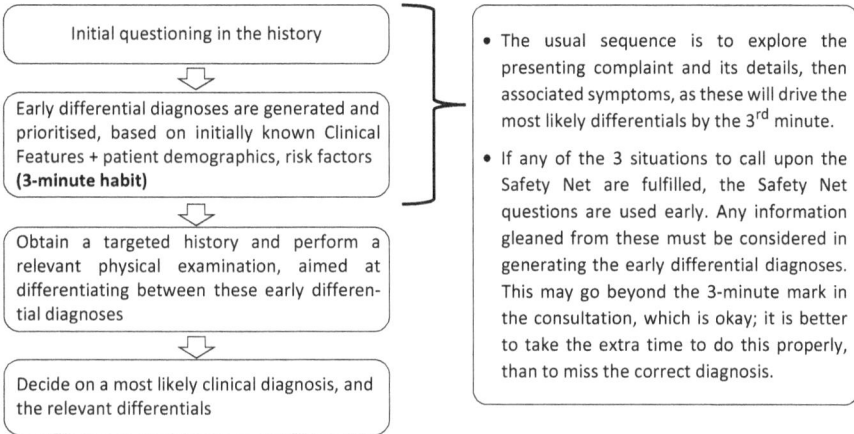

Initial questioning in the history

⬇

Early differential diagnoses are generated and prioritised, based on initially known Clinical Features + patient demographics, risk factors (**3-minute habit**)

⬇

Obtain a targeted history and perform a relevant physical examination, aimed at differentiating between these early differential diagnoses

⬇

Decide on a most likely clinical diagnosis, and the relevant differentials

- The usual sequence is to explore the presenting complaint and its details, then associated symptoms, as these will drive the most likely differentials by the 3rd minute.
- If any of the 3 situations to call upon the Safety Net are fulfilled, the Safety Net questions are used early. Any information gleaned from these must be considered in generating the early differential diagnoses. This may go beyond the 3-minute mark in the consultation, which is okay; it is better to take the extra time to do this properly, than to miss the correct diagnosis.

You may ask: 'What is the basis for those 3 situations that invoke the Safety Net?'

The answer is based on a combination of reasoning and the relevant diseases. See the next figure for the breakdown and the specific Risk Factor questions.

The specialities/systems clinically involved in the Safety Net

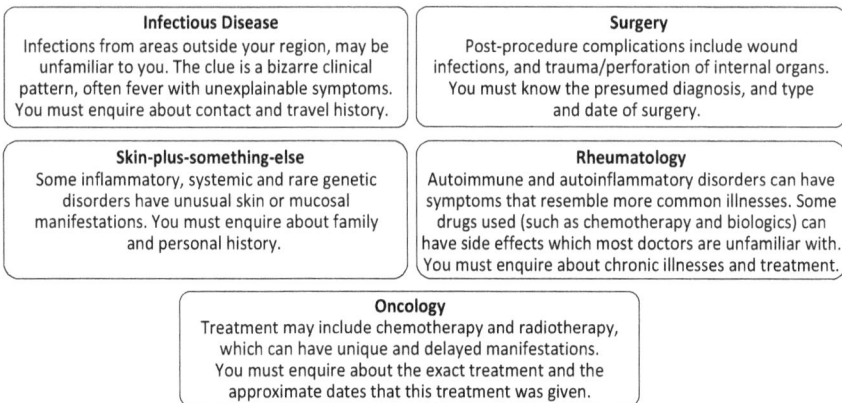

Infectious Disease	**Surgery**
Infections from areas outside your region, may be unfamiliar to you. The clue is a bizarre clinical pattern, often fever with unexplainable symptoms. You must enquire about contact and travel history.	Post-procedure complications include wound infections, and trauma/perforation of internal organs. You must know the presumed diagnosis, and type and date of surgery.

Skin-plus-something-else	**Rheumatology**
Some inflammatory, systemic and rare genetic disorders have unusual skin or mucosal manifestations. You must enquire about family and personal history.	Autoimmune and autoinflammatory disorders can have symptoms that resemble more common illnesses. Some drugs used (such as chemotherapy and biologics) can have side effects which most doctors are unfamiliar with. You must enquire about chronic illnesses and treatment.

Oncology
Treatment may include chemotherapy and radiotherapy, which can have unique and delayed manifestations. You must enquire about the exact treatment and the approximate dates that this treatment was given.

Though it may seem easier just to specify the specialities in your initial differentials, and then call upon only the questions relevant to each speciality, the speciality of the patient's diagnosis is often neither apparent nor guessed correctly if you must invoke the Safety Net.

The Safety Net helps to ensure that you do think of the relevant differential diagnosis. It does not mean that the Safety-Net-suggested differential diagnosis will be the correct diagnosis. The risk factors in the Safety Net do not override Rule #1 of clinical reasoning: the entirety of the patient's clinical features.

Use of Safety Net questions at other times

Safety Net questions may be useful if the patient's subsequent progress surprises you.

Surprises include:

- Test results you did not expect
- The development of new symptoms or signs, and
- Failure of the patient's existing symptoms and signs to change over time as you had expected.

These developments challenge the fundamental assumption you made: your diagnosis.

After all, if your diagnosis was right, you should not be getting surprises.

Since your diagnosis is now in question, all the steps you took to reach that diagnosis, should be restarted and re-checked with extra caution.

Some 'diagnostic dilemmas' can be solved rapidly and clinically, because the necessary risk factor is detected in the Safety Net and considered appropriately. Failure to record or consider these risk factors can lead to tragedy. Consider Cases #7 and #8.

CASE #7: Tom

Tom is a 55-year-old man presenting with breathlessness on exerting himself, for a week.

This breathlessness occurs only on climbing two or more flights of stairs. He has to rest for 5 minutes to recover fully.

There are no other symptoms.

The vital signs are normal. On examination, there are crepitations and rhonchi bilaterally. Air entry is equal and normal bilaterally. There is no dullness to percussion.

--

Differential diagnoses that were considered:

- Exercise-induced asthma
- Chronic obstructive pulmonary disease
- Pneumonia

A chest X-ray demonstrated an opacity over the right lower hemithorax.

Tom was treated for all of the above diagnoses. None of the treatments worked.

Over the next few days, Tom deteriorated, developed respiratory failure, and was then sent to the Intensive Care Unit.

--

Crucial information from the Safety Net (which was known, but ignored): Tom had had cancer of the lower lobe of the right lung, and received chemoradiotherapy in the past 1 year.

The correct diagnosis was radiation pneumonitis.

CASE #8: Delia

Delia is a 9-year-old girl presenting with itchy skin over her calves and backs of her knees, for the past 1 month.

She has no other symptoms.

Her mother mentions Delia also has iron deficiency and is on iron supplements. Delia is following up with another doctor for the problem of iron deficiency.

The vital signs are normal. On examination, the rash feels slightly dry, with some excoriations. There are no other signs on examination.

--

Delia was diagnosed with eczema. Moisturisers were recommended. However, the moisturisers had no effect on her symptoms.

--

Crucial information from the Safety Net (which was not asked early on):

Delia's mother had celiac disease.

Delia turned out to have dermatitis herpetiformis. This is a rare manifestation of celiac disease.

The previous doctor who saw Delia had been concerned about the unexplainable 'iron deficiency' her mother had mentioned. The doctor had known about the itchy skin, but had been unable to think of a diagnosis that explained both the iron deficiency and the itchy skin.

Revelation of the family history — her mother had celiac disease — highlighted the correct diagnosis, which explained both her rash and the iron deficiency anaemia.

If risk factors are important in some diagnostic situations, why not put these on equal footing as clinical features?

Clinical features directly manifest from and therefore point to the correct diagnosis. Risk factors cannot make the same claim and thus, are less important than clinical features.

Poor reasoners tend to argue that symptoms may be subjective or imagined, then argue that subjectivity is the same as being totally unreliable, and then argue that the patient's inconvenient clinical features are unreliable and should be ignored. The chain of poor reasoning can go like this: 'Anything is possible. Therefore, the patient may be providing inaccurate information. Therefore, I can believe whatever I want.'

These arguments are self-serving and deceitful. Most patients do not lie about their symptoms.

If the information the patient provides is confusing, the doctor needs to ask themselves if they have asked the right questions, instead of impugning the patient's words.

If we were to apply the same argument of 'subjectivity' to risk factors, risk factors are even more subjective than clinical features:

- The patient may not know they have the risk factor, so they cannot tell you about it. For example, the adult patient had an allergic reaction to a food they ate during infancy, but their parents never told them about it and they have never eaten that food since. If you asked such a patient 'do you have food allergies?', the answer could be 'no.'

- Some patients know their risk factors for their disease, such as sexual intercourse, alcoholism or recreational drug abuse, but deny these out of fear of embarrassment or punishment. Some patients eventually admit to having these risk factors, days or weeks later. Meanwhile, the correct diagnosis was not made and optimal care was not provided, because the doctors never considered the correct diagnosis due to an insistence on the presence of risk factors (which the patient initially denied) for that diagnosis.

The next weakness of risk factors lies in the statistics. Statistically, most risk factors are inaccurate in predicting the correct diagnosis. From a reasoning perspective, the question is 'how much does the presence of this risk factor increase the likelihood of this disease compared to the differentials, and how much does the absence of this risk factor decrease the likelihood of this disease compared to the differentials?'

Many studies describe the prevalence and severity of the risk factors in people who <u>already have the disease</u>. The conclusions of these studies cannot be used for diagnostic purposes, because the studies did not analyse the diagnostic accuracy of the risk factors.

A diagnostic study requires a group of patients who have the disease and another comparator group who does not have the disease.

Consider this analogy: you are peering into the yard of a prison. Everyone in the yard is a hardened criminal. Most of the criminals have 2 arms and 2 legs:

- Do most imprisoned criminals in the yard have 2 arms and 2 legs? Yes.

- Does this mean that having 2 arms and 2 legs is the cause of becoming a criminal? No.

The prevalence of having 2 arms and 2 legs is high in criminals. This is unsurprising; how many robbers and murderers would try to commit crimes without having the use of 2 arms and 2 legs?

To argue that having 2 arms and legs is a risk factor for being a criminal in comparison to non-criminals, you would need to compare criminals and non-criminals. Looking only at criminals does not tell you about the non-criminals. Looking only at the number of arms and legs in criminals, does not tell you about the number of arms and legs in non-criminals.

Diagnostic studies that analyse the ability of risk factors to discern between different diseases, show a uniformly abysmal picture. Most risk factors have poor likelihood ratios regardless of whether they are present or absent. To put it simply, neither the presence nor absence of risk factors significantly changes the likelihood of most diagnoses for a specific time point, which is the exact scenario the doctor faces in a doctor–patient consultation.

When doctors prioritise risk factors over 'explain all clinical features', they often cherry-pick 1 risk factor from the patient's information, and then ignore the entirety of the patient's clinical features and the other risk factors. This behaviour often leads to them making the wrong diagnosis.

Consider the next 3 cases.

CASE #9: Jim

Jim is a 70-year-old man with a past medical history of cystitis. He comes with the Presenting Complaint of right-sided abdominal pain, nausea and fever for 1 day.

There are no other symptoms.

His temperature is 38 degrees Celsius. The other vital signs are normal.

On examination, Jim refuses to allow the right side of the abdomen to be palpated, pushing the doctor away when the doctor tries to palpate the abdomen.

--

The doctor says, 'Jim has a history of urinary tract infection. Therefore, this must be a urinary tract infection. Since the pain is on the right side, the diagnosis must be an infection of the right kidney: acute pyelonephritis. The kidney is part of the urinary tract, so infection of the kidney fits the risk factor. Treat him with intravenous antibiotics for a kidney infection.'

--

The doctor had fixated on the risk factor of cystitis, and then ignored the implications of the patient refusing the palpation of their abdomen. Severe pain to the extent that palpation is refused, is a crucial detail of this clinical feature. The pain of acute pyelonephritis is usually not

(*Continued*)

(Continued)

severe enough for patients to refuse palpation. Some other diseases, such as acute appendicitis, do have patients refusing palpation.

Acute appendicitis was an obvious clinical diagnosis. However, the doctor's fixation on the risk factor of cystitis, blinded them to the obvious diagnosis.

Jim had acute appendicitis.

He worsened whilst receiving intravenous antibiotics for a presumed pyelonephritis. A few days after the initial encounter, by which point he was in even more pain, the correct diagnosis was made. He underwent an appendectomy. He was very unhappy with the initial doctor who misdiagnosed him.

CASE #10: Lyla

Lyla is a 16-year-old girl being seen in the Psychiatry clinic of a hospital, for a follow-up of her panic attacks. During the consultation, she becomes upset over the discussion of her triggers, and complains of severe chest pain and breathlessness.

There are no other symptoms.

--

The doctor says, 'Lyla has had panic attacks in the past. Therefore, this must be another panic attack.'

--

The doctor had fixated on the known medical history of panic attacks, and then failed to consider other relevant differential diagnoses for Lyla's symptoms.

(Continued)

Lyla was told to calm down, breathe into a paper bag, and sent home. Her parents became more concerned as she did not improve over the next few hours. They sent her back to the hospital the same night.

The history taken by the doctor in the Emergency Department revealed that her chest pain was more severe than her usual 'chest discomfort from a panic attack'.

There was hyper-resonance on percussion of her chest.

The diagnosis of spontaneous pneumothorax was clinically obvious.

A chest X-ray demonstrated the extent of the pneumothorax.

Lyla underwent thoracocentesis.

Lyla complained, 'I told my psychiatrist the pain was worse than usual, but she did not listen! She just said it must be a panic attack! She did not ask more questions or examine me at all!'

CASE #11: Theron

Theron is a 3-year-old boy who came to the Emergency Department with his parents, for the presenting complaint of cough and fever up to 38 degrees Celsius for 1 week. There were no other symptoms. His appetite and activity were normal.

His parents said there was no witnessed choking on food or putting toys in the mouth.

The vital signs were normal. On examination, there was decreased air entry over the right side of his chest, with no adventitious sounds and a resonant percussion note.

--

Theron was diagnosed with pneumonia despite the absence of clinical signs of consolidation.

(Continued)

(Continued)

The chest X-ray seemed unremarkable. The absence of radiological consolidation, which would have been expected in pneumonia, was explained away as 'radiological lag'.

Theron was treated with oral antibiotics for presumed pneumonia. The fever disappeared for a few days whilst the cough continued. Once the 1-week course of antibiotics was complete, the fever recurred 3 days later.

--

The reviewing doctor in the clinic was puzzled by the entire clinical picture and the recurrence of the fever, and asked a colleague (non-respiratory specialist) for suggestions. This colleague listened to the description of the symptoms and signs, and then stated that the child had inhaled a foreign body into the lungs.

The respiratory specialists were informed immediately. An urgent bronchoscopy plucked a peanut out of the right main bronchus. Theron recovered fully soon afterwards.

--

When asked why a foreign body inhalation was never considered, the response by the previous doctors was 'because there was no risk factor in the history to support foreign body inhalation'.

The previous doctors had fixated on the absence of the risk factor for the correct diagnosis, and therefore insisted that diagnosis was impossible.

They had then chosen a diagnosis that did not explain the child's entire clinical picture.

At the teaching round for this case, the audience of doctors was reminded: 'You cannot insist on the presence of subjective risk factors as a requirement to make the diagnosis'.

Capsule summary

- Information in the category of Epidemiology/Risk Factors can add value to the diagnosis and patient's care.

- In certain situations, Safety Net questions help to avoid missing the correct diagnosis.

- Fixation on Epidemiology/Risk Factors to ignore Rule #1 of Clinical Reasoning, invites disaster.

Frequently asked questions

Q: Like Universal Clinical Features, are there Universal Risk Factors?

A: Yes. Some diseases can only be present when the risk factor is present. However, memorising universal risk factors is almost useless.

For example, one could argue that you should only think of traumatic brain injury if there is a history suggesting major trauma to the head.

Requiring the presence of this risk factor in history is often unnecessary. In most cases of traumatic brain injury, there are obvious signs of major trauma to the head, even before enquiring about the history of a fall or heavy blow to the head.

Even when there are no obvious signs of major trauma, the circumstances in which such patients are found often prompt the thought of major head trauma anyway. If a patient was found unconscious and alone, even if there was no club lying next to his or her head, would the absence of a history of head trauma stop any sensible doctor from considering traumatic brain injury as a relevant differential diagnosis?

Once you apply all the above arguments to other diseases, you will probably reach the same conclusion I did.

Some diseases do have universal risk factors. However, those diseases are often obvious upon obeying the basic diagnostic reasoning requirement. Thus, knowledge of the universal risk factor is unnecessary.

If you discover a disease where you absolutely must rely on the presence of the universal risk factor to think of that disease despite following the steps in this book, please let me know.

PUTTING IT ALL TOGETHER: THE MOST LIKELY DIAGNOSIS

At this point, you have obtained the relevant diagnostic information for your patient.

To recap, the correct diagnosis has 3 elements. The correct diagnosis should:

1. Explain all the patient's Clinical Features…(if 'all' is not possible, at least 'most'…while you learn more to try to explain 'all')

2. …with a Disease/Illness…

3. …and include your impression of the Severity of the illness

The first part of this chapter will focus on the first 2 elements.

Summarise the information within their respective diagnostic categories (Clinical Features and Epidemiology/Risk Factors). This summary will focus your thoughts and reduce the cognitive load.

Write down the summary for every patient, until you can visualise the entire summary mentally or present the patient using this summary without missing any crucial bits.

The figure on the next page is a template for a basic diagnostic summary.

DIAGNOSTIC SUMMARY: TEMPLATE

(Insert patient name) is a (insert brief demographics: age, gender, race). He/she comes with the Presenting Complaint of (insert all symptoms of presenting complaint)

The symptoms are…(insert relevant details of the symptoms of the presenting complaint)

The other symptoms are…(insert other known symptoms and their relevant details)

The significant negatives (symptoms relevant to my differential diagnoses, which are absent) are…(insert significant negatives among symptoms)

The known risk factors are…(insert any risk factors relevant to your differential diagnoses)

Other information includes (insert other risk factors that seem irrelevant to the current diagnosis)

The vital signs are…(insert vital signs)

The signs on physical examination are…(insert signs found)

The significant negatives (signs relevant to my differential diagnoses, which are absent) on physical examination are…(insert significant negatives among signs)

--

My differential diagnoses are (order of descending likelihood):

1. (Insert most likely). How likely is this in absolute terms?

2. (Insert next most likely). How likely is this in absolute terms?

3. (Insert next most likely). How likely is this in absolute terms?

4. …and so on.

The patient's name and demographics allow you to visualise the patient mentally and thus, come first. The Presenting Complaint comes next.

Subsequent information after the Presenting Complaint is in descending order of importance. In this sample template, I placed vital signs and physical examination after the history, to match the chronology of a commonplace consultation.

Vital signs and physical examination findings are clinical features. Priority wise, they should be placed above risk factors. Thus, a common variation of the basic template puts all the clinical features in the history and physical examination up front, and then places the risk factors after the clinical features.

If so desired, alter this template to suit your style. I call upon my personal, universal template mentally the moment the consultation begins, filling the template as the consultation proceeds. My template uses all 3 Rules of Clinical Reasoning, so it is different from the basic template.

I will discuss my templates later in this chapter. For now, let us focus on the fundamentals of deciding the likelihood of differential diagnoses.

Stepwise mental weighing, and arguing for and against your diagnoses

You have assembled the information on the patient and organised it into categories.

You have your relevant differentials.

Start with the most likely diagnosis. Apply these 2 steps to that diagnosis:

1. Look at the clinical features, and then apply Rule #1 of clinical reasoning. Which and how much of these Clinical Features and their details, cannot be explained by this diagnosis?

2. Then look at all the information on Epidemiology/Risk Factors and ask yourself: which of the information in this category, are arguments for and against this diagnosis?

Once you have completed these 2 steps for the first diagnosis, apply the 2 steps to the next-lower-likelihood differential diagnosis in line, then the next-lower-likelihood differential diagnosis after that, and so on.

If the patient's Epidemiology/Risk Factors do not seem to distinguish between the differentials, consider the general prevalence of the differentials in the population.

By the end of this exercise, you will have assembled your arguments regarding each diagnosis. Let us illustrate this with Case #12.

CASE #12: Xiao Bei

Xiao Bei is a 35-year-old lady who came to your clinic. She complains of severe upper central abdominal pain and fever (maximum 38 degrees Celsius) of 2 days' duration. The patient reports her pain score is 8/10. The pain is worse with meals and does not radiate.

There are no other symptoms.

She drinks 1 can of beer every day. She eats 3 regular meals a day. She does not skip meals.

Her body temperature is 38 degrees Celsius. Her other vital signs are normal. Weight and height are normal. On examination, she has marked abdominal tenderness, just superior to the umbilicus. There is no abdominal guarding or rebound tenderness. The bowel sounds are normal. There are no other signs on examination.

--

Your 2 main differentials are acute pancreatitis, and peptic ulcer disease.

(*Continued*)

You start with acute pancreatitis:

1. Clinical features: this diagnosis explains all the patient's clinical features.

2. Epidemiology/Risk Factors: this disease is common in patients with these demographics. She has a supporting risk factor: she drinks beer daily.

You then consider peptic ulcer disease:

1. Clinical features: this diagnosis fails to explain the patient's fever. The abdominal tenderness cannot be explained unless she has a perforated ulcer.

2. Epidemiology/Risk Factors: this disease is common in patients with these demographics. She has a supporting risk factor: she drinks beer daily.

As the patient's demographics and known risk factors do not argue strongly for 1 diagnosis over the other, you consider the prevalence of these differentials in the population. You realise that peptic ulcer disease is more common than acute pancreatitis.

You then rank your differentials based on likelihood. How is the ranking decided?

A commonplace way is to assign 'points' without regard to the information categories, and then add the points up for each diagnosis. The diagnosis with the highest score is usually deemed to be the correct diagnosis. Applying this 'point' system to Case #12:

- Acute pancreatitis: fever (1), upper central abdominal pain worse with meals (1), abdominal tenderness (1), drinks beer (1), fits demographics (1) = 5 points total.

- Peptic ulcer disease: fever (0), upper central abdominal pain worse with meals (1), abdominal tenderness (surprising, but not impossible. Maybe give it 1 point? Or half a point?), drinks beer (1), fits demographics (1), more prevalent than pancreatitis in the general population (1) = 4 points plus up to 1 more point for abdominal tenderness.

The 2 differentials seem close.

If you decided that marked abdominal tenderness gets the full point in peptic ulcer disease, you would assign a total of 5 points to this diagnosis.

When the 2 differentials are close or appear equal, you would be stuck. You would then be tempted to order diagnostic tests for both diseases, trying to differentiate between them.

This common, unprioritised point system does not recognise the relative importance of Clinical Features over Epidemiology/Risk Factors. This point system fails the basic diagnostic reasoning requirement and increases the chance of mistakes. Thus, I do not use this point system.

Let us try this again, my way.

Clinical Fit has the highest priority. A disease that cannot explain all of the clinical features in the patient, will be less likely than a disease that does. Information in the category of Epidemiology/Risk Factors has lower priority than Clinical Fit.

The ranking then becomes clearer. From most likely to least likely, it is:

1. Acute pancreatitis: does not fail Rule #1. Risk factors and demographics: no surprises there.

2. Peptic ulcer disease: fails Rule #1 in terms of inability to explain fever; the abdominal tenderness is surprising, though not impossible. Risk factors and demographics: no surprises there.

The most likely diagnosis would be acute pancreatitis, merely by applying Rule #1.

The patient did have acute pancreatitis.

Let us suppose you considered a 3rd differential, biliary colic. Applying Rule #1, the ranking from most likely to least likely is:

1. Acute pancreatitis: does not fail Rule #1. Risk factors and demographics: no surprises there.

2. Peptic ulcer disease: fails Rule #1 in terms of inability to explain fever; the abdominal tenderness is surprising, though not impossible. Risk factors and demographics: no surprises there.

3. Biliary colic: fails Rule #1 in terms of inability to explain fever and abdominal tenderness. Risk factors and demographics: no surprises there.

If you argued that biliary colic or peptic ulcer disease is much more common than pancreatitis in the general population, you are right. You are right in your description of the population.

However, your duty is to the patient in front of you. Thus, your arguments must focus on the patient instead of everyone else. If you tried arguing that the patient's disease must be the most common disease in the population, a decent reasoner can rightly reply:

- Are you diagnosing everyone else, or this patient?

- Are you ignoring the patient's symptoms and signs in their entirety?

Let us illustrate with another case, ramping up the risk factors:

CASE #13: Xiao Pan

Xiao Pan is a 15-year-old girl who came to your clinic. She complains of severe upper central abdominal pain of 2 days' duration. The abdominal pain is scored as 8/10, and radiates to the back.

There are no other symptoms.

She has been eating only 2 meals a day for the last 4 months. She says she is intentionally skipping meals because she is trying to lose weight.

She has a history of systemic lupus erythematosus diagnosed 1 year ago, with frequent symptomatic flares requiring titration of her

(Continued)

(Continued)

immunosuppressant medication in the last 6 months. Her most recent flare was 1 month ago. She claims compliance to her immunosuppressants.

Her vital signs are normal. Weight and height are normal. Physical examination of her abdomen is unremarkable. Her joints appear unremarkable. There is a faint rash over the bridge of her nose. She says her rheumatologist told her that her rash was due to her lupus. She mentions that her rash gets worse during some of her flares of lupus.

--

Your 2 main differentials are acute pancreatitis, and acute gastritis.

You start with acute pancreatitis:

1. Clinical features: this diagnosis explains all the patient's clinical features, except for the rash. The rash is explainable by the concomitant uncontrolled lupus.

2. Epidemiology/Risk Factors: this disease is uncommon in teenage girls. However, she has systemic lupus erythematosus, which seems uncontrolled. Uncontrolled lupus is a risk factor for pancreatitis.

You then consider acute gastritis:

1. Clinical features: this diagnosis fails to explain the pain radiating to the back, and also fails to explain the rash. The rash is explainable by the concomitant uncontrolled lupus.

2. Epidemiology/Risk Factors: she skips her regular meals. Furthermore, this disease is common in patients with these demographics.

As the demographics and risk factors do not really argue strongly for 1 diagnosis over the other, you consider the prevalence of these differentials in the population. You realise that acute gastritis is more common than acute pancreatitis.

Applying the common but flawed 'point' system to Case #13:

- Acute gastritis: upper central abdominal pain but radiates to the back (half a point?), skips meals (1), fits demographics (1), more prevalent than pancreatitis in the general population (1) = 3.5 points total.

- Acute pancreatitis: upper central abdominal pain radiating to the back (1), has supporting risk factor of uncontrolled lupus (1) = 2 points total.

Using the common point system, you would say the correct diagnosis is acute gastritis.

Even if you decided that the upper abdominal pain would not be worth any points for acute gastritis, the total score for acute gastritis would still be 3 points, which is higher than the score for acute pancreatitis.

By deciding the correct diagnosis is acute gastritis, you would be wrong. This patient had acute pancreatitis.

Let us do it my way. Apply the reasoning priorities and Rule #1. From most likely to least likely, it is:

1. Acute pancreatitis: does not fail Rule #1. The rash is explainable by uncontrolled lupus. Risk factors and demographics: she has uncontrolled lupus erythematosus, which can predispose her to acute pancreatitis.

2. Acute gastritis: fails Rule #1 in terms of inability to explain the pain radiating to the back. The rash is explainable by uncontrolled lupus. Risk factors and demographics: no surprises there. She skips her regular meals! Acute gastritis is more common in the population than pancreatitis, too.

Using the basic diagnostic reasoning requirement, the conclusion would be acute pancreatitis. This conclusion would be correct.

The knowledge of having uncontrolled systemic lupus erythematosus is reassuring when making the diagnosis of acute pancreatitis, as even a robust reasoner might hesitate to make this diagnosis of acute pancreatitis in a teenager without supportive risk factors.

However, with these clinical features, a robust reasoner would consider and act on the diagnosis of acute pancreatitis even if there were no risk factors supporting acute pancreatitis.

As explained in the previous chapter, risk factors may not be known at the time of presentation. For example, the teenager could have had asymptomatic gallstones (a risk factor for pancreatitis) without being aware of it. The patient cannot tell you about the risk factor if they do not know of its existence. Thus, insisting on the risk factors for acute pancreatitis being present before you would consider the diagnosis of acute pancreatitis, would be a mistake.

Epidemiology/Risk Factors cannot be used to ignore clinical features

Imagine that the bank nearest your home was robbed yesterday at lunchtime. The masked robbers escaped. The bank staff described them as big, brown-skinned men who spoke broken English. You have just finished viewing this news report with your family on television.

Your father is sitting beside you. He says: 'I bet our neighbour was one of the robbers!'

You blink.

Your father's accusation is surprising to you. The neighbour was having lunch with your family yesterday at the time of the robbery. Your father was present at the same meal and saw your neighbour, but did not speak to your neighbour. You have long suspected that your father is prejudiced against people of other races or backgrounds.

Carefully, you say: 'Uh, Dad? Wasn't he eating lunch with you and me yesterday when the robbery took place? And he left the meal after the time that the news says the bank robbers had left the bank? How could he have robbed the bank?'

Your father declares: 'He is male, brown-skinned and speaks broken English! He was previously convicted of petty theft over 10 years ago! He has all the risk factors and demographics that fit the news report!'

You have long known that your father can be illogical. This is partly because he does not listen to others and does not follow up to see if his arguments were proven right. He insists that he is always right, so there is no need to find out what happened after each assertion he makes.

This short story may seem comical and unreal.

However, a glaring absence of logic is not uncommon in humankind. Prioritising risk factors over direct proof to the point of ignoring the proof, can be accompanied by declarations of 'anything is possible' and a refusal to follow up to discover the truth.

Direct proof of the disease comes from its clinical features. Arguing that risk factors allow the doctor to ignore direct proof, is illogical.

I have sat in on countless arguments between doctors from many specialities, about the patient's diagnosis. Doctors sometimes rejected the most likely diagnosis, which was evident from the clinical features. Instead, they would use a single data point in Epidemiology/Risk Factors to argue in favour of another diagnosis, and then argue that the inconvenient clinical features that did not fit their favoured diagnosis should be ignored.

The usual arguments include:

- 'Common things happen commonly. This disease is rare in the general population even though it explains all the patient's symptoms and signs. Instead, another more common disease should be more likely, even if it does not fit the patient.'

- 'This disease is less common in the patient's (insert demographic group) even if it explains all the patient's symptoms and signs. Instead, another more common disease should be more likely, even if it does not fit the patient.'

- 'The patient has a risk factor for another disease that does not explain all the clinical features, unlike the disease that explains all the patient's clinical features but lacks a supporting risk factor. The risk factor is more important than explaining all of the patient's symptoms and signs.'

I have never seen a doctor who argued in this way, turn out to be correct in the end.

When asked if they followed up on the patient to check the final diagnosis and their assertions, these doctors often say, 'No, I am too busy.'

Recall the arguments at the end of Tina's case:

CASE #2: Tina

Tina is a 13-year-old Chinese girl with a past medical history of cystitis (this is a lower urinary tract infection). She consults you with the Presenting Complaint of headache and fever for 3 days.

--

Clinical reasoning-based mental process: The patient has symptoms of fever and headache lasting 3 days. These are direct clues to the current diagnosis.

Next course of action: You tell the patient, 'Please tell me more (about the headache and fever).'

--

In this example, there is the patient's name, age, gender, race, and past medical history. These fall under Epidemiology/Risk Factors.

Though this information is 'nice to have', is it more important than exploring the Clinical Features? No.

Do you <u>need</u> to pursue the Clinical Features to make the diagnosis? Yes.

Would any of these sentences be sensible or logical?

- Tina has a disease because she is female. Her gender caused the illness.

(*Continued*)

- Tina has a disease because she is a child. Her age caused the illness.
- Tina's current disease must be due to her history of cystitis. The past always predicts the future.

Certainty of each diagnosis being present in your differentials

After ranking the differential diagnoses, it is important to decide on 2 more factors:

- Your certainty of each diagnosis being present in the patient
- The severity of each diagnosis, if that is indeed the patient's diagnosis.

Certainty can be expressed either mathematically, or by 'rough estimate'.

If you are estimating the certainty of each diagnosis mathematically, assume the total certainty of your differential diagnoses adds up to 100%. Split this total of 100% among your differentials, the proportions being based on your certainty for each differential in that patient.

For example, in Case #12, the ranking and justification were:

1. Acute pancreatitis: does not fail Rule #1.
2. Peptic ulcer disease: fails Rule #1 in terms of inability to explain fever; the abdominal tenderness is surprising, but not impossible.
3. Biliary colic: fails Rule #1 in terms of inability to explain fever and abdominal tenderness.

Therefore, your % certainty might be:

1. Acute pancreatitis: does not fail Rule #1 — 70%.
2. Peptic ulcer disease: fails Rule #1 in terms of inability to explain fever; the abdominal tenderness is surprising but not impossible — 20%.

3. Biliary colic: fails Rule #1 in terms of inability to explain fever and abdominal tenderness — 10%.

I never mentioned Rules #2 and #3 in deciding the diagnosis or the proportion of certainty of each differential.

This omission was intentional, as applying Rules #2 and #3 requires more proficiency in this method than applying Rule #1. Applying Rules #2 and #3 would have significantly altered the certainty and accuracy of each differential, such as increasing the certainty of acute pancreatitis in both cases #12 and #13 to above 90%. In turn, these additional Rules would facilitate more rapid and confident diagnoses and decision-making.

Clarity when assigning certainty to each differential, matters because excellent decision-making employs decision thresholds.

A vague 'more likely than the rest' declaration about one diagnosis is insufficient for accurate, decisive and efficient action. Decision thresholds and their relationship with clinical certainty are further explained in Section 2.

When the doctor is uncertain about the most likely diagnosis, confidence in their decision-making drops. A common reaction to uncertainty is to become more defensive, ordering a battery of tests and treating for several diagnoses at once. This is a reflexive and incorrect response, and is explained in the next chapter.

Instead of assigning percentages, you may prefer to use rough descriptions of 'certainty levels'. If so, I suggest the following breakdown to match % certainty:

- 90–100%: Very certain
- 70–89%: Certain, but some concern about being wrong. Consider rule-in and rule-out diagnostic testing in some situations.
- 31–69%: Uncertain. Consider diagnostic tests.
- 6–30%: Unlikely. May warrant 'rule out' testing in some situations.

- Less than 6%: Very unlikely. Doing anything for this diagnosis would require a strong justification.

The severity of each diagnosis in your differentials

Estimating severity clinically

Severity decides the intensity and urgency of all decisions you make, with and for the patient. Thus, discerning severity rapidly is crucial in emergencies.

The basic clues to severity include the quantitative scoring of the symptoms the patient reports, such as the pain score if they are in pain, or the number of times they have vomited each day.

The impact on the patient's current function (such as impact on drinking ability and daily activities) is a significant help in this assessment. The more severe the disease, the greater the impact on function.

In addition to the patient's current ability to function, consider the velocity at which the patient's function deteriorated. Examples include:

- Did their leg pain worsen so rapidly that they were able to walk when it began, were limping 2 hours later, and were refusing to move or allow you to touch their legs by the time they saw you at the 4-hour mark? This implies a severe disease.
- Did this deterioration occur over 2 weeks? This implies a less severe disease than someone who deteriorated within 4 hours.
- If their drinking ability went from 100% to about 5% of their usual intake, was this over the span of 1 day, or 1 week? The patient who deteriorated dramatically in 1 day is likely to have more severe disease than if they had deteriorated to the same extent over 1 week.

The greater the velocity of deteriorating function, the greater the disease severity.

Estimation of disease severity requires awareness of the difference between severity and activity. Disease severity (what you must get) is not always the same as disease activity (what you see):

- Disease activity refers to the symptoms, signs and test results at that time point. These markers of disease activity may have been suppressed (masked) by treatment.

- Thus, the true severity of the disease is equal to disease activity when there was zero masking, and greater than disease activity when masking has occurred.

- This distinction is crucial because overall management must match each patient's disease severity.

However, commonplace medical training often teaches doctors that disease activity is equal to disease severity, and then teaches that decisions are based on that disease activity.

Assuming activity is equal to severity predisposes doctors to underestimate the true magnitude of danger in their patients. Decisions based on this mistaken assumption, lead to unnecessary errors and tragedy. The crucial distinction between disease activity and disease severity and the many uses of this distinction, is taught in the chapter 'Diagnosis: disease, severity and treatment'.

Some patients with a severe disease do not 'look sick' by commonly used standards, descriptions or monitoring of vital signs. However, robust reasoners can recognise the severity of the disease in these patients by applying various concepts in this book. The combined application of Rule #1 and at least 1 other skill, such as mastery of Physical Examination Level 2 or recognition of the distinction between disease severity and disease activity, enables the immediate recognition of such patients.

Matching management to the severity

Early recognition of the disease severity allows you to immediately match the intensity and urgency of your management decisions to that patient.

Matching is necessary for optimal outcomes in emergencies and non-emergencies.

The 5 main areas of management are:

1. Tests
2. Treatments
3. Disposition
4. Monitoring
5. Counselling

If tests are indicated, patients with more severe diseases tend to require more tests, more often and sooner, than those with milder diseases. In some severe diseases, the ability to recognise the severity of the disease clinically can save the patient from permanent harm or death, because the results of the tests will not return in time for the doctor to save the patient. For example, in a patient who has a tension pneumothorax, immediate needle decompression is warranted even if the chest X-ray has not been performed.

Overall treatment intensity must at least match the severity of the disease.

Disposition refers to decisions regarding where the patient goes, whom they see, and when. Examples include:

- If the patient has an acute disease or flare-up of a chronic disease, should they be hospitalised or managed in the clinic/Emergency Department alone?
- If they are hospitalised, can they be managed in the general ward, or do they require Intensive Care?
- Can the general practitioner handle the disease, or should the patient be referred to a specialist?

Monitoring refers to decisions on the type and frequency of checks on the patient's status. Examples include:

- How short should the intervals be between follow-up visits, even if the disease seems controlled?

- Does the patient need focused monitoring of heart rate and oxygen saturation continuously? Or is checking these vital signs every 8-hourly, sufficiently safe?

Counselling involves the provision of information to the patient and a discussion with the patient. Greater disease severity requires more intensive management, which must be explained to and discussed with the patient. If the patient disagrees with the doctor's recommendations, the effort the doctor spends on persuading the patient to reconsider, should match the disease severity. The deadlier the disease, the more effort should be expended.

Diagnostic approach and template, using all 3 rules of clinical reasoning

This subsection demonstrates how the rules of clinical reasoning may change your personal template.

I use all 3 rules of clinical reasoning for all consultations, from the start of the consultation to the end of the clinical diagnostic process.

I have 3 templates. There is a base diagnostic template that I start with for all patients.

There are 2 options for the subsequent add-on template after my base template is used. One of these 2 templates is chosen as the add-on, based on the outcome of applying all 3 rules of reasoning in the base template.

I place vital signs and physical examination above risk factors, as I prefer to place information of the same priority level together.

The choice of the add-on template depends on the final check at the end of the base template. The base template identifies the most likely diagnosis in almost all patients. Thus, the primary add-on template is used for most patients.

The secondary add-on template is used when the 3 rules of clinical reasoning, applied in 1 pass in the base template, are not sufficient to identify the single, most likely diagnosis.

Think of these as proficiency-required templates. Do not use them until you are proficient in all 3 rules of clinical reasoning.

This is the base template:

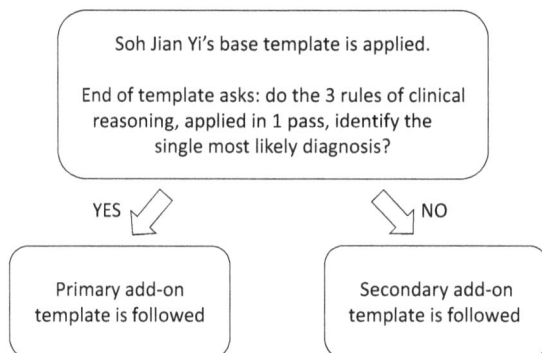

DIAGNOSTIC SUMMARY (Soh Jian Yi's base template for all patients):

1. (Insert patient name) is a (insert brief demographics: age, gender, race). He/she comes with the Presenting Complaint of (insert all symptoms of presenting complaint).

2. My early differential diagnoses that fit the entire presenting complaint are:

   A. (Insert most likely)

   B. (Insert next most likely)

   C. (Insert next most likely)

3. If not yet mentioned by the patient, I ask for Universal Clinical Features for each differential. The absent Universal Clinical Features are (insert Universal Clinical features which were absent). This absence eliminates (insert the corresponding early differentials with those Universal Clinical Features that were absent).

(Continued)

(Continued)

4. For each remaining differential, I then ask for the Secondary Specific Clinical Features of each differential diagnosis, starting with the highest remaining differential. The secondary specific clinical features are (insert Secondary Specific Clinical features).

5. I ask for any other symptoms. They are (insert all other symptoms).

6. I check the vital signs and perform the physical examination, looking for the same absence of universal clinical features and presence of secondary specific clinical features for each remaining differential. They are (insert presence and absence of signs that are universal, or secondary specific for each differential).

7. I check other relevant systems for my other differentials. At this point, is there clearly **1** most likely diagnosis?

8. If 'Yes', then self-check: does this diagnosis explain all the symptoms and signs so far? (Am I fulfilling Rule #1 of clinical reasoning?)

If there is 1 most likely diagnosis by the end of the base template, I move to the primary add-on template:

DIAGNOSTIC SUMMARY (Soh Jian Yi's primary add-on template):

(Condition for use: the 3 rules of clinical reasoning point to a single most likely diagnosis with at least 90% certainty)

1. The most likely diagnosis is (insert most likely diagnosis). Certainty of this diagnosis is (insert % certainty).

2. This is because the patient has (insert presence of secondary specific clinical feature — symptom or sign), and this diagnosis also explains all the symptoms. (Check: am I fulfilling Rule #1 of reasoning?)

3. Less-likely differentials are (List up to 2.). They are less likely than the most likely diagnosis because (insert why each differential fails

(Continued)

to fulfil Rule #1). Chance of each differential diagnosis will be (100% subtracting the % certainty of the most likely diagnosis, split between any remaining differentials).

4. The known risk factors for the differentials are (insert any risk factors relevant to my differential diagnoses).

5. Other information includes (insert other risk factors such as chronic diseases that seem irrelevant to the current diagnosis).

6. Final check for diagnosis: do any risk factors or patient demographics challenge the order of these differentials?

The primary add-on template leaves the risk factors information to the last. By the time all the rules of clinical reasoning are fulfilled, the most likely diagnosis is clear.

The risk factors are usually an afterthought, diagnosis-wise. They may still be useful for adjusting treatment or anticipatory care (anticipatory care is discussed later in this book).

Occasionally, the patient has more than one top differential diagnosis of equal likelihood, even after applying all 3 rules of clinical reasoning. I then call upon the secondary template:

DIAGNOSTIC SUMMARY (Soh Jian Yi's secondary add-on template):

(Condition for use: the 3 rules of clinical reasoning did not identify a single most likely diagnosis)

1. There is still more than 1 top diagnosis of equal likelihood, based on all 3 rules of clinical reasoning! They are (insert relevant diagnoses, which are equal because they either fulfilled Rules #1 and #2 of Clinical Reasoning, but Rule #3 was not fulfilled; or none of them fulfilled Rule #1).

(Continued)

(Continued)

2. If the patient has an unusual or prolonged fever, or neurological symptoms/signs, I ask myself if I have checked the perineum thoroughly.

3. I now ask the Safety Net questions. The answers are (insert information on risk factors).

4. Answers to the Safety Net questions may prompt reranking of the differentials and new differentials. If the answers to all Safety Net questions are negative, I now review all the risk factors.

5. After all, this, I re-generate the differential diagnoses afresh (order of descending likelihood):

   A. (Insert most likely)

   B. (Insert next most likely)

   C. (Insert next most likely)

6. I repeat the search for universal and secondary specific clinical features of any new differentials, and the answers are (insert answers for the new differential's clinical features).

7. I ask for other risk factors for the differentials. They are (insert any risk factors relevant to your differential diagnoses).

8. Other information includes (insert other risk factors that seem irrelevant to the current diagnosis).

9. After adding in the risk factors and patient demographics and any new clinical information, my differential diagnoses are (order of descending likelihood):

   A. (Insert most likely). (Insert % certainty)

   B. (Insert next most likely). (Insert % certainty)

   C. (Insert next most likely). (Insert % certainty)

When the most likely diagnosis is not obvious after applying all 3 rules of clinical reasoning at 1 pass, this is a diagnostic puzzle. The subsequent steps in my secondary add-on template reflect this situation.

The optimal handling of diagnostic puzzles is discussed in the next chapter.

Capsule summary

- The 3 elements of the correct clinical diagnosis are used to decide the most likely diagnosis and differentials.

- Of the 3 Rules, the most important is Rule #1: Try to explain all Clinical Features.

- When added to Rule #1, Rules #2 and #3 of Clinical Reasoning significantly enhance your diagnostic speed, accuracy and certainty.

- The accuracy and certainty of each diagnosis will influence the confidence and accuracy of your decisions.

Frequently asked questions

Q: It is often said that thinking of differential diagnoses is important. There is no unified agreement on the number and relevance of the differentials. Some teachers say you should try to generate as many differentials as possible. Others insist that only relevant differentials should be mentioned. What would you recommend?

A: I would recommend a minimum of 2 (meaning, 1 most likely diagnosis and 1 differential) and a maximum of 3 differential diagnoses. This recommendation is based on both reasoning and decision thresholds.

Applying the basic diagnostic reasoning requirement will usually leave you with 1, sometimes 2, and very rarely 3 diagnoses of relevance. The likelihood of all other diagnoses plunges so dramatically after 2 to 3 differentials, that any differential beyond a third is often academic. Even mentioning a 3rd differential diagnosis for the sake of doing so, will feel like an afterthought sometimes. Doctors who are fully proficient in all 3 rules of clinical reasoning are often left with only 1 relevant diagnosis after using the 3 Rules; mentioning a 2nd differential diagnosis feels like an afterthought to them.

It is important to avoid tunnel vision, which is why thinking broadly initially and through to the end of the consultation, is a must. Robust reasoners do think broadly. However, thinking broadly does not mean it is sensible to insist on meeting an arbitrary quantity (3, 4, 5 or more) of differential diagnoses by the end of the consultation. It is illogical to assume a fixed quantity of differentials is more important than the relevance of those differentials and the practical decisions to be made around these differentials.

If you are a senior physician leading a team of junior doctors, explain the dangers of tunnel vision and the need to think broadly at the start of the consultation. Junior doctors who see you leap to a single diagnosis clinically, may copy you without realising the dangers of premature closure.

For teaching purposes, I frequently discuss 1–2 differentials other than the most likely clinical diagnosis even when these differentials are very unlikely, then go through the 3 rules of clinical reasoning to demonstrate the potency of the 3 Rules.

Q: Is the most likely clinical diagnosis, going to be the correct diagnosis all the time?

A: No. However, this method compels you to make high-yield decisions and hones your diagnostic skill simultaneously. When you become proficient in this method, the most likely clinical diagnosis is going to be the correct diagnosis in almost all of your patients.

If the most likely clinical diagnosis is not the correct diagnosis, either your clinical evaluation missed something, or your analysis of the clinical information was flawed, or both. In this situation, your robust reasoning and your vigilance will help you. You will be surprised by something: unexpected test results, new clinical features, the patient failing to improve as expected, and so on. These surprises will warn you that the diagnosis you made may not be the correct one, prompting you to recheck your clinical evaluation and analysis.

Conversely, if you are inattentive or reasoning poorly, you often do not notice any surprises until much later. Noticing surprises much later is not ideal, partly because patients dislike their time and money being wasted, and partly because a late surprise can be a disastrous event, such as a collapse.

Q: Some patients will be puzzling because they have 2 simultaneous diseases. How should these situations be approached?

A: When you encounter a patient who seems puzzling when you try to reach a single unifying diagnosis, the plausible scenarios are:

- The patient has only 1 current and active disease. You do not have enough information in your illness scripts to explain all the patient's clinical features.

- The patient has only 1 current and active disease. However, you are not following the technique shown here, e.g. you insist on explaining all the patient's risk factors with your diagnosis.

- The patient has 2 concurrent diseases. You have detailed illness scripts for multiple diseases. You just need to consider the combinations of 2 concurrent diseases that would, together, explain all the patient's clinical features.

Therefore, to instantly recognise the rare patient with 2 concurrent diseases, you need robust clinical reasoning and detailed illness scripts.

If you have adhered to the technique and undertaken the learning journey described thus far, you will build up detailed illness scripts for multiple diseases. When your illness scripts contain all the clinical features for the patient's concurrent diseases, the basic diagnostic reasoning requirement compels you to accept that you cannot explain all of the patient's clinical features with 1 disease. Explaining all of the patient's clinical features by using the combined illness scripts for 2 diseases, now allows you to fulfil the basic diagnostic reasoning requirement.

Conversely, if you did not undertake the necessary learning journey, you probably lack the detailed illness scripts and the technique to be clinically accurate for just 1 disease.

How are you going to accurately figure out whether the patient has two or more concomitant diseases when you cannot diagnose even 1 disease accurately?

Here are 2 conversations to illustrate the need for reasoning and detailed illness scripts when handling patients with 2 concomitant diseases.

Conversation #2 (this took place in 2022)

A colleague says: 'Hey, I have a case I am unsure about. I have a middle-aged man with fever, right-sided colicky right upper abdominal pain with positive Murphy's sign, nausea, vomiting, and severe unremitting left flank pain. All this has been going on for a week. There are no other symptoms or signs.'

'Going by Rule #1, I would have to diagnose both acute cholecystitis and pyelonephritis coexisting at the same time, right? Slightly more than half of the clinical features are explained by acute cholecystitis, which does not explain the other clinical features. Those other clinical features are explained by pyelonephritis, which does not explain most of the first half of the clinical features that acute cholecystitis would. Thus, the patient probably has both diagnoses to "explain all clinical features". The alternative is a single unifying diagnosis, but I cannot think of one.'

Me: 'That's right. The patient has both diseases.'

Later, the colleague says: 'Hey! We did the tests, and the patient did indeed have both of those diagnoses simultaneously! And we treated both right away! The decisions were perfect!'

Conversation #3

A professor was conducting the morning rounds of the children who were hospitalised for various illnesses. She was going from bed to bed, discussing each child's information and the likely diagnosis with the team of junior doctors following her. I was part of the team of junior doctors.

Another junior doctor, Doctor Q, comes up and says: 'Professor, an 18-month-old boy has just been admitted for 2 weeks of fever and cough. There is mild tachypnea and there are crepitations on auscultation. No one else at home was sick. The Emergency Department said it was pneumonia. The chest X-ray was reported as "infiltrates".'

The professor says: 'Okay, what would you do?'

I speak up. 'Hold on. What was the exact duration of each of the fever and cough, respectively?'

Doctor Q looks abashed. 'I did not ask. I just asked the child's mum about the fever and its duration. The fever was there for 2 weeks. I then assumed the duration of the cough was also the same.'

Many doctors ask for the duration of one of the main complaints, then assume the duration of every other symptom is not relevant to the diagnosis. This omission prevents the recognition of simultaneous diagnoses and the development of time-based illness scripts.

Me: 'Please go and ask that question. The answer is crucial.'

Doctor Q returns a minute later: 'The cough has been there for the past week.'

I nod. 'Thank you. Send off the stool culture.'

At this point, the rest of the team looks confused. The unspoken sentiment is: 'What?! What has the stool test got to do with the apparently respiratory system problem?'

The professor frowns and replies in annoyance: 'Do you know how rare 2 simultaneous diagnoses are?'

Factually speaking, she is correct. However, the patient always takes priority over the common population rules mentioned in textbooks.

Me: 'Have you ever seen a patient with pneumonia who had a cough starting only on the 8th day of fever?'

To her credit, the professor does not ignore my suggestion because of my youth. She thinks for a few seconds, and her frown vanishes.

She says quietly: 'Good point.'

Then, she tells Doctor Q: 'Do as he says. Send the stool culture. Do not treat yet.'

We went to review the patient soon afterwards. There were bilateral crepitations but no clinical signs of consolidation. The child was mildly tachypneic. There were no other physical signs. The chest X-ray looked normal.

We agreed the child had bronchiolitis as one of the current diseases. Everyone waited to see what the stool culture would show.

A few days later, the stool culture returned with the result I expected: Salmonella enteritidis.

My thought process had been: the child has a fever for 2 weeks, with no localising symptoms for the first week. There is no single disease that explains the child's entire clinical picture. Thus, the child probably has two or more diseases. The respiratory symptoms and signs are probably manifestations of 1 disease: bronchiolitis would fit the clinical picture for the 2nd week of illness, but not the 1st week. The child was probably functional most of the past 2 weeks, as he was admitted only on the 14th day of illness instead of much earlier on. For the 1st week of isolated fever in a functional preschooler in our local context, the common but non-obvious pathogen is non-typhoid salmonella infection. Though non-typhoid salmonellosis often has 'intestinal symptoms' like vomiting and diarrhoea, infection with a minority of these species may result in prolonged fever without any diarrhoea.

Knowing which non-typhoid Salmonella species is present in this scenario of fever-with-apparently-nothing-else, requires following up on patients.

When the patient's sibling was hospitalised a few days later with vomiting and diarrhoea for 1 day, this patient's stool culture result helped with their sibling's diagnosis.

Q: When we suspect 2 simultaneous diseases in the patient, do we then go for 2 simultaneous diseases, or 1 unifying diagnosis first?

A: Given that the patient with 2 simultaneous diseases is a rare situation, you should always strive to make a single unifying diagnosis of 1 disease.

By the time you are facing 2 simultaneous diseases versus 1 rare and unifying disease, the 'unifying diagnosis' (Disease X) is often a dangerous disease whereas the 2 simultaneous diagnoses (Diseases Y and Z) are common illnesses in the population. If both possibilities of Disease X alone versus Diseases Y and Z together are equally plausible based on the rules of reasoning, respect both possibilities. You cannot ignore disease X, which is likely to cause major harm if present but ignored. Nor should you be fixated only on disease X, ignoring diseases Y and Z. Sometimes diseases Y and/or Z also require immediate treatment.

There are 3 circumstances where 2 simultaneous diseases occur:

- By association. Both diseases tend to co-exist more frequently than unrelated diseases, but there is no direct cause-and-effect between them. For example, the patient presenting with concerns over symptomatic eczema also has active asthma.

- One disease is a complication of the other. By definition, a complication is another disease that often requires separate management from the original disease. Complications tend to occur when the original disease has been inadequately treated or is uncontrolled for a sufficiently long period. Complications can occur after the onset of acute as well as chronic diseases. Examples include Pott puffy tumour from acute sinusitis and the eye-and-renal-diseases from uncontrolled diabetes mellitus.

- Coincidence. Both diseases have no relationship whatsoever with each other. In places where diagnostic accuracy is very low, this coincidence seems to happen more often. When diagnostic accuracy is low, the patient's initial disease is often completely missed. The patient continues to suffer and then develops a second unrelated disease, prompting another consultation for the new symptoms.

Q: Some have said that clinical reasoning is not important for surgeons, and claim that surgeons only need skill in performing surgery. What do you think?

A: The argument 'clinical reasoning is not as important for surgeons' is a fallacy. This fallacy is commonly believed by poor reasoners: both surgeons and non-surgeons, of any age and rank.

The best doctors, including the best surgeons, completely disagree with this fallacy.

Diagnostic accuracy and reasoning do matter to surgeons. Gross errors, patient deaths and lawsuits occur with alarming frequency, partly because surgeons get the diagnosis wrong. These mistakes occur at:

- The initial diagnosis. The surgeon did not make the correct diagnosis initially, and therefore made suboptimal decisions.
- The post-operative diagnosis. After the operation, the patient develops a complication of the initial disease or a problem from the operation itself. The surgeon misses this diagnosis.

The best surgeons realise that skill with their hands and mastery of 'Anatomy' is not enough for excellent care. Surgical skill matters little if the surgeon fails to operate on the right patients at the right time, and fails to save patients who develop problems after the operation.

The best surgeons see patients personally, carefully, and frequently (usually at least once or twice a day, on all or almost all days of the patient's hospitalisation). Their vigilance is not a coincidence. This vigilance directly contributes to their superior outcomes. This vigilance arises from their superior reasoning. These surgeons routinely make optimal decisions, just like the best non-surgeons.

The fallacy about clinical reasoning not being important to surgeons, often accompanies another stereotype: surgeons are inattentive to patients, and rush through their patient reviews to go to the operating theatre.

Major harm arises from humans believing that stereotypes idealise or justify behaviour. Thus, the stereotype about surgeons being inattentive, unreasoning and hasty can become a personal truth: the surgeon knows the stereotype and then decides that they should be inattentive, unreasoning and hasty towards patients outside the operating theatre. It is unlikely that such surgeons have seen (or if they have seen, they have ignored) the best surgeons in action.

Clinical reasoning affects clinical attention and diligence. Paying attention to the hospitalised patient before and after surgery, is necessary to know:

- Is the patient deteriorating and needs surgery?
- Is the response to surgery adequate?
- Is the wound healing adequately?
- Are there complications?

The poorly reasoning doctor is habitually inattentive to patients. On top of the increased frequency of disasters due to poor reasoning, the disasters are compounded by this habitual inattentiveness towards angry patients and their families. The disastrous chain of dominoes can look like this:

1. Suppose a patient is hospitalised for a disease that can be treated with drugs, or surgery. The surgeon is the primary doctor. Drugs are tried first. The patient is observed.

2. The patient is not reviewed personally, properly and regularly by the poorly reasoning primary doctor. Instead, this doctor delegates the job entirely to junior doctors, nurses, or other subordinates. This doctor seems uninterested in the patient in general. This inattention is copied by the subordinates, who may delegate the job of checking the patient even further down the hierarchy. Sometimes, these subordinates 'push' the job to the ward nurses or allied health practitioners, and do not pay attention to the patient themselves.

3. There is a lack of transparent communication with the patient and their family. Patients can assume that everything is fine: 'If there was bad news, they would tell me, right?' The real reason for the lack of clear communication, however, is the inattention of the healthcare team.

4. The drugs are insufficient to treat the disease. The patient begins to deteriorate. Inattentiveness towards the patient by the entire healthcare team, often means any deterioration may not be noticed until much later. Even when noticed, this news may not be promptly conveyed to the patient and their family. Sometimes, faulty reasoning contributes to the delay in communication: 'Even if I told them, they may not understand anyway. Maybe the problem will go away on its own. Maybe if the patient gets better, we do not have to tell them now that anything is going wrong.'

5. The patient's condition continues to deteriorate. Finally, the patient and their family are abruptly told 'major surgery is needed'. This message comes as a shock because there was no bad news in the preceding days. The patient has often noticed that they are not improving or slowly worsening, but the absence of communication had them thinking that the doctors knew what was going on, and that everything was going to be fine.

6. When the surprised patient and their family ask how the decision for surgery was made, they are now told about the deterioration, which was noticed days back. This sends a disastrous message: 'We knew about the deterioration earlier, but we did not tell you. We do not care about updating you, and we do not care about how you feel. We want you to sign consent for surgery. We are not here to listen to you. If something goes wrong after the surgery, do not expect us to tell you either. We will tell you if and when we feel like it.'

7. When the unhappy patient and their family request or attend a family conference with the doctors, poor reasoners may be late or send their junior doctors to speak for them instead. This behaviour shows the patient and their family that they are not considered important enough for the poor reasoner to be punctual or attend in person. This unspoken message does not help the mood of the unhappy patient and their family.

8. The patient and their family ask relevant questions about the patient's condition over the past few days to weeks. Poorly reasoning doctors and their juniors come unprepared because they have never paid attention to the patient. They struggle to answer these patient-centred questions. Instead, they can evade the questions. They can try to use textbook answers, hoping the patient and the family do not notice that they are still evading the question. Such evasion does not fool listeners who can reason.

9. Apologies or genuine attempts at empathy are rare. The doctors focus on what they want to say. They can pretend to listen to the patient's unhappiness, then go back to talking about the operation, thereby demonstrating that they are not listening. Some poor reasoners mistakenly believe that an apology is an automatic admission of wrongdoing; therefore, they never apologise for their mistakes.

10. When the doctors demonstrate their inattention and poor communication are deliberate, habitual and unchanged, even the rare apology is obviously insincere. Actions and outcomes speak louder than words. It only takes one half-reasoning listener (patient or family member) to realise that if the patient remains under the care of these doctors, they can expect more disasters and more of the same behaviour towards the patient afterwards.

My former students have complained about colleagues in surgical teams who conduct 'paper/computer rounds'. These rounds are conducted by looking at numbers (vital signs, intake and output, lab results, etc.) on the computer screen instead of the patient. The patient's clinical review is minimal or nonexistent. Decisions are based on the numbers, not the patient.

This behaviour is unsafe. Dangerous post-operative problems may not cause derangements in vital signs or other numbers until the patient is about to collapse.

Sometimes, disaster is averted by just *one* doctor who bothered to clinically check, and discovered a sign of a dangerous post-operative problem.

The junior doctors are sometimes told by their seniors to do paper/computer rounds, just like the seniors do. The robust reasoners refuse and insist they will see the patient clinically.

Q: You have stated that the correct clinical diagnosis helps to focus all subsequent decisions on the appropriate options: 'what to do'. How about what *not* to do?

A: The correct diagnosis and differentials drive appropriate decision-making. Options that do not apply to that patient's diagnosis and differentials, are irrelevant to that patient. Choosing irrelevant options (such as batteries of tests and polypharmacy) creates additional problems, such as confusing the situation or lulling the doctors into a false sense of complacency. These additional problems are discussed in the chapters 'Common mistakes in testing' and 'Common mistakes in treatment'.

In addition, some tests and treatments are contraindicated in certain diseases. Contraindicated tests and treatment are often dangerous to the patient (or in a pregnant woman, the foetus). You must recognise these diseases early enough to avoid ordering contraindicated tests and treatment. An example is a diagnostic hysteroscopy, which is contraindicated for pelvic infections, genital herpes, and cervical cancer.

Q: Does having or showing greater confidence, help?

A: No. Studies have shown that the confidence levels of doctors did not correlate with their accuracy. Many doctors and students can be eloquently confident as they argue in favour of their wrong diagnosis and make inappropriate decisions. Flawed arguments lack patient-centredness, solid logic or understanding of human biology. Having great confidence without any solid foundation, logic or genuine skill may be useful for swindlers, but has no place in excellent healthcare.

Between the cautious-sounding doctor who is thinking, versus the apparently confident doctor, students are most easily impressed by outward confidence. Some may think 'the senior is so confident, so he or she must be correct. The other doctors who disagree, must be wrong'. Students who never follow up on the patient, never discover the truth about the outwardly confident but inaccurate doctor.

Patients do want their doctors to show some confidence. However, appropriate confidence must be balanced with caution. This balance varies with each patient and the degree of uncertainty.

Genuine, deserved confidence must be earned. This comes from studying patients closely to determine the final correct diagnosis, learn your strengths and weaknesses, and hone your skills in diagnosis and decision-making. Actions and outcomes speak louder than words.

DIAGNOSTIC PUZZLES: HOW TO HANDLE THEM

A diagnostic puzzle/dilemma is a situation where the most likely diagnosis is not obvious by the end of a targeted clinical evaluation.

This label should only be applied after proper clinical evaluation and reasoning have been undertaken for the patient. Robust reasoners rarely encounter genuine diagnostic puzzles.

Failure to evaluate and think logically often tempts poor reasoners to label the patient as a 'diagnostic puzzle'. Poor reasoners often encounter diagnostic puzzles because they tend to:

- Skimp on the clinical evaluation.

- Have no idea what a diagnosis is, do not try to make a diagnosis, or both.

- Generate differential diagnoses based on 1 symptom or sign at a time, then get stuck with a long list of differentials.

- Generate differential diagnoses based on 1 patient demographic or risk factor at a time, then get stuck with a long list of differentials.

- Assume all information is equally important, and then get overwhelmed while trying to process everything equally.

In this chapter, I will focus on the puzzles that still exist after applying the requirement of basic diagnostic reasoning.

What is a significant diagnostic puzzle?

The significant diagnostic puzzle is the scenario where there is a significant chance of preventable harm, should there be a delay in making the correct diagnosis or providing appropriate management. All subsequent mention of the phrase 'diagnostic puzzle' refers to this definition.

Diagnostic puzzles despite following the basic diagnostic reasoning requirement

There are 2 situations:

1. No apparent diagnosis that makes sense, or
2. There are two or more seemingly equal diagnoses which almost obey Rule #1

The 'no apparent sensible diagnosis' scenario involves a bizarre pattern of clinical features that cannot fit neatly into the doctor's illness script for any disease. Any single illness script often explains less than 60% of the patient's clinical features and their details.

If a doctor has scant illness scripts, the doctor must build these illness scripts up to the patient-centric standard. However, the patient often expects immediate action from the doctor. The doctor cannot mumble 'sorry, I gotta go read' and then disappear for the next few days, leaving the patient hanging.

The two-or-more-equal-diagnoses situation involves differentials that explain between 80% and 90% of the entire clinical picture. Thus, they match each other in almost fulfilling Rule #1, but neither completely fulfils Rule #1.

Violating Rule #1 invites the significant possibility that the patient has another unthought-of disease.

The more detailed the robust reasoner's illness scripts are, the more uneasy that reasoner would feel in these situations. For good reason (pun intended), too: robust reasoners with detailed illness scripts readily recognise most illnesses.

By extension, the inability of a robust reasoner to fulfil Rule #1, means that the likelihood of the patient having a rare and potentially dangerous disease increases in proportion to the richness of that doctor's illness scripts and reasoning ability. The likelihood of recognising this situation also increases in proportion to this doctor's reasoning ability, which is why robust reasoners often become extra careful and summon help in this situation.

It is possible to have two or more diagnoses that fully fulfil the basic diagnostic reasoning requirement. However, this is not a significant diagnostic puzzle because there are no other differentials to miss.

Let us examine the appropriate reactions to both situations. The reaction sequence is mostly the same in both situations, with a slight variation at the step of 'Get help'.

Appropriate reactions to diagnostic puzzles, chronological order of execution:

No sensible diagnosis	Two or more somewhat-feasible diagnoses, none of which fully obey Rule #1
Emergency: resuscitate based on vitals and physical signs	
If febrile or neurological, check the perineal region thoroughly	
Recheck risk factors, especially Safety Net questions	
Get help	Get help. Consider diagnostic testing for the most likely differentials, while keeping a wary eye on the patient clinically
Empirical treatment is instituted only if necessary	
Follow up on the patient closely	

<u>**Emergency:**</u> If the patient's life is in immediate danger, such as an unwitnessed collapse or the presence of severe haemodynamic compromise,

resuscitate the patient first. If necessary, contact the relevant family member/ witness for the corroborative history. A proper clinical evaluation should be undertaken early, sometimes concomitantly with resuscitative efforts, to get the correct diagnosis. Some diseases can kill rapidly if missed, and resuscitation alone cannot avoid this tragedy.

If febrile or neurological, check the perineum thoroughly: Examination of this region is often neglected because many doctors feel uncomfortable about examining the areas near the genitalia. However, some infectious diseases that cause prolonged fever or have seemingly bizarre neurological symptoms, have cutaneous signs that may be present only on the patient's perineum and nowhere else. Examples include eschars and chancres. Hair may need to be shaved away and skin folds moved aside to allow proper inspection of the entire area.

Recheck risk factors: The Safety Net questions are employed. Should the Safety Net be insufficient, go over the entire list of risk factors with the patient. The time window of enquiry may need to be expanded, such as asking about all travel and activity history for the past 6 months instead of 1 month.

Some infectious diseases may be symptomatic only several months after exposure. For example, you are puzzled about the bizarre fever along with other bizarre symptoms and signs. As rare autoinflammatory syndromes and exotic infections outside your experience are both plausible, you call upon the Safety Net questions. Autoinflammatory syndromes may be apparent on checking the family history. Exotic infections may be more likely after scrutiny of the travel and activity history.

Get help: Ask yourself 2 questions:

- Which speciality do I suspect this patient's diagnosis to fall within?
- Who is the best reasoner available?

Ask any or all of those colleagues for help.

If the scenario involves two or more diagnoses that mostly obey Rule #1, diagnostic testing can be attempted to differentiate between the 2 diagnoses. If attempting diagnostic testing in this situation, be careful. Recall the chain of dominoes: the skill driving clinical diagnostic accuracy is also the same skill that enables the accurate choice of tests and interpretation of the test results for that patient.

If the doctor could not figure out the correct clinical diagnosis for a particular patient, that doctor's skill may be insufficient for choosing the correct tests and interpreting them correctly for that patient. Therefore, 'reassuring' test results may be irrelevant or interpreted wrongly, and are not truly reassuring. Hence, robust reasoners are doubly careful about ordering and interpreting tests when they encounter a diagnostically perplexing patient.

Empirical treatment is instituted only if necessary: By definition, empirical treatment is a treatment that is commenced based on a clinically educated guess, without necessarily having the full picture:

- 'Clinically' is based on a proper clinical evaluation and deciding the most likely diagnosis for that patient.
- 'Educated' requires having some knowledge of the likely pathogen and site.
- 'Not necessarily having the full picture' is not an excuse to skimp on the clinical evaluation!

If the diagnosis is not certain, then empirical treatment should be commenced only if the benefit is likely to outweigh the harm. An example is a septic-appearing patient whose clinical picture suggests septic shock due to an unknown source. This patient receives broad-spectrum intravenous antibiotics while the doctors strive to uncover the source and the pathogen.

However, poor reasoners often succumb to the temptation of starting treatment based on 'common things happen commonly', biases and personal fears. Commencing treatment without robust reasoning or a proper clinical evaluation is wild guessing, not empirical treatment.

The usual mistake is commencing antibiotics in a patient because 'by population-level statistics, the most common disease is infection' and 'I do not want anything to go wrong', without reasoning or a proper clinical evaluation.

Commencing empirical or wildly guessed treatment when the diagnosis is unknown in a seemingly stable patient, can predispose to 2 unhappy consequences:

1. Complacency, and
2. Masking the correct diagnosis.

Poor reasoners who indiscriminately prescribe treatment, such as antibiotics for 'anyone with fever/high fever/fever beyond 5 days', usually succumb to both consequences.

1. *Complacency*

Sometimes, doctors feel safe after commencing treatment, and then become complacent. They stop paying attention to the patient.

The most common example is starting antibiotic treatment for a patient with a fever. This treatment can fall short in:

- An infection of greater intensity than the treatment can cure
- A different infection (pathogen or site) that the treatment cannot address
- A non-infection, such as an autoimmune disease or cancer.

In the next 2 to 5 days after starting treatment, if the patient does not improve or worsens, the complacent doctor often insists 'the treatment needs more time to work' instead of pausing to consider if they could be wrong.

If the patient has new symptoms or signs, the doctor either fails to notice these clinical features because of inattentiveness, or dismisses the new information: 'There is something new, but I have labelled this patient as "sepsis" and I think sepsis can cause anything including this new clue. Give the antibiotics more time to work.' In this example, there are 3 extra mistakes: the doctor did not commit to a specific disease, is ignorant of 'sepsis', and continues to guess wildly about 'sepsis'. Sepsis does not 'lead to anything'.

2. *Masking the correct diagnosis*

When treatment is instituted and the patient seemingly improves over time, many doctors want to believe the treatment is the only possible explanation for the patient's improvement.

However, there are 3 possible explanations:

1. The medications are curing/controlling the disease (which of the medications is doing this?), or

2. The disease is resolving spontaneously instead of responding to the treatment, or

3. The disease activity is waning spontaneously (see the chapter 'Diagnosis: disease, severity and treatment', subsection on the Law of Central Tendency) but the disease will persist. The disease activity will worsen later.

Close follow-up must continue for at least 2 weeks after completion of all treatment.

If the disease responds to the treatment, problems arise if the treatment is insufficient. Treatment can mask disease activity: the subsequent symptoms, signs and results of most tests (e.g. blood cultures). This masking can delay the recognition of the correct disease or its severity, with the recurrence of the clinical features after treatment is stopped.

If the patient develops more symptoms or signs subsequently, are these due to the treatment or the current, unknown diagnosis? The uncertainty and thus, the difficulty of deducing the correct diagnosis, increases. Since getting the correct diagnosis is important for excellent healthcare, this increased uncertainty and difficulty can be counter-productive to excellent healthcare. Some signs, such as a rash, predispose doctors to consider drug allergy; subsequent actions such as referring to a specialist in allergy, could have been avoided by withholding unnecessary treatment.

Masking creates problems for every other doctor who becomes involved in the care of this patient. By masking the true disease and the disease activity, other doctors are misled and are more likely to make mistakes. This is a pet peeve of robust reasoners who are often asked to solve diagnostic dilemmas. If you are unable to get the correct diagnosis, promptly getting help is more desirable than doing something that makes the job of clinching the correct diagnosis, even harder for the next doctor. To put it simply: if you cannot get it right, do not make the situation worse.

In addition to antibiotics, other drugs can mask potentially dangerous diseases. Systemic steroids can mask inflammatory disorders and leukaemia. Proton pump inhibitors can mask chronic gastritis and eosinophilic oesophagitis. The list goes on.

Follow up on the patient closely: New clinical features and changes in existing clinical features can help you to deduce the correct diagnosis. If the patient seems unstable, hospitalisation can enable closer monitoring and appropriate resuscitation. This is discussed in more detail in the chapter 'Follow-up', in Section 4.

Inappropriate reactions to diagnostic puzzles

Doctors may make poor decisions out of fear and ignorance.

When faced with a puzzle, the robust reasoner often has sufficient reasoning, wisdom, willpower, and foresight to avoid rushing into tests and treatment. In contrast, poor reasoners often lack the reasoning, situational awareness, self-discipline and foresight to realise the dangers of 'only fools rush in'. Thus, poor reasoners often cannot get the clinical diagnosis, and then compound their initial mistakes by rushing into poor decision-making.

The frequency and extent of these inappropriate reactions are influenced by the doctor's degree of fear and insecurity. The temptation to prematurely rush into action can be countered by clinical reasoning to some extent. Even so, robust reasoners can be tempted to 'do everything now to avoid missing anything'.

The common inappropriate reactions are:

- Test for everything
- Treat for everything
- Ask everyone else
- Wait and see what happens, relying on arbitrary numbers or clues.

Test for everything: This manifests as ordering a battery of tests: laboratory, imaging, you name it. These tests may be superficially justified by vague labels such as 'pyrexia of unknown origin', 'sepsis', '(insert symptom) for investigation', and so on. This behaviour often accompanies inattention to the patient's clinical features. Sometimes the tests target every differential in the long list of unprioritised and mostly (or totally) irrelevant differential diagnoses.

Ordering many tests inflicts significant discomfort and extra costs on patients, and produces an overwhelming list of results. Lacking robust reasoning and understanding of the clinical context, the doctor struggles to interpret the results correctly. When overwhelmed, the poor reasoner cherry-picks and treats individual results instead of the patient. The classic example is 'the total white cell count is high. It must be a bacterial infection, nothing else. Now that I have decided something, I do not have to pay attention to the other results. I will prescribe antibiotics'.

Treat for everything: Polypharmacy usually involves antimicrobials, antipyretics and other medications for 'symptomatic treatment'. As part of the disastrous chain of dominoes, 'treat for everything' tends to accompany 'test for everything'. Complacency often accompanies polypharmacy: 'if I treat for everything now, the patient will probably get better and nothing can go wrong'.

Ask everyone else: The doctor refers the patient to every specialist whose speciality is superficially perceived to be related to each symptom, sign, and test result abnormality. In this fashion, multiple referrals are often made. Examples include:

- Fever lasting more than 5 (or any other number) days: refer to Infectious Disease
- Chest pain: refer to Cardiology
- Weight loss: refer to Oncology
- Vomiting or diarrhoea: refer to Gastroenterology
- Rash: refer to Dermatology or Allergy
- Limb pain: refer to Rheumatology or Orthopaedic Surgery
- Neutropenia: refer to Immunology
- Hyponatremia: refer to Renal or Endocrine.

Poor reasoning predisposes to inappropriate communications. The referral letter may insist the receiving specialist focus on only the organ system involved. A common request is to exclude 1 disease. The referral letter often omits crucial information, such as the details of the patient's clinical features and the clinical diagnosis.

This can create the disastrous situation of 'too many cooks spoil the broth'. If the patient has multiple poorly written referrals that ask the specialists to focus on different parts of the patient in isolation, every specialist may do exactly that. Each specialist focuses on only 1 tiny part of the patient's picture, ignores the rest of the picture, and makes inappropriate decisions. No doctor looks at the patient in their entirety to realise the correct diagnosis. The doctors argue with each other over 'whose test or treatment to schedule first'. After a significant expenditure of time and money, the correct diagnosis remains unknown.

Wait and see what happens, relying on arbitrary numbers or clues:
The doctor may give instructions like 'come back to see me only if your temperature exceeds 39 degrees Celsius, you cannot walk or you have not gotten better after 7 days'. The doctor may order the patient's vital signs to be monitored, setting arbitrary cutoffs such as 'inform me if the patient's

temperature goes above 38 degrees Celsius or the heart rate climbs above 110 beats per minute'.

'Wait and see', also known as watchful waiting, can be useful and safe if employed by a robust reasoner. The robust reasoner considers all relevant differentials, and then decides on a monitoring plan that targets those differentials. The robust reasoner also accounts for any new information that can change the differentials.

For example, when one of the less likely differentials for a patient is acute appendicitis, serial abdominal examinations within the next 12 hours can be undertaken. The other relevant differentials are considered, and the monitoring plan accounts for these. Any new symptoms or signs are crucial clues and thus, must be immediately reported to the doctor.

Conversely, when 'wait and see' is performed without knowing the relevant differentials, it is difficult to accurately predict the specific red flags that would identify those diseases in time to prevent major harm to the patient. It is unwise to assume that your personal preferences, such as 'red flags' you want to look at or vital signs you consider important, are sufficient to avoid disaster. If you rely purely on arbitrarily monitoring numbers or specific symptoms, it is easy to ignore everything else about the patient. This mistake accounts for some preventable collapses and deaths.

Though most diseases do have changes in the vital signs just before collapse or death, some do not. When the diagnosis is unknown, you must continue trying to obey Rule #1, which means following up on all the clinical features and checking for new clinical features. Any new clinical feature and change in existing clinical features can be the clue that points to the correct diagnosis.

Capsule summary

- The better your illness scripts and reasoning are, the more careful you must be with a diagnostic puzzle.
- Only fools rush in. Respond appropriately to uncertainty.

PATHOPHYSIOLOGY IN REASONING

Pathophysiology refers to the disruptions in the normal structure, function, and development of the human body and the natural, detrimental changes with ageing.

Pathophysiological understanding is central to expert performance. Every expert I have met was a master of pathophysiology in their field and affirmed its importance when I asked.

The 3 areas of

1. Disease knowledge,

2. The pathophysiological basis underpinning disease knowledge, and

3. Clinical reasoning,

synergise with each other. This synergy is most evident when the patient's clinical presentation does not match the classic 'textbook example' (common disease knowledge). The expert calls upon their pathophysiological understanding to explain the variation from the textbook pattern, and then applies their reasoning to this explanation. Thus, all 3 areas should be developed concurrently.

This chapter will focus on the role of pathophysiology in acquiring disease knowledge, clinical reasoning, and performance.

Pathophysiology in learning

Why bother?

'This is so boring.' This is the common refrain from medical students who are handed basic science textbooks on Anatomy, Biochemistry, Physiology, Histology, Embryology, Immunology, and so on. Much of the content of these textbooks does not seem directly relevant to healthcare.

Some have argued that skipping these subjects is viable. Start the students on clinical medicine and surgery right away. Why learn all this boring stuff?

The answer lies in this analogy: A house of bricks needs a solid foundation to support the structure, and enough cement to hold the bricks and other components of the structure together. If you want a long-lasting house that can be huge and strong, you need lots of bricks and the necessary support for those bricks: the foundation and ample cement.

The structure in the doctor's mind is the knowledge from basic science, disease, and anything else of potential use for healthcare. Each 'brick' is a piece of knowledge: symptoms, signs, relevant tests, test results, treatment, and so on. The pathophysiology of the disease is the foundation and the cement linking and supporting each brick. If you want your house of knowledge about the disease to be huge, strong and long-lasting, you need lots of support.

This foundation and cement will help you understand the location of each brick and the disease itself. Understanding something allows better retention, retrieval and application of knowledge than rote memorisation. This concept applies to many skills, such as swimming. When you first start learning how to swim, even remembering how to move your arms and legs correctly, takes effort. Conversely, seasoned swimmers have gone beyond rote memory to understand how to swim, and thus do not need to think about basic movements. Champion-level swimmers understand the basis for the movements and their effect better than everyone else, which helps them to perform better than everyone else.

Without solid support, your bricks easily fall off and the house collapses readily. Mentally, this leaves you confused and wondering about the disease soon after you had studied it to build the 'house'.

To know what is abnormal, you must know what is normal.

If you wish to master the abnormal (disease), you must know the normal human body: structure, function and development as well as the natural, detrimental changes with ageing. Therefore, I recommend the study of the basic sciences. However, I am not encouraging the sweeping study of every bit of knowledge in all the basic sciences. Instead, I recommend prioritised study, which will be discussed next.

How do students and doctors often study, when acquiring disease knowledge?

In most textbooks describing diseases, each disease has a dedicated entry. The pathophysiology subsection is often a short, single paragraph at the start of each disease entry. The usual subsections immediately after the pathophysiology subsection are devoted to clinical features and risk factors. Most of the entry is devoted to the clinical features, abnormal results on testing, treatment options, complications, and so on.

Since many learners (mistakenly) assume that the relative proportion of each disease entry's subsections corresponds to its relative importance for that disease, they skip or glance briefly at the initial pathophysiology subsection, then labour to memorise the rest of the entry.

Seven days later, much of the knowledge acquired from studying the disease entry has been forgotten.

Soon after I began teaching, I noticed that students who struggled with getting the correct clinical diagnosis and proper clinical reasoning, also struggled with questions on the pathophysiology of the disease. Noticing this correlation between clinical performance and understanding of pathophysiology, I asked medical students how much time they spent on the pathophysiology subsection. Most said they did not look at it or spent a short time on it. When asked to estimate the percentage of time they spent on that subsection in proportion to the total time spent on the entire disease entry, the answers usually ranged from 0 to 5%.

The few students who spent 10% or more of their total time on that pathophysiology subsection, were invariably the students who were stronger clinically than most of their peers.

Every student was mystified that I would bother to enquire about such a seemingly trivial matter. Things became clear to them once I explained the potency of understanding pathophysiology during the learning process.

Pathophysiology dictates the symptoms, signs and variations of these in the disease. The same pathophysiology also dictates the abnormal results on testing and the basis for all effective treatment, including 'symptomatic treatment'.

If you fully understand the pathophysiology of a disease, everything about the disease is easy to retain, recall and apply clinically.

You might wonder about my observation that students who struggled with clinical performance and clinical reasoning, also struggled with pathophysiology. What does reasoning have to do with this process? The answer: clinical reasoning is an offshoot of overall reasoning, which is used during studying or before studying. Overall reasoning refers to the ability to apply reasoning to general situations and surprises. Robust clinical reasoners probably have enough overall reasoning to recognise the importance of understanding pathophysiology. Poor reasoners seem to lack the overall reasoning to recognise the importance of pathophysiology.

What I recommend when studying disease theory

In the earliest years of medical school, before I built up my illness scripts and understanding of pathophysiology, I spent at least 60% of the total time devoted to each disease entry on fully understanding the tiny pathophysiology subsection. It did not matter if the disease was in the medical or surgical specialities; the proportion of time remained the same.

This 60%-or-more would involve going sentence by sentence through the pathophysiology subsection, mentally recalling the relevant basic human science (such as anatomy, physiology, embryology, biochemistry, histology, and so on) as I read the words. Where I could not remember the basic science offhand, I would pick up the basic science textbook and seek the information I lacked. Having plugged the hole in my knowledge of the normal human body, I would return to the pathophysiology subsection, look at the sentence that had stopped me, and ensure I understood the meaning and implications of the entire sentence. I would then move on to the next sentence, and repeat the same process.

I completed the entire subsection on pathophysiology in this fashion.

The aim of this initially slow and painstaking process was to prepare the 'cement' and support for the mental house of knowledge of that disease. Though many students goggled at the revelation of a minimum of 60% of the time being spent on the tiny pathophysiology subsection, the reasoning became clear once I explained the analogy of the house of bricks.

Before starting to build the house, I spent extra time and effort preparing a special cement. This cement had unique tagging devices mixed into it. I was then pouring this cement over the pile of bricks, ensuring every brick was coated with ample amounts of the cement. The tags in the cement would adhere tightly to each brick, thereby allowing me to locate and identify each brick afterwards. I had not begun scrutinising the bricks yet. The cement remained fluid and non-sticky until I began building the house.

Once I began building my house of knowledge and looking at the 'plan' to build the house (this plan being the rest of the disease entry), I only had to put each brick in its place, then take up the next brick and put that brick in place, and so on. The house would be rapidly built and stay intact, and I would be able to locate any brick I desired.

This rapid process of building the house of knowledge, mirrored the analogy of the house of bricks. After fully understanding the pathophysiology, I would read the rest of the disease entry. The reason behind everything else in the entry — clinical features, tests, treatment, complications, and so on — became clear. I could speed through the remainder of the entry, understanding everything with no difficulty.

Though I had spent significant time understanding the pathophysiology subsection, this initial effort to build a solid foundation and prepare lots of special cement for my 'house of bricks of knowledge' paid off. This understanding of pathophysiology dramatically reduced the total amount of time spent studying the disease entry by about 50 to 70%, compared to trying to memorise the entire entry without pathophysiological understanding.

The huge difference in speed was amply demonstrated on the rare occasions I was studying with classmates. The others would often glance at or skip the Pathophysiology subsection completely, moving on to the clinical features much earlier than I did. Meanwhile, I would plod through the Pathophysiology subsection.

When I finished this subsection, my classmates were often stuck halfway through or at the end of the subsection on clinical features, trying to remember all of these. Having understood the Pathophysiology subsection, I would smoothly complete reading and understanding the rest of the disease entry.

By the time I finished studying the first disease entry, my classmates were often still stuck at the subsection on clinical features. This was evident from some highlighting the words in that subsection with marker pens, or saying those words aloud in their 5th, 7th or 10th attempt to remember the symptoms and signs. Those who gave up and went to the next subsection, Tests, ran into the same difficulties trying to remember the tests and abnormal test results that were described.

Whenever I suggested looking at the basic science books, my suggestion was rejected. The usual reply was: 'That is too much work.' After the 2nd or 3rd such reply, I stopped making those suggestions.

Being able to study effectively at double to triple the conventional speed, was only the initial efficiency of this method.

When first undertaken, mastery of pathophysiology took the most time out of all the subsections in each entry, because I had to keep checking the relevant basic science books. Having to read only clinically relevant parts of the basic science books revealed the exact bits that were relevant across most diseases. These bits took up between 0.1 and 1% of each basic science book for 1 disease, and about 3 to 10% of the entire science book when studied in this manner for virtually all diseases.

Thus, this process revealed the answer to the question, 'which small bits in which parts of the basic science books, are important for understanding pathophysiology across all diseases?'

This answer is valuable:

- The individual student often wants to know the relevant bits for clinical understanding and exams, instead of having to study everything.

- Many medical schools aim to reduce curriculum time devoted to studying, to free up time for clinical postings and the learning of other important areas such as communication skills, humanism, medical technology usage, and so on.

If medical schools knew this answer, and focused their teaching and exams on basic science to target the 3 to 10% of each science book that is crucial to understanding pathophysiology, students and teachers would be much happier.

After a while, retrieving the basic science books became a rare event, because the same bits from repeated revisions had been permanently 'cemented' into my memory. For example, the function of the lobes of the brain and the blood supply for each lobe does not change regardless of whether one is studying the many stroke syndromes, vasculitic disorders that can affect the brain, or traumatic brain injury.

At this point, studying diseases often meant the pathophysiology subsection was mostly or totally understood, instantly. The entire disease entry could often be read and understood without needing to pick up any other book. The speed factor for completing each entry went from the initial double-to-triple to *quintuple-to-octuple*.

If that were the only benefit alone, this process would be worth it. Medical students frequently complain about spending lots of time studying. I complained too. Initially.

However, there are more benefits. Mastering the pathophysiology of each disease meant retaining and easily retrieving the contents of each disease entry for years, without needing more than the occasional (once in many years) refresher. As I sometimes remark to students, 'If you do not want to have to rush through 10 or more textbooks in the short time before your final exams because you forgot everything after a week of studying in the preceding years, mastering pathophysiology will help. A lot.'

Such proficiency allows superior performance even in obscure areas. For example, an exam question on a particular stroke syndrome could ask, 'which of these (obscure) options is not a symptom or sign of this type of stroke?' Since each of the dozen-or-more syndromes had over a dozen symptoms and signs, many students had to wildly guess the answer, because it was virtually impossible to memorise the details of the many stroke syndromes and keep the information about each syndrome separate from the other syndromes, in one's head.

With pathophysiology, one could easily recall or derive the pathophysiology-based clinical features. If I was not sure of my answer, I only had to recall the pathophysiology paragraph for each stroke syndrome and the relevant lobes of the brain, their function, and the blood supply. I could then derive the answer through that process. Going back to the analogy of the house of bricks that had been built with tagged bricks, I was activating the homing device that would indicate the exact bricks of knowledge I needed. I could locate any of the bricks whenever I wanted.

As I transitioned to the patient-centric standard of acquiring disease knowledge, studying from the recommended reference textbook alone became insufficient. I still needed the pathophysiological understanding as 'cement' because the bricks of knowledge for the patient-centric standard, acquired from subspecialty textbooks, journal articles and other sources, far outnumber the bricks from the standard textbook alone.

Without this pathophysiological 'cement' for the much larger patient-centric house of bricks, understanding each brick and thus keeping the house intact, would be more difficult.

Pathophysiology and its role in illness scripts

The learner who has understood pathophysiology is better able to understand and recall their illness scripts, than the learner who lacks pathophysiological understanding. Retaining any additional information for an illness script is likewise facilitated by an understanding of pathophysiology.

The learner who keeps the patient logs recommended in the earlier chapter 'Targeted evaluation: history' and fully understands the pathophysiology for each disease, has a lot of cement to build many long-lasting houses of knowledge.

Pathophysiology during the diagnostic journey

Being able to rely on pathophysiology to understand each patient's symptoms and signs, increases the doctor's certainty and accuracy.

The best teacher I have ever seen in employing pathophysiology to understand clinical features is Professor Yeshwant Amdekar (an internationally renowned clinician and teacher). He has put video recordings of some of his lessons, on Youtube.

Expert diagnosticians employ pathophysiology as a backup for patient encounters. The priorities and rules of clinical reasoning are applied first. When a patient requires a non-standard dose or type of treatment, understanding the disease pathophysiology enables the safe usage of non-standard treatment.

Without understanding pathophysiology, doctors are more reluctant to offer or use treatment outside their everyday routine. If the patient requires non-standard treatment, these doctors often struggle with providing such treatment.

Combining the basic diagnostic reasoning requirement with mastery of pathophysiology enables the recognition of diseases the robust reasoner has never encountered before, which is especially useful when the patient has a rare and dangerous disease.

In the chapter 'Generating early differentials: the 3-minute habit', Cases #5 and #6 demonstrated the utility of expert-tier illness scripts. Pathophysiology played a big role in both cases.

In Case #5, Ash had no visible discomfort. Pathophysiological understanding enabled the expert to understand the 'weird' clinical features and instantly deduce the most likely diagnosis. This enabled a relevant, targeted clinical evaluation and the subsequent decisions to be optimal.

In Case #6, understanding the pathophysiology behind different patterns of pain, helped the expert to deduce the disease. The optimal decisions then became obvious.

The following case is another example.

CASE #14: Tommy

Tommy was an 8-year-old boy who had been having proptosis of both eyes and headaches for months. He underwent an MRI scan of the brain, which revealed a large intracranial mass.

Two needle biopsies of the mass had been performed. The first showed spindle cells. The doctors were baffled by this finding. A second biopsy was performed, which showed multinucleated cells. The doctors were even more baffled.

Tommy was given systemic steroids for 1 year, with no improvement in his symptoms. A repeat MRI scan of the brain had not shown any improvement near the end of the steroid treatment.

He came to Singapore for a second opinion. A third needle biopsy was performed, which revealed fibroblasts.

Everyone was baffled by the differing results of the biopsies.

(Continued)

His case was brought up for discussion. This took place in a large room. The abovementioned information, along with images of the MRI scans, was presented to the audience: dozens of specialists from different specialities, and junior doctors.

Since the results of the biopsies differed from each other, the senior doctors concurred that at least some of the biopsies (possibly all) had not been performed accurately. The debate raged around subsequent testing: perhaps a battery of blood tests to screen for various disorders? A fourth biopsy? Another MRI scan?

The correct clinical diagnosis is required for all healthcare decisions to be excellent.

Recall the first element of the correct clinical diagnosis: Rule #1 of clinical reasoning, which requires explanation of all clinical features.

At this point, the only description of Tommy's clinical features had been the abovementioned single line about headaches and proptosis, with no details. The discussion had focused on testing and test results.

The discussion was going nowhere.

I was a young doctor sitting in the room and listening quietly. I was unsurprised by the impasse. Without enough information about the clinical features, how could one nail the correct clinical diagnosis to allow good decision-making?

Just as I was about to ask about the clinical features, a senior consultant, Doctor K, said loudly to the doctors in the room: 'I happened to see him too. He is interesting. He had a xanthoma on his forehead, too! Very strange! His parents did not have a xanthoma!'

In my head, the clinical features clicked together instantly. The reason for the seemingly bizarre test results instantly became clear. I asked loudly, 'Can we see the child's face?'

(Continued)

(Continued)

The picture was brought up on the huge screen in front of the room. The picture showed bilateral proptosis and a xanthoma over the forehead.

I nodded. 'Thank you.'

I turned to my handphone, typed in the name of the disease I suspected, and nodded in satisfaction.

Then I waited to see if someone else would recognise the significance of my request, and figure out the correct diagnosis.

The next 5 minutes returned to the previous debate on testing. It was as if the clinical features had never been mentioned.

Finally, I gave up waiting.

I said aloud, 'The child has a cerebral xanthogranuloma. The scenario points to a slowly growing intracranial mass causing headaches and proptosis. There is a xanthoma on the child's face, which is probably from the same intracranial mass that is near the eyes and infiltrating the skin. The xanthoma cannot be explained by risk factors such as a family history.'

'Furthermore, the biopsies all show different cell types. In Histology (a subject routinely taught in medical school), the name of the tissue with different cell types is a "granuloma". Therefore, putting everything together, the child must have a xanthoma-granuloma, or xanthogranuloma.'

The room had fallen silent. At the end of the explanation, the sound of hundreds of fingers tapping on their handphones to look up the disease, filled the room. Doctor K turned to me and said, 'You are right!'

I nodded. 'You are welcome.'

With the most likely diagnosis now known, the decisions were straightforward.

This case demonstrates the reliance of pathophysiological knowledge upon the basic diagnostic reasoning requirement, and the synergy between both. If one has never seen a disease before, pathophysiology greatly helps in figuring out that disease.

I was not as intelligent or experienced as many of the other doctors in the room. I am not an oncologist. I had never heard of or seen a xanthogranuloma before.

Why was the discussion going down the wrong path and thus, stuck at an impasse? Why were the results misinterpreted by many doctors?

1. Proper interpretation of test results requires the clinical context.

2. An open mind and attention to the patient's entirety are required. However, doctors often dismiss inconvenient patient information, such as clinical features that they cannot explain. By extension, it becomes easy to dismiss test results they cannot explain.

3. 'Groupthink' could have contributed. Groupthink refers to the situation where people in a group state their agreement with a proposed opinion, even when they mentally disagree. This apparent agreement comes from ignoble motives such as 'wanting to fit in'. This outward agreement by everyone creates the impression that that opinion is unanimous and therefore must be correct.

4. Many doctors assume (wrongly) that seniority automatically equates to accuracy. Thus, when senior doctors state their opinion, many junior doctors agree because they assume their seniors are automatically correct. The junior doctors stop thinking.

Fulfilling the basic diagnostic reasoning requirement, and then trying to 'explain all the puzzling test result information', opened the window to calling upon pathophysiology.

Always start with the principles and rules of clinical reasoning, and the clinical evaluation.

Pathophysiology for significant diagnostic puzzles

Understanding pathophysiology helps the doctor to understand unusual symptoms and signs. Recognising the basis for unusual symptoms and signs is useful for improving diagnostic accuracy.

The expert diagnostician pauses whilst considering the unexplainable clinical feature(s). They review their illness scripts. They may mentally revisit the pathophysiological process for each differential.

The expert asks:

- Can these differentials explain this unusual clinical feature?

- If not, what might be the pathophysiological process for this clinical feature?

- How would that process then explain all the other clinical features in this patient?

Recall the 3 Rules of Clinical Reasoning. Employing all 3 rules proficiently is no mean feat. Answering the abovementioned questions correctly to be safe enough to make the correct decisions for the patient when Rule #1 has not been fulfilled, is even more difficult.

Only someone who has thoroughly mastered pathophysiology across the entire human body can stake the patient's health on pathophysiology-based reasoning, with any reasonable chance of success. Such an expert is not foolhardy. 'Reasonable chance of success' is not the same as being certain of success. Thus, these experts often call upon other measures simultaneously.

Thus, though pathophysiology-based reasoning can be used for diagnostic puzzles, I left this reasoning out of the recommended sequence of reactions to a diagnostic puzzle (the previous chapter):

- If you are not a pathophysiology expert, relying on your deficient pathophysiological understanding to make decisions, is dangerous.

- If you are an expert in pathophysiology as well as clinical reasoning, relying on pathophysiology alone to make decisions, should worry you.

Pathophysiology during decision-making

If you have fully understood the pathophysiology of each disease, the tests and treatments appropriate to that disease are often obvious. Likewise, a full understanding of the pathophysiology that explains the results of testing, helps you to understand and interpret these results.

Capsule summary

- Understanding pathophysiology reaps tremendous benefits when acquiring knowledge about diseases.
- Relying on pathophysiological understanding alone when the basic diagnostic reasoning requirement has not been met, is potentially dangerous.

RULING OUT:
WHEN, WHY AND HOW

Ruling out (the synonym is 'excluding') refers to the process of excluding a less-likely differential. However, ruling out a less-likely differential is not the first fundamental job of any doctor.

Ruling in the most likely diagnosis is the first fundamental job.

The occasional patient may require a rule-out test after ruling in the most likely diagnosis has been performed.

Ruling out is often performed inappropriately: by ruling out a disease or list of diseases <u>o</u>nly, <u>a</u>lways or <u>f</u>irst (ruling out OAF).

The proper method of ruling out will be discussed first. Thereafter, I will discuss ruling out OAF.

When is ruling out, potentially indicated?

The disease must fulfil 3 criteria. The disease:

1. Is dangerous

2. Explains most or all of the patient's clinical features

3. Is not the most likely diagnosis

The disease is dangerous: This is the main concern that drives many doctors to rule out diseases. When a patient has a dangerous disease, the risk of major harm is significant. Doctors want to 'catch' dangerous diseases early, to promptly commence appropriate treatment. However, ruling out a disease that does not fulfil the other 2 criteria, often becomes ruling out OAF.

The disease explains most or all the patient's clinical features: All clinical features point to the current diagnosis. The more clinical features of the patient that you cannot explain with a disease, the less likely it is that the patient has that disease. If you intend to rule out a disease, that disease should have a significant chance of being present, instead of being virtually impossible.

Pursuing any disease whose probability is less than 3%, is often futile. If there is a 100% total chance of having any disease, going after the 2% possibility of a disease instead of considering the disease(s) that makes up the remaining 98% probability of the correct diagnosis, wastes time and resources.

Since clinical probability depends on the clinical fit of the entire patient's picture to a disease, it is absurd to cherry-pick 1 symptom, sign, or test result abnormality of the patient, then pick a disease 'to rule out' that can have that symptom or sign, and then ignore the fact that this disease cannot explain the other 30–90% of the patient's clinical features.

Suppose a patient presents with generalised pain. The poor reasoner decides to rule out a brain tumour because there is a headache, rule out acute myocardial infarction because there is chest pain, rule out acute appendicitis because there is abdominal pain, rule out deep vein thrombosis because there is calf pain, and so on. None of those diseases come close to explaining the entire clinical picture and thus, are virtually impossible. A robust reasoner would have pursued diseases that cause generalised pain.

The disease is not the most likely diagnosis: The disease to rule out cannot be the most likely clinical diagnosis. The most likely clinical diagnosis must be ruled in instead of being ruled out. If tests are needed, the tests for ruling in a disease can be different from the tests for ruling out that disease.

Ruling out a disease requires clinical information or tests with strong negative likelihood ratios.

Without this understanding, doctors often misuse information and tests to mistakenly conclude that they have 'ruled out' a disease. At best, the doctor wastes some money. At worst, the doctor misses a dangerous disease because they chose tests unsuited to rule out that disease, then misinterpreted the test results, and then concluded wrongly that the patient did not have that disease.

Why ruling out is occasionally necessary

In emergencies where information is scant and delays in appropriate care can be lethal, ruling out can make a huge difference. This is the basis for the focused physical examination and certain bedside procedures.

It may be tempting to always appear supremely confident and make 1 diagnosis, whilst ignoring all others. This is dangerous when such behaviour leads to flatly ignoring differentials.

Robust reasoners often nail the most likely diagnosis without needing to rule out anything. They adapt to each unique patient and will rule out when required.

Ruling in, and then ruling out only if necessary

The first step is clinical. Targeted history taking and physical examination are undertaken, aiming to rule in the most likely diagnosis first.

You should rule in first, because:

- If your reasoning was robust enough for that patient's disease, the most likely clinical diagnosis is usually the final correct diagnosis.

The efficient doctor goes for this diagnosis first, rather than go after less-likely differentials with correspondingly lower yields.

- If your reasoning was inadequate for that patient's disease, it may not matter which diagnosis you pursue because you are unlikely to choose the next steps or tests correctly.

- Since it is not always clear if your reasoning is robust enough for each unique patient's disease, you should pursue the most likely clinical diagnosis. If your reasoning is poor, you should improve your reasoning instead of resorting to ineffective measures like ruling out OAF.

Rule #3 of clinical reasoning is useful for ruling in; the presence of secondary specific clinical features strongly suggests 1 specific disease in the patient.

The doctor should strive to rule in the most likely diagnosis to the point that its certainty is over 97%. Once the diagnosis is at least 97% certain, the combined chance of any other diagnosis being present is (100% minus the certainty of the most likely diagnosis) = less than 3%. At less than a 3% chance of any other diagnosis, trying to rule out the differentials is often unnecessary.

If the doctor cannot rule in the most likely diagnosis with such certainty, then ruling out clinically is undertaken. Rule #2 of clinical reasoning is employed for the disease that is being ruled out.

If there is significant diagnostic uncertainty, watchful waiting can be a viable option. As discussed in the chapter 'Diagnostic puzzles: how to handle them', watchful waiting is safe if the doctor has obeyed the basic diagnostic reasoning requirement, thereby anticipating all relevant diseases and their respective red flags. The classic example is performing serial abdominal examinations in a patient whose most likely diagnosis is gastroenteritis, but acute appendicitis is the next most likely differential and has a significant chance of being present.

Finally, if the clinical measures are insufficient, diagnostic testing comes into play. As with the clinical evaluation, ruling in the most likely diagnosis should be attempted first. If you can rule in this diagnosis with 97% or higher certainty, then any other diagnosis is very unlikely. If the most likely diagnosis cannot be ruled in with near-100% certainty, then the rule-out test for the dangerous differential that fulfils the 3 criteria for ruling out, should be employed.

There is 1 exception to this recommended sequence. In emergencies where:

- There is a differential that fulfils the 3 criteria to rule out,
- Major harm or death would occur if the dangerous-but-less-likely-diagnosis was correct but the doctor did not act promptly,
- There is no clinical information that can 'rule in' the most likely diagnosis with near-100% certainty, and
- The rule-in test for the most likely diagnosis would take more time than is prudent whilst
- The rule-out test for the dangerous differential would provide results in time to avoid major harm or death,

then performing an immediate rule-out test is required.

An example of this exception would be a lady with a most likely diagnosis of acute appendicitis, but the differential diagnosis is an ectopic pregnancy with a ruptured fallopian tube. She has no clinical evidence that would make ectopic pregnancy with a ruptured fallopian tube, more likely than appendicitis.

In this rule-out-ectopic-pregnancy scenario, the rule-out tests to consider would be a human chorionic gonadotropin test, urine pregnancy test, and/or ultrasound scan. The prudent doctor would order rule-in tests for acute appendicitis, the appropriate rule-out-ectopic-pregnancy test, a complete blood count (to look for a sudden drop in the serum haemoglobin level compared to any previous results, if available), and pre-operative blood tests in expectation of surgery. These pre-operative blood tests are 'tests for adjusting treatment', which are discussed in Section 2.

'Diagnosis of Exclusion'

Some diseases are called a 'Diagnosis of Exclusion'. These diseases are common, and benign.

Examples of diagnoses of exclusion include:

- Costochondritis, in a person presenting with chest pain
- Simple febrile seizure, in a child presenting with a seizure whilst being febrile.

Some dangerous diseases can mimic the presentation of a Diagnosis of Exclusion.

By definition, before concluding a Diagnosis of Exclusion is the most likely diagnosis, you must think of other differential diagnoses that can mimic the patient's current presentation.

The definition reminds the doctor not to be target-fixated in any way, such as arbitrarily deciding 'the most common diagnosis I usually see, must always be the diagnosis'. This definition reminds the doctor that the relevant differentials are patient-centred, instead of a textbook list. This definition echoes some of the principles of patient-centred reasoning: explaining all clinical features and generating relevant differential diagnoses.

For example, if you suspect a patient with chest pain has costochondritis, you need to ask yourself: 'What are the relevant differentials for this unique patient's presentation?' Always explain all clinical features. An unexplained clinical feature may suggest a differential that is not on the standard list for 'causes of chest pain'.

What about the rest of the name, i.e. 'of Exclusion'? Do you have to exclude all the other differentials? This is where the common misunderstanding comes in. Many doctors mistakenly assume that the name 'diagnosis of exclusion' means that they must 'exclude all dangerous diagnoses'. This mistaken assumption results in them performing ruling out OAF.

For example, if a child is suspected to have a simple febrile seizure, the doctor must take a careful history and perform a physical examination to look for clues of the differential diagnoses, such as bacterial meningitis. The doctor is not required to perform a lumbar puncture on every child with a febrile seizure.

A diagnosis of exclusion can be the most likely clinical diagnosis.

Ruling out OAF

Ruling out OAF usually occurs when the doctor fixates on the disease(s) they fear missing. This usually results in attempts to rule out dangerous diseases (the 1st criterion for ruling out) whilst ignoring the 2nd and 3rd criteria for ruling out: the patient's entire clinical picture, and the real-world effect of probability on decision-making.

The fallacy behind ruling out OAF is: if you rule out a fixed or arbitrary list of diseases, you will be a safe doctor regardless of the patient's presentation or actual diagnosis.

Since the safest doctors are the doctors who pay attention to the entirety of the patient to make the correct diagnosis, this fallacy encourages the exact opposite of being a safe (or effective, or efficient) doctor.

Why, then, is ruling out OAF so widespread?

The historical (irrational) basis behind ruling out OAF

The historical basis behind ruling out OAF explains its genesis, persistence, and continued contribution to poor healthcare outcomes.

Appropriate defensiveness accepts uncertainty, and prompts sensible decisions to account for this uncertainty whilst ignoring nothing about the patient.

Inappropriate defensiveness occurs when the doctor is consumed by fear of uncertainty. The fear of the unknown, combined with the fear of missing dangerous diseases that will harm the doctor's career, drive irrational thinking and behaviour. Instead of accepting that the best way to address uncertainty is to be effective and attentive, inappropriate defensiveness is often arbitrary and narrow-minded: focusing on dangerous diseases only, always or first, to the exclusion of the patient. Thus, inappropriate defensiveness drives ruling out OAF.

The phrase 'defensive medicine' usually refers to inappropriate defensiveness.

Irrational behaviour that does not address the real problem, will not solve the problem. If you cannot recognise a dangerous disease, how does ruling out a fixed or arbitrary list of dangerous diseases ensure you do not miss a dangerous diagnosis outside that list?

Instead of addressing the real problem by teaching proper clinical evaluation and reasoning, an easier solution is to target the 'dangerous diseases'. This solution manifested as writing defensive guidelines and protocols.

These defensive documents describe one or more symptoms and signs, and then suggest a fixed list of dangerous diseases to rule out. This ruling out often involves testing. Reliance on these defensive documents is tempting to poor reasoners for 2 reasons:

1. There seems to be no need to think or pay attention to the entirety of the patient.

2. The focus on dangerous diseases implies that excluding these diseases will keep the doctor and the patient, safe.

As these documents became more widespread, more and more doctors practised according to the documents' apparent premise: if you rule out some diseases through tests always or first, you will be safe.

Doctors who heard of other doctors following these documents, might also jump on the bandwagon and follow these documents. The basis for copying the other doctors may be one or both of:

1. Wanting to 'fit in' with the common behaviour of other doctors.

2. The assumption that other doctors must be following these documents because the documents taught them how to provide excellent, defensible healthcare.

These documents do not address the real problem in their intended audience and thus, usually ignore the entirety of the patient. Unfortunately, a mistaken belief that these documents describe everything the doctor needs, leads to 2 common assumptions by poorly reasoning readers:

1. Paying attention to the entirety of the patient is not important, and

2. Doing anything else outside of the document is not important.

With these assumptions, it is easy to decide 'since paying attention to the entire patient and doing anything else is not important, it is unnecessary to bother with a proper clinical evaluation or reasoning. I only need to rule out diseases on this list, and my job is done! No thinking is required.'

The combination of fear, poor reasoning, mistaken assumptions, and inattention towards the patient predisposes to defensive obsession. A common manifestation of defensive obsession is to rule out OAF.

When poor reasoners believe that there is no need to think or pay attention to the entirety of the patient, ruling out often becomes ruling out Only, Always *and* First. This is the most extreme and harmful form of ruling out OAF. Ruling out OAF (only, always *or* first) was already bad enough.

Is ruling out OAF, based on defensive obsession alone? No. Worse is to come

If the doctor knows the patient's diagnosis and can reason properly, ruling out OAF becomes difficult to justify. Try either of these arguments:

● 'I know your diagnosis, but I should rule your diagnosis out anyway. Let us pretend you do not have the diagnosis. I will now perform steps and suggest tests to show this diagnosis is unlikely.'

- 'I know your diagnosis. Instead of managing the disease you probably have, let me rule out something else you obviously do not have.'

These arguments are difficult to make if the doctor knows the patient's diagnosis. This difficulty demonstrates how the doctor who performs ruling out OAF, has no difficulty with ruling out OAF because they do not know what is going on. This doctor does not dare to admit their bafflement to the patient, their colleagues, and often, to themselves.

Thus, the frequency with which a doctor rules out OAF, inadvertently reveals the frequency with which they are baffled by their patients, the extent of their ignorance and their surrender to their fears.

Many of my students have independently concluded the same: ruling out OAF occurs when the doctor does not know the patient's diagnosis and does not want to admit this to the patient, their colleagues, or themselves. They are horrified when their seniors or colleagues perform ruling out OAF in most or all of the patients. Many of the patients then have poor outcomes.

These frequent displays of ruling out OAF across the entire spectrum of patient presentations, in patients whose common diseases are clinically obvious to the students (but not to their seniors and colleagues), demonstrate how little these seniors and colleagues know and think, despite their experience.

Hearing these seniors and colleagues tell them 'experience is important' whilst witnessing how these same doctors have wasted their experience by seemingly learning nothing useful, is ironic and drives home the points cited earlier in this book: experience is important as an opportunity to learn, but wanting to believe that experience automatically confers skill, is a harmful self-deception.

Realising that these seniors and colleagues can see their consistently poor outcomes but do not seem interested in acknowledging the outcomes or improving themselves, allows the students to conclude that these seniors and colleagues are being deliberately inattentive, care little or nothing for their patients, and are not even listening to themselves when they say 'experience is important'.

The students can make these conclusions independently because the doctor's clinical evaluation, their documentation, and what the doctor says when pressed, all point to the same conclusions.

The documentation reflects the scant clinical evaluation. There is no diagnosis, or the doctor uses a vague label: 'sepsis', 'chest pain for investigation', and so on. The plans demonstrate ruling out OAF, with a glaring absence of decisions that target or treat the most likely diagnosis.

When pressed, the conversation between the observer (who may be an astute medical student) and the doctor can go like this:

Student: 'Why do you want to rule out pulmonary embolism?'

Doctor: 'The patient complained of breathlessness. In a breathless patient, you must always rule out pulmonary embolism.'

Student: 'How about all the other symptoms? The patient also complained of fever of 39 degrees Celsius, and chest pain.'

Doctor: 'Yes, so I must also rule out myocardial infarction. Because the patient had chest pain.'

Student: 'Uh, myocardial infarction and pulmonary embolism should not cause such a high fever.'

At this point, the doctor either ignores the student because the doctor cannot logically defend their behaviour, or uses a fallacy such as 'you must choose the most important information to use' to imply that the doctor can ignore any information as they please, regardless of its importance.

Rarely, the doctor quietly admits, 'I do not know what the patient has.'

After ruling out OAF and still having no idea of the correct diagnosis, the doctor has 3 options:

1. Hope the patient's disease goes away spontaneously

2. Treat the patient for a random disease, hoping the treatment cures the patient

3. Refer the patient to someone else, hoping the next doctor is better and does the job this doctor was supposed to do

The doctor should get help when they do not know what is going on. Knowing when to get help does not require medical training or genius. Many children and adults know they must get help when they need help. What stops many humans from getting help, is their ego and poor reasoning: they do not want to admit they need help.

Getting help does not always require a formal referral. Picking up the phone to call someone reliable for advice, is viable. Of course, if a doctor needs to call for advice very often, this points to huge flaws in knowledge and reasoning.

To an observer who has even a bit of overall or clinical reasoning, the doctor who refuses to get help when help is needed, has no clinical reasoning, no courage to admit the truth, and no empathy. The doctor is willingly wasting the patient's money and time, and delaying the appropriate care.

The observer who sees the doctor treat for random diseases or numbers on the test results, can wonder: Is this doctor wildly guessing and treating the numbers, instead of managing the patient or the correct disease? The observer quickly realises that the answer to their question is 'Yes'.

Is it dangerous to admit ignorance of the correct diagnosis to the patient? No, if you do this early instead of attempting multiple tests and treatments. Honesty to the patient, combined with a concrete plan to seek help, goes a long way in building trust.

Virtually all patients want their doctor to tell them the truth, instead of trying to hide it behind a fusillade of actions, which wastes the patient's time and money. Furthermore, many patients notice when the doctor fails to get the correct diagnosis and institute appropriate treatment for them, because they continue to suffer! However, poor reasoners are often inattentive to human beings (including themselves), and so tend to underestimate their patients.

Does ruling out OAF increase safety for the patient and the doctor's career? Probably not

A doctor who relies solely on ruling out a fixed or arbitrary checklist of dangerous diseases is not safe.

Their tunnel vision causes them to miss the forest for the trees.

They are so busy excluding all the easier-to-remember diagnoses, that they cannot see the entirety of the clinical picture pointing straight at the dangerous diagnosis that is not on the list.

The patient runs out of time and money as test after test returns negative. Sometimes the patient runs out of time by deteriorating rapidly and disastrously. Another doctor then makes the diagnosis. At this point, there will usually be some explaining for the original doctor to do, be it to the colleague who takes over the care of the patient who has collapsed, or the angry members of the patient's family.

If there is an official complaint or lawsuit, this doctor is in a poor position. A staple of legal or disciplinary investigations is the opinion of another doctor in the same field. The defensiveness-obsessed doctor cannot expect support for ruling out OAF. No colleague is going to defend this doctor before the court, review committee or disciplinary tribunal with any version of 'taking action to rule out your fears whilst ignoring the patient's information, is perfectly professional and acceptable'.

For example, acute cholecystitis can cause chest pain, but is not on many lists of 'common causes of chest pain'. A patient with acute cholecystitis causing chest pain often has other clinical features pointing to cholecystitis.

Suppose a patient with acute cholecystitis sees the doctor complaining of a few symptoms, with 1 symptom being chest pain. The doctor fixates on the symptom of chest pain, ignores the rest of the clinical picture, and goes through their list of 'dangerous causes of chest pain'. The patient stays for days, undergoing test after test.

The diagnosis of cholecystitis is discovered much later, sometimes after the patient has deteriorated due to a perforation of the gallbladder. The perforation occurred due to a failure to make the correct diagnosis in time. The patient is furious because their time and money were wasted as the doctors ruled out OAF, and even more furious because their poor outcome was avoidable if the doctors had paid attention to their complaints. Doctors have been sued for making this exact mistake: ruling out OAF and thus, missing acute cholecystitis in the patient who had chest pain *and* other symptoms and signs that point to the correct diagnosis.

Doctors, like all other professionals, do make mistakes. Healthcare is not perfect. Thus, missing a diagnosis whilst being attentive, logical and generally competent is often insufficient to lose a lawsuit.

Missing a diagnosis because you ignored the patient's information to behave illogically, which the robust reasoner would not have done, brings in two of the elements necessary to lose a lawsuit.

If ruling out OAF gets it right once in a blue moon, does this mean we should rule out OAF?

Proponents of defensive obsession, who routinely order batteries of rule-out tests in patients, occasionally encounter a patient who truly has a dangerous disease, with matching test results. These anecdotes are trotted out to justify 'ruling out OAF' across all patients, whilst withholding any mention of the clinical picture. Meanwhile, these doctors rule out OAF in vain in many of their patients, often missing the correct diagnosis in those patients.

Even a stopped clock is right twice a day.

I would be horrified to be right only twice a day, and be wrong the rest of the day.

In my experience, in the patients for whom the defensive test 'got it right' once in a blue moon, the entirety of the clinical features, even when scantily documented by poor reasoners, often points to the dangerous diagnosis being likely and among the top 2 differentials. Thus, ignoring the clinical context to claim that ruling out OAF revealed the correct diagnosis is illogical, wasteful, often delays appropriate care, and is nothing to boast about.

In some patients who were subjected to ruling out OAF, the documentation is so scant that I cannot assert the correct clinical diagnosis could be made. The doctor's complete skimping on the clinical evaluation has ensured that they, and anyone else reading their notes, are unable to make the diagnosis clinically. The poor reasoner has put themselves into a self-created situation: failure to make the clinical diagnosis because of inadequate clinical evaluation, then insisting on ruling out OAF because of the inadequate clinical evaluation, and then being left without the correct diagnosis after ruling out OAF. The poor reasoner ends up wildly guessing the diagnosis, or saying the patient 'has no dangerous disease' and then hopes that the patient truly has no dangerous disease.

When the patient has a dangerous disease that is listed in the defensive document, the decently reasoning doctor will perform better than the defensive doctor. This is because the decent reasoner often figures out and takes appropriate, prompt action on the dangerous diagnosis. The defensive doctor often ignores the clinical picture and waits for test results, leading to delays in the appropriate care.

The safest doctor is the one who is the most accurate across all diagnoses. Thus, a decent reasoner is safer, quicker and more accurate for every patient. In contrast, a doctor who rules out OAF is consistently slower, sloppier, more wasteful, and more dangerous for every patient.

Can a junior learner rule out OAF while trying to become a good doctor? Probably not

It is impractical, if not impossible, to expect junior learners (medical students and young doctors) to:

1. Try to apply knowledge,
2. Listen fully to the patient,
3. Fully focus on making the correct diagnosis, and
4. Fully focus on a list of diseases with their corresponding 'red flags' to rule out,

all at the same time.

Now, add in the time constraints of a patient encounter, tutorial or exam scenario.

Should teachers demand learners do many things simultaneously (and badly), or accept that learners need to prioritise fewer and more important tasks and do these well?

Of the 4 tasks on the list, the 4th is the least important. This task relates to ruling out OAF.

As another of my students, Ting Yu, observed for the umpteenth time, it was easier and clearer to pay attention to the entirety of the patient, nail the correct diagnosis and manage appropriately when she was not burdened with the 4th task. It is difficult to undertake the first 3 tasks whilst simultaneously trying to remember a mental list of dangerous diseases, symptoms and signs to look for.

We cannot expect anyone, including junior learners, to be right all the time. However, it is an entirely different matter to suggest, even indirectly, that it is not important to try to be right about the patient's clinical diagnosis. To teach ruling out OAF is to make this inappropriate suggestion.

Results do matter. Patients do not care much about your processes if they suffer a poor outcome. Doctors have been sued for missing a dangerous diagnosis after the patient suffered for days while the doctors ruled out OAF, such as the earlier example of missed cholecystitis.

Conclusions about ruling out OAF

In summary, it is impossible to justify 'ruling out OAF'. The unnecessary, unempathetic test-related pain, risk and expense are unjustifiable because there is a superior alternative: ruling in the correct diagnosis. Ruling out OAF has no advantage compared to ruling in the correct diagnosis, unless the doctor decides the absence of thinking is an advantage and is willing to sacrifice everything else along the way for this 'advantage', including the patient.

Ruling in versus Ruling out OAF

The next table compares ruling in first, versus ruling out OAF.

Factors	Ruling In first	Ruling Out only, always or first
Emotions vs. Probability	Emotions balanced with Probability	Emotions (such as fear/excitement) usually override Probability
Information-gathering	Proper	Can be sloppy
Attention to clinical features	Must put everything together	Can readily ignore anything
Reaction to clinical features that do not 'fit' the patient	React appropriately	Ignore
Effort required	More mental effort initially, but then less effort thereafter once you have figured out the diagnosis	Almost zero mental effort initially, but then have to chase remote possibility after remote possibility until you give up
Skill that you are honing	Getting the correct diagnosis	Looking for what you feel like looking for

The next table shows the major fallacies that drive ruling out OAF, with the corresponding facts:

Fallacy	Facts
If I rule out all the dangerous diseases in my mind, I am safe	• The safest doctors are the most accurate doctors in getting the correct diagnosis. • When you fixate on your personal list and ignore the patient, you will miss every dangerous diagnosis outside that list.
Ruling out is faster than ruling in	• You will become faster at whichever skill you choose to hone. • A doctor proficient in ruling in, will always be faster than the doctor who rules out. And more often correct, too! • No matter how fast you become at ruling out, you must still rule in the correct diagnosis if you want to be safe. Excluding diseases #3–8 does not automatically tell you if the patient has disease #1, #9 or #12.
Anything is possible, therefore I should rule out everything I want	• Excellent decisions are based on probability, not 'Anything is possible'.

Ruling out OAF is for oafs.

Consider the following conversations:

Conversation #4

Sarah is an 18-year-old lady who presents to the Emergency Department with a headache for 2 days.

Doctor V is the junior doctor seeing Sarah.

Doctor V: 'Okay, so you have had a headache for 2 days. Is it the worst-ever headache of your life?'

Sarah: 'No. Doctor, it goes away with sleep.'

Doctor V: 'Do you have weakness or numbness in your body?'

Sarah: 'No. Doctor, I do see some funny lights when I get the headache…'

Doctor V interrupts: 'Does the headache wake you up at night?'

And the consultation goes on in this fashion.

Doctor V is ruling out OAF.

Afterwards, Doctor V presents to the senior doctor on duty: 'My patient does not seem to have raised intracranial pressure. There was nothing on history and physical examination. However, we should do a CT scan of the head to rule out causes of raised intracranial pressure, to be sure.'

The senior doctor replies, 'Ruling out is not your job. *Ruling in the correct diagnosis is your job.* What is her diagnosis?'

Doctor V looks blank.

The senior doctor waits for 30 seconds, then continues, 'I overheard the history. The diagnosis was obvious if you were listening. Your patient sounded very annoyed as you were leaving the room because you told her: "You probably do not have raised intracranial pressure." Patients want you to figure out what they have, not what they do not have!'

'Please go back to her, apologise, take a proper history, listen to her, and think.'

Sarah had classic migraine with aura; her answers to Doctor V's initial questions already pointed to the correct diagnosis.

However, Doctor V was target-fixated and ruled out OAF, so he was not listening to her answers.

He would have continued with a CT scan of the head if not stopped. If the CT scan had been performed, it would probably have been normal. The CT scan would have wasted money, increased Sarah's chance of some cancers in the future, and helped no one. Doctor V would still have no idea of the correct diagnosis or management.

Conversation #5

Dora, a 22-year-old female medical student attends the Emergency Department in a hospital in Singapore. She complains of fever and rash, both of 4 days' duration. The fever goes up to 38 degrees Celsius. The painless, non-itchy rash is present only over her cheeks and over the bridge of her nose. There are no other symptoms.

Her vital signs are normal. On physical examination, there is a macular erythematous rash over the bridge of the nose and part of both cheeks, and nothing else.

The first doctor who sees her, says: 'It is a malar rash and fever! This must be systemic lupus erythematosus!'

Going by the basic diagnostic reasoning requirement, the most likely clinical diagnosis is not lupus.

Dora: 'Huh? Er, okay...'

The lupus panel, complete blood count and other tests are sent off.

The lupus panel comes back negative. The full blood count shows neutropenia (neutrophil count: 0.9×10^9 cells/litre) and thrombocytopenia (platelet count: 60×10^9 cells/litre).

At this point, with a suggestive complete blood count and this clinical picture of an adult in Singapore, the diagnosis is even more obvious...if trying to 'Rule In' the diagnosis.

The correct diagnosis is not made. Instead, Dora is hospitalised for further workup of 'abnormal full blood count results for investigation'.

The next doctor reviews her and says: 'You have cell line involvement on the blood count! Your platelets were low! We must rule out leukaemia! Let us do a bone marrow aspirate!'

A bone marrow aspiration is an invasive procedure. It hurts afterwards, even if you sedated the patient during the procedure.

Dora says: 'I came in with fever and rash! What does leukaemia have to do with this?! No! I refuse!!'

Angrily, she thinks: 'Why are you ignoring my symptoms to justify what you want to rule out?!'

Clearly, Dora is a better reasoner than the doctors.

A third doctor reviews her a day later and says: 'Hang on. Fever, rash, this full blood count result. This is dengue fever.'

Dengue fever is a common infectious disease in tropical Singapore, usually presenting with a few days of fever and rash. This would have been obvious by Ruling In initially. Every doctor in Singapore is familiar with dengue fever. Clearly, this familiarity with dengue fever did not help the previous doctors who saw Dora.

The third doctor orders a dengue serology. The dengue serology comes back positive.

Conversation #6

A 35-year-old man walks into the allergy specialist's clinic.

He is holding a referral letter from a nephrologist.

The allergy specialist opens the envelope and reads the letter:

'Dear colleague,

This man has been complaining of itching for over 6 months. He has known chronic kidney disease with marked uremia, over 30 mmol/L for the past year. Please rule out other causes of itching before we treat him.'

Shocked, the allergy specialist reads the letter a second time to ensure he read everything correctly. Then he looks up at the patient sitting before him.

Doctor: 'What did the kidney specialist tell you?'

Patient: 'He said he does not know why I am itching. He said he would refer me to a specialist in itch to figure it out.'

The allergy specialist is thinking: chronic kidney disease with marked uremia for at least 1 year, with matching symptoms such as itching, is known to medical students. Such patients are routinely handled by kidney specialists every day. What kind of kidney specialist does not recognise symptomatic uremia in a patient with kidney disease?

The allergy specialist evaluates the patient clinically and determines there is no clinical feature to suggest any other likely cause of the chronic itch. The allergy specialist tells the patient the diagnosis of chronic kidney disease, then writes a short reply letter to give to the kidney specialist:

'Dear colleague, this man has symptomatic uremia due to his chronic kidney disease. The uremia is causing the itch. Please initiate dialysis and treat his disease. When the cause of his symptoms is known, you should treat it. Thank you.'

Before the patient leaves, the allergy specialist says to him, 'By the way, you may want to find another kidney specialist to treat you.'

The allergy specialist has realised the danger to the patient if he returns to see that kidney specialist.

Would you trust a specialist who cannot be logical?

Conversation #7

The junior officer, Doctor B, is presenting a patient to the senior doctor, Doctor J.

Doctor B: 'This 60-year-old man has been having breathlessness and swelling of the legs for 2 weeks. He has been vomiting every week for the last 7 months. On examination, he is hypertensive with a blood pressure of 220/120 mmHg. His oxygen saturation is 93% on room air. He has findings of anasarca and crepitations in both lungs. He is on follow-up with Nephrology for chronic kidney disease, with progressive uremia for over a year. They did not specify the stage of kidney disease in their notes. He is not on dialysis.'

Doctor J: 'Odd. What was Nephrology's impression for this admission?'

Doctor B: 'Fluid overload for investigation, and vomiting for investigation. Separate issues. They tried antacids for the last few months, which made no difference to the vomiting.'

Doctor J: 'Huh? Putting all the symptoms and signs together, what is the diagnosis?'

Doctor B: 'Symptomatic uremia in end-stage renal failure. Differentials like liver failure are unlikely, as the patient does not have the encephalopathy or jaundice that would have accompanied or preceded these symptoms. They also tried to rule out acute myocardial infarction. The troponin levels came back elevated. The ECG was normal.'

Doctor J: 'Troponin levels would be elevated in end-stage renal failure. And the clinical picture points to the first diagnosis you said. Neither liver failure nor acute myocardial infarction explains the entire clinical picture. They must commence urgent dialysis! Why wait for months?'

Doctor B: 'Well, they want to refer to Gastroenterology first to rule out other causes of vomiting, and Cardiology to rule out causes of raised troponin levels.'

Doctor J (shocked): 'What? Are there other symptoms or signs to suggest other diseases?'

Doctor B: 'There are no symptoms or signs to suggest other causes of vomiting. I do not know if they will commence dialysis urgently. They may ask to rule out "central nervous system causes of vomiting" with a CT or MRI scan of the brain, or refer to Neurology for that purpose. They said to increase the doses of oral antihypertensive medication and start intravenous diuretics first.'

Doctor J: 'Those medications will not be enough. I will speak to the nephrologist now.'

--

These conversations demonstrate the tunnel vision of ruling out OAF. The patient's clinical features are ignored whilst the doctors fixate on a feared diagnosis or fear of the unknown, and then make irrelevant decisions.

The fear of missing dangerous diseases can induce such tunnel vision that even when the second doctor looked at the test results for Dora, they fixated on the most dangerous diagnosis on their arbitrary list.

Fear of the unknown can predispose to ruling out OAF. The doctor wants to be sure there is only 1 cause of the patient's symptoms and signs. Thus, even when the diagnosis is obvious, they withhold appropriate treatment from the patient whilst waiting for other specialities to affirm 'there is no other diagnosis'. The delay in proper care increases the patient's suffering and the risk of complications. The doctor who indulges in such behaviour often shows no remorse or compassion for the patient.

Ruling out OAF often leaves the doctor seemingly blind and deaf. They are clueless as to the correct diagnosis because they ignored the entire clinical picture. After ruling out everything on their list, there is still no diagnosis.

Sometimes, with no diagnosis in mind and all dangerous diseases ruled out whimsically, the doctor's next assumption is 'there is no dangerous problem'. The truth is 'I do not know what is going on', but what they tell themselves is something different: 'There is no danger'. The doctor tells the patient 'There is no dangerous problem' instead of 'I do not know what you have'. The doctor then prescribes 'symptomatic treatment', which is often ineffective because the doctor does not know the diagnosis. Sometimes, symptomatic treatment can mask symptoms that would have warned the next doctor of the correct diagnosis, misleading the next doctor too.

In contrast, the moment you have ruled in the correct diagnosis, there is often nothing else rational to consider. You have automatically ruled out everything else!

Years ago, I was asked to 'rule out immunodeficiency' for a teenage patient with bronchiectasis. I must have been temporarily insane; I did just that, and only that. The tests for immunodeficiency came back negative. I then kicked myself, realising what I had just done. Further evaluation revealed the patient had cystic fibrosis.

That was the first and last time I ruled out OAF.

Ruling out OAF: How teachers encourage it (unthinkingly)

Ruling out OAF can be encouraged by senior doctors, teachers and authors. This occurs partly because many people are loosely flinging the phrase 'rule out' around when they meant 'rule in'. Unfortunately, using 'rule out' and 'exclude' frivolously only reinforces the impression that ruling out OAF is appropriate.

Ruling out OAF is sometimes deliberately encouraged by teachers and authors. The author of the journal article, protocol or guideline is a teacher too; they are teaching the reader of their document. Many documents encourage ruling out OAF.

The teacher says or writes, '**You** must rule out disease X!'

The teacher either cannot or will not teach how to rule in the correct diagnosis.

Sometimes, the teacher literally means those exact words. There are no unwritten or unspoken words. The teacher routinely rules out disease X because he/she cannot rule in the correct diagnosis. Thus, the teacher instructs learners to do the same.

At other times, there are unwritten or unspoken words. The teacher's actual meaning (I will put the unspoken words in italics) was '*I think you are incompetent. You cannot make the correct diagnosis. Maybe I could have, but I did not see the patient myself. Therefore,* **you** must rule out disease X!'

Notice the difference in meaning once the italicised text is put in. However, since the italicised text may offend the learner and may lead to complaints or 'lower teaching scores', many teachers only say or write a misleading fraction of the entire sentence. Thus, it is easy for learners to think they should rule out OAF.

If the teacher can and is willing to teach their learners how to make the correct diagnosis, they should do exactly that. A good teacher aims to teach the incompetent learner how to become competent, not offer ineffective substitutes for competence.

To avoid being misleading, authors who encourage ruling out OAF should have added this preface: 'The doctor's main job is to rule in the correct diagnosis. Ruling out a rigid list of diagnoses without paying attention to the patient, is not ideal and does not automatically make you a safe doctor'.

To be able to write this preface, the author must have sufficient reasoning to realise the truth and the importance of telling the whole truth. However, an author who had enough reasoning to realise the truth would be unlikely to encourage ruling out OAF in the first place. Thus, the absence of this preface while simultaneously encouraging the reader to rule out OAF in the same document, is unsurprising.

Capsule summary

- Ruling out is potentially indicated if the 3 criteria are fulfilled: dangerous, explains most or all the patient's clinical features, and is not the most likely diagnosis.

- Ruling out a less-likely disease is best accomplished by trying to rule in the most likely disease first. Ruling out immediately is sometimes necessary, such as in emergencies.

- When ruling in or ruling out, clinical steps are usually undertaken before considering the need for tests.

- Diagnoses of exclusion require you to think of relevant diseases for each unique patient's presentation, and then act appropriately.

- A diagnosis of exclusion can be the most likely clinical diagnosis.

- Ruling out OAF is for oafs. Do not be an oaf.

COMMON MISTAKES IN THE CLINICAL APPROACH

Common mistakes that directly affect the clinical approach can be divided into

1. Diagnostic mistakes during the consultation, and

2. Mistakes in learning, which predispose to mistakes in the clinical approach.

The previous chapters fully described some of the mistakes that occur when doctors are not applying the optimal approach to patients. To avoid repetition, those mistakes are not discussed in detail in this chapter.

Common Mistakes in clinical approach

Diagnostic mistakes during the consultation	Mistakes in Learning
A. Target fixation / premature closure B. Ruling out only, always or first C. Tests adequately compensate for lack of reasoning D. Guidelines/protocols adequately compensate for lack of reasoning	A. What I've (bothered to) read, are the only possible differentials B. 'My teachers are always right' C. 'My teachers describe their thought process fully'

1. Diagnostic mistakes during the consultation

A. *Target fixation / premature closure*

Target fixation refers to fixating on a single disease to the exclusion of all others: 'tunnel vision'.

Premature closure refers to the situation where one stops thinking prematurely, thereby closing off their mind. Thus, premature closure usually occurs simultaneously with target fixation: the doctor fixates on 1 disease and then refuses to analyse all other information that challenges this fixation. When target fixation or premature closure occurs, the doctor is tempted to skimp on the clinical evaluation and ignore inconvenient information.

To stop gathering information and ignore inconvenient information, feeds target fixation, and premature closure: no other diagnosis is considered, so no evaluation for other diagnoses is performed and no information for other diagnoses is accepted. Hence, there is little or no other information that challenges the doctor's belief.

These mistakes tend to occur when the doctor picks:

1. The disease they or someone close to them has
2. The disease they have recently read about in the textbook
3. The disease that must be in their speciality
4. The dangerous disease they are most afraid of missing
5. The disease that they see most often in everyone else

Examples include:

- **I (or someone I know), have this:** The doctor has gout, which causes pain in her joints. Thus, she decides that gout must be the diagnosis for most patients presenting with pain in their joints.
- **I just read about this:** The doctor recently read about leukaemia and its symptom of weight loss. In the next 1 week, this doctor proceeds to diagnose almost every patient with weight loss, as having leukaemia.

- **The only diseases that exist, are in my speciality:** The orthopaedic surgeon who often manages broken bones and other mechanical injuries. When a patient consults this surgeon with pain in their fingers, the surgeon only thinks of the usual illnesses they see.

- **I never want to miss this disease:** The psychiatrist who is afraid of discovering that one of their patients with 'psychosis' turned out to have systemic lupus erythematosus. Thus, this psychiatrist insists that all patients with potential psychoses require the exclusion of lupus through tests, and may refuse to treat these patients until all the test results return.

- **The most common disease I see in everyone else with this symptom:** The doctor who decides that anyone coming with cough and rhinorrhea, must have a viral upper respiratory tract infection.

The usual decisions afterwards involve testing and/or treating for the chosen disease.

B. *Ruling out only, always or first (ruling out OAF)*

Ruling out OAF: the clinical approach

Ruling out OAF tends to manifest as a long list of questions posed to the patient. Each question looks for symptoms and 'red flags' of dangerous diseases.

The evaluation of the patient's presenting complaint is often lacking. The doctor asks a few cursory questions about the presenting complaint, and then launches into their list of questions for the dangerous diseases.

Regardless of the answers to the doctor's questions, the doctor remains fixated on the diseases they fear. Thus, history-taking can be pointless because the doctor may not listen to the patient's answers. The doctor usually proceeds to order unnecessary tests to rule out OAF.

At the end of the consultation, despite all the questions and tests, the doctor often does not know the patient's diagnosis.

The full discussion on ruling out OAF was covered in the previous chapter.

C. *Tests adequately compensate for a lack of reasoning*

This fallacy suggests that tests will decide the diagnosis and management of the patient; reasoning is unnecessary. Since reasoning drives a proper clinical evaluation, the fallacy also suggests that a proper clinical evaluation is unnecessary. Poor reasoners favour this fallacy, because it allows them to skimp on the clinical evaluation and avoid confronting their weaknesses.

However, tests are tools.

If you were a carpenter who had many tools for the many tasks you must accomplish:

- How good would you be if you did not know the exact purpose of each tool?

- How safe would you be if you did not know how to wield the tool properly?

- Would such a carpenter be a master who somehow did not bother to learn the basics? Or an amateur who thought that carpentry only involved copying what they saw other carpenters do, without learning the how and the why, and without checking the competence of the carpenters they were mimicking?

Every tool requires skill to be used well. A tool is of little use or even dangerous to the unskilled in any profession. Healthcare is no exception. The tools of our profession, such as tests, are often useless and sometimes dangerous when used by poor reasoners.

Poor reasoners usually choose tests illogically. Examples include:

- All patients with fever need a complete blood count. Some variations of this insert a number ranging from 1–5 days of fever.

- In all patients with pain in the limbs, order an X-ray of those painful areas.

In the next step of the disastrous chain of dominoes, the test results tend to be misinterpreted. Proper interpretation requires the clinical context, which the poor reasoner has failed to obtain and often ignores anyway.

D. *Guidelines/protocols adequately compensate for a lack of reasoning*

There are 3 categories of guidelines and protocols: defensive, neutral and best-care.

1. Defensive: These documents focus on avoiding missing a fixed list of dangerous diseases. They tend to be long documents focused on ruling out diseases through tests and averting disaster. The format and content of these documents imply the intended audience is doctors who are any of the following:

   - Cannot make the correct diagnosis

   - Are ignorant

   - Have poor or zero reasoning

   - Have questionable or nonexistent clinical skills

   - Need tests to substitute for presumed weaknesses in competence, knowledge or reasoning

   - Cannot provide excellent care. Thus, averting disaster becomes the goal of care instead

   - Evidence from studies, if cited, tends to be interpreted in defensive ways to justify recommendations.

2. Neutral: These documents focus on standard care. The target audience is broad. Evidence from studies, if cited, tends to be interpreted objectively.

3. Best care: These documents are rare. The target audience is decent reasoners with adequate knowledge. These documents aim to provide above-average care. Evidence from studies, if cited, tends to be high-quality and carefully curated.

These documents cannot evaluate and analyse each unique patient in their entirety.

Guidelines and protocols are tools and thus, are subject to the same limitations as all tools. Poor reasoners tend to favour defensive documents because they want to believe these documents make them safe. Ironically, the defensive documents that are supposed to help poor reasoners, are often misused because poor reasoners lack the reasoning to use them properly.

2. Mistakes in learning (that predispose to diagnostic mistakes)

A. 'What I have (bothered to) read, are the only possible differentials'

Textbooks and references are often organised into disease entries, each entry listing symptoms and signs. Thus, those who only study disease entries often can think of only one or two diseases that include a particular symptom or sign.

Often, many diseases can cause each symptom and sign. Looking up the differentials for a symptom or sign would have required the learner to ask themselves: 'Are there other diseases that have these clinical features?' Rule #1 compels learners to ask themselves this question.

When learners do not look up other diseases causing a symptom or sign, their differential list is often grossly deficient. This deficiency can show up in clinical care and tutorials. Consider this example.

Tutor: 'What are the common causes of exudative tonsillitis?'

The usual response is: 'Streptococcus throat infection. Epstein–Barr Virus infection causing infectious mononucleosis.' Most references that describe these 2 diseases, mention 'exudative tonsillitis' in their disease entries.

The tutor waits for another 15 to 30 seconds. No other responses are forthcoming. The students realise there are more answers.

Tutor: 'Only two? What are the others?'

B. *'My teachers are always right'*

This fallacy manifests as 2 common assumptions:

- My teachers always teach the correct information
- My seniors are always right in their decisions.

Any student who bothers to check both assumptions, will rapidly discover that the assumptions are wrong.

Teachers do not want to mislead students. However, teachers may not be up to date with the latest knowledge. Teachers may have incorrect knowledge that they had never verified themselves. When challenged with tough questions, some teachers are too embarrassed to admit they do not know the answer, so they fabricate an answer on the spot. If the teacher's reasoning is poor, their explanations reveal their weakness.

Students who want to believe their teachers and seniors are always right, are often confused when reality shows them the truth: their teachers and seniors are wrong, and the patient's outcome is poor. Despite reality asserting itself, many students cling to this fallacy.

Students should:

1. Periodically and objectively verify what they were taught, such as checking updated and reliable sources of information.
2. Keep an open mind towards their seniors instead of unthinkingly assuming everything they see and are taught, must be correct.
3. Request explanations, and be wary if their teacher/senior has no or illogical explanations.
4. Follow up on patients to discover the final diagnosis, and then reflect on the patient's clinical course and test results to teach themselves.

Though I found it tiresome to keep checking the accuracy of my teachers' lessons independently, this additional work was preferable to wholesale copying of misconceptions and mistakes, which would harm my future patients, my career, and my reputation. In this fashion, I learnt which teachers could teach properly.

I recommend identifying and learning from excellent teachers. Hallmarks of excellent teachers include:

- Willingly saying 'I do not know', and then working with the learner to find the answer

- Freely admitting and discussing their mistakes. The best teachers include a lesson on the optimal reasoning process to prevent such mistakes in future

- Having robust reasoning (such as applying the concepts in this book consistently).

C. 'My teachers describe their thought process fully'

It is difficult to fully describe one's thought process. In an earlier chapter, I described how the teaching of 'common things happen commonly' is often distorted. To recap: Upon hearing a student mention rare diseases and nothing else, the teacher may have admonished them with 'you should always think of common diseases first'.

However, clinically competent teachers who say this, often do not follow their own advice and fail to recognise that their teaching did not match their thought process. Thinking of common diseases was the 3rd or 4th step in their thought process.

The 1st step was listening to the patient and generating the relevant differentials based on the clinical features.

The 2nd step was generating the mental Venn diagram.

Since the teacher did not describe their first 2 steps, their students may mistakenly think the teacher always thought of common diseases first.

Capsule summary

- Common mistakes in diagnosis occur due to poor reasoning.
- Suboptimal learning and copying others' mistakes, predisposes to diagnostic mistakes.
- Target fixation often goes hand in hand with premature closure and 'ruling out OAF'.
- Tools, including tests and defensive documents, cannot compensate adequately for poor reasoning. Poor reasoners usually misuse these tools.

Frequently asked questions

Q: Can physician behaviour due to poor clinical reasoning, such as ruling out OAF, lead to burnout?

A: Yes. This is most evident in hospitals.

Robust reasoners often make the correct clinical diagnosis, and then make optimal decisions for the patient. Daily entries about the patient are succinct, yet comprehensive. Everyone knows what is going on, and does not document irrelevant information, unrealistic differentials, or irrelevant 'red flags to look out for'. Presentations about the patient mirror the daily entries. The ward rounds and handovers are focused and succinct. Deteriorations and collapses are rare; thus, frantic, unnecessary resuscitations and discussions on poor outcomes are infrequent.

The patient is hospitalised for a shorter duration, has an optimal outcome, and goes home sooner and happier. Since patients are diagnosed and treated properly, readmissions for an unrecognised disease are rare. The total number of patients for each team is lower because patients are being properly managed and discharged appropriately, without needing to revisit the hospital for missed diagnoses. The workload is as little as is necessary for optimal patient care.

Poor reasoners often do not understand what is going on, and dare not admit this to their colleagues or patients. Ruling out OAF is often used to try to compensate for a lack of reasoning. Batteries of tests and treatments are often ordered, many or all of which will be irrelevant. The excessive testing and treatments strain the hospital facilities. The strain becomes apparent through running out of medication stocks and frequent delays in testing for many patients. Daily entries about the patient are either confused or encyclopaedic (or both). Presentations about the patient mirror the daily entries.

Ward rounds drag on for hours because the doctors keep discussing random pieces of patient information, often-irrelevant tests, and treatments. Handovers are unfocused and can be completely off: 'This patient will be fine for the next 12 hours' at handover is the patient who collapses unexpectedly 2 hours later. Without appropriate care, patients stay longer or deteriorate, requiring more updates to the patients and their families. A prolonged stay with slow or no improvement upsets many patients: 'Are the doctors wasting my time and money?'

Some doctors routinely tell patients 'You will get worse before you get better' whilst secretly hoping the tests give them the answers or the treatments they are frantically cycling through eventually work, not because the patient's disease really gets worse before it gets better. Deteriorations and collapses occur with alarming frequency, so frantic resuscitations and lengthy discussions on poor outcomes are likewise frequent. The patient eventually goes home or unhappily seeks a second opinion. Readmissions for missed diagnoses are frequent.

The total number of patients for each team is huge because the patients are being mismanaged and readmitted due to prior mismanagement. When faced with long-staying patients due to mismanagement and a shortage of beds, some doctors try to 'force' the patient to go home. 'Forcing' patients to go home can take various forms, such as prematurely referring the patient to step-down care facilities, or suggesting to the patient that since they are not rapidly worsening, they can continue taking the medications at home. Inattention to the home environment and caregivers compounds mistakes in the hasty and inappropriate discharge plans, which infuriates the patient and their family.

In hospitals, junior doctors do most of the abovementioned work, including:

- Typing the entries in the medical record
- Presenting the patients
- Ordering tests and tracing the test results
- Ordering treatments
- Making referrals
- Updating patients and trying to explain the plans of their seniors to the patient,
- Handling collapses at any time of the day, any day
- Preparing the presentations for Morbidity and Mortality rounds for patients who deteriorated or collapsed.

Thus, when the senior doctors are robust reasoners, the junior doctors have less work, and more time to relax and learn on the job.

When the senior doctors have poor reasoning, much of the greatly increased burden is shouldered by their unfortunate juniors. Junior doctors end up expressing various sentiments such as feeling like 'secretaries' and being tired all the time. Ironically and tragically, one of the sentiments expressed by both junior and senior doctors in this situation is 'having no time to think'. Without thinking, there is even more work, more unhappiness, and a higher chance of burnout because the unhappy situation continues.

Robust clinical reasoning is necessary to break the vicious cycle of increased work, unhappiness and burnout.

When the junior doctor works like this for years, not thinking and observing the mindlessness of their seniors, poor reasoning and sloppy clinical evaluation become habituated. These juniors often become the same kind of doctor as their seniors.

Even when junior doctors make valuable suggestions, senior doctors with poor reasoning often ignore the junior doctors because of:

1. Projection. The senior doctor assumes that others are like them, and therefore cannot be better than them: 'I cannot get it right, so you cannot either.'

2. Inattention. The senior doctor habitually ignores inconvenient information. The junior doctor's suggestions require the senior doctor to think, or to consider the possibility that they were wrong all this while. The senior doctor deems thinking or admission of mistakes to be inconvenient, and thus ignores the suggestions.

Robust reasoners rapidly realise that their poorly reasoning seniors see and treat them as mindless drones.

Robustly reasoning seniors do not readily dismiss suggestions. Skilled seniors are open to different perspectives, learning and admitting their mistakes. When one admits one's mistakes, one can then learn from these mistakes.

Poor reasoners often do not admit or tackle their mistakes, and thus improve slowly or not at all.

GATHERING ADDITIONAL INFORMATION TO MANAGE PATIENTS

In the first chapter, I described an optimal approach to the consultation:

1. Recognise the reality behind the patient's presentation, which drives effective questioning and the accurate use of patient information

2. Use each piece of initial information, according to its importance

3. Shape and prioritise the information-gathering to match each clue's importance to our task

4. Organise all the information according to their importance

5. Analyse the information according to their importance

6. Mentally decide the most likely diagnosis and reasonable alternative diagnoses

7. Gather additional information to understand the patient as a whole

8. Combine the additional patient-unique information with general medical knowledge, to make decisions with and for the patient

The first 6 steps were covered in the previous chapters.

Steps 7 and 8 will be covered in this chapter.

If you condensed the 8 steps into 'jobs', there are 3 fundamental jobs the doctor must accomplish for all patients:

1. Make the most likely clinical diagnosis (Steps 1 to 6 of the 8 steps)

2. Gather additional information needed for optimal management of that patient (Step 7 of the 8 steps)

3. Make optimal healthcare decisions in partnership with the patient (The last step of the 8 steps)

The 3rd job is the application of the same reasoning and mindfulness necessary to perform the first 2 jobs well.

This is the chain of dominoes all over again. The robust reasoner will understand the patient's perspective, perform the first 2 jobs well, and then do the same for the 3rd job. In contrast, the poor reasoner will fumble or omit the first 2 jobs and then fumble the 3rd job.

Step 7: Gather additional information to understand the patient as a whole

The most likely diagnosis decides the potentially feasible options for management. The clinically estimated severity of the disease suggests the best choices among the potentially feasible options.

You have decided on the most likely diagnosis and thus, have a tentative management plan. More information is needed for patient-centred decisions.

To quote Sir William Osler: 'The good physician treats the disease; the great physician treats the patient who has the disease.'

Understanding the patient to treat *the patient and the disease* as a whole, separates the best (doctors) from the rest (of the doctors).

At this Step, you strive to understand your patient better. Your questions should target specific information about the patient that will help you decide whether you can use your tentative management plan, or need to modify the management plan further to suit the patient. For example, asking the patient for drug allergies when your management plan does not involve prescribing drugs, is silly.

The additional information needed to understand the patient, comes from the patient's:

- Comorbidities and status effects
- Recent treatment
- Perspective: situation, values, expectations and preferences
- Potential caregivers.

Comorbidities and status effects

Concomitant (usually chronic) diseases and status effects can affect routine testing or treatment. Some of this information is available from the patient's medical record. Examples include:

- Drug allergy: It is usually unsafe to administer this drug and the other drugs that can cross-react to the culprit drug.
- Pregnant: CT scans of the abdomen/pelvis are potentially dangerous to the foetus. Drugs that are likely to harm the foetus should be avoided.
- Significant kidney injury: Nephrotoxic drugs are often discouraged. Drugs excreted through the kidneys may require dose adjustment for the degree of kidney injury.

Recent treatment

Recent treatment includes medications and procedures.

Recent treatment can 'mask' the true severity of the illness by reducing or removing symptoms, signs, and test-based markers of disease activity. The masking effect is troublesome when the treatment is relevant but inadequate. The result is a patient who seems less sick than they truly are, yet the treatment is insufficient to cure or control the illness. Missteps in subsequent management are likely unless the doctor understands this masking effect. Details of the masking effect are discussed in the chapter 'Diagnosis: disease, severity and treatment'.

The patient may be taking medication that can interfere with the function or metabolism of the drugs you intend to prescribe. Ascertaining this information helps you to decide whether to change the type or dose of the drug you intended to prescribe, or make changes to the existing medication the patient is taking.

Perspective: Situation, values, expectations, and preferences

The patient perspective includes the situation, values, expectations, and preferences.

Understanding each unique patient's perspective helps the doctor to make recommendations that appeal to the patient.

Situation includes the residential conditions, setup of the household, financial stability, social support, and occupation. These may be motivators to seek healthcare, or barriers to effective healthcare. For example:

- Consider the patient whose disease causes pain on walking. If this patient must climb the stairs to the 4th floor of a building to get home each day, he/she would be highly motivated to control the disease. Conversely, staying in a remote area that requires them to walk a few hundred metres each day to reach a vehicle that can take them to the hospital, can discourage these patients from travelling to the hospital every week for treatment.

- If the patient is the caregiver for dependents such as young children, or a sick or elderly family member, this burden of care may motivate the patient to recover quickly so that they can resume their caregiver duties. However, if these patients are the sole caregiver and hospitalisation would take them away from their dependents, some patients may be more reluctant to be hospitalised for treatment.

- Personal wealth affects the ability of the patient to afford expensive tests and treatment. Poverty can render even basic healthcare unaffordable.

- The needs of an occupation and the patient's passion for that occupation can affect their healthcare. The footballer with an injured leg will want to recover quickly. The passionate baker who develops 'baker's asthma' (an allergy affecting the airways) may be reluctant to find another job.

Values are the principles the patient considers important. One example is productivity: a patient proclaims they want to get back to work as soon as possible. Another example is self-reliance: the patient prefers to change their diet to control their mild hypercholesterolemia instead of taking drugs.

It is easy to confuse prejudices with values. Prejudices are an opinion, often preconceived, with no basis in reasoning or experience. Prejudices often manifest as the patient proclaiming an illogical and unhealthy view. For example, the patient may feel that all drugs are undesirable because they 'are artificial and therefore must be harmful to me'. The doctor must try to counter the patient's prejudices. Logic and reasoning may not work well, because many prejudices arise from poor reasoning. The wise doctor will call upon more than logic when trying to overcome prejudices.

Expectations are the outcomes the patient desires. Knowledge of the patient's expectations will allow the doctor to correct any unrealistic expectations.

Preferences are a liking for one option over the other. Often, there are two or more viable options for healthcare, each having pros and cons. The patient's situation, values and expectations will influence their preferences.

After an adequately informed discussion, the final preference of the patient should be solicited.

Potential caregivers

Potential caregivers include other adults in the same household, family or friends who can help the patient during their recovery. Without these caregivers, activities of daily living and complying with treatment can be dangerous or impossible. For example:

- A toddler with severe eczema needs moisturising of their skin several times throughout the day. Someone must be available to perform this task.

- A young adult with dengue fever is feeling very dizzy. Sending this person home may not be safe when there is nobody else to support and monitor them. Dizziness while trying to walk to the toilet or dining table, can be dangerous.

Step 8: Combine the additional patient-unique information with general medical knowledge, to make decisions with and for the patient

This step is the equivalent of the 3rd fundamental job: to make optimal healthcare decisions in partnership with the patient.

In brief, this entails:

1. Telling the patient about the clinical diagnosis.
2. Explaining each relevant management option that seems suitable, given the additional information you gathered from Step 7. This explanation and discussion revolve around the pros, cons, costs, risks and predictable results of each option.

These explanations and discussions are part of the shared decision-making style, which is generally superior to the top-down dictatorial style. These styles are detailed in Section 3.

How this all comes together: Example

Let us illustrate how having additional information about the patient, and mindfully planning for the treatment in advance before even seeing the patient, can significantly help with the management. This example will discuss immunotherapy, a cutting-edge treatment for food allergies in 2023.

Food allergies are common. The spectrum of severity ranges from mild to severe for each food allergy. The severity level inversely correlates with the patient's 'Threshold of Reactivity' (ToR). Developing an allergic reaction requires exposure to an allergen dose that meets or exceeds that ToR. The greater the exceeding of this threshold, the more severe the allergic reaction. The ToR concept explains observations for various allergies (food and non-food) such as:

- People who tend to have more frequent and more severe allergic reactions than others, usually react to smaller quantities of allergen exposure than others with allergies.

- Patients who have mild allergic reactions to significant quantities of food, often can eat lower quantities of that same food with no or milder reaction.

- People with house dust mite allergy often have mild symptoms of allergy because of superficial and limited exposure to the mites. Upon exposure to a megadose of dust mites through ingesting these dust mites by accident (called 'pancake syndrome', which occurs through eating foods prepared with mite-contaminated wheat flour), the patient has a severe allergic reaction.

Patients with food allergies are often told to avoid the food. This is easy to say but much harder to execute:

- Accidental exposure is common because some allergens, such as eggs, cow's milk, wheat, and peanuts, are commonly hidden in many dishes and processed foods.

- Being perpetually vigilant with everything you eat and buy, is tiring.

- Even if the patient and family are vigilant, everyone else who does not have a food allergy (such as friends, school teachers, and staff of eateries) may not be vigilant. Thus, other people may unknowingly offer these allergens to the patient. Sometimes, when the patient asks 'does this food contain (the allergy I have)?', other people may say 'no' instead of admitting 'I do not know'.

Thus, accidental exposures and allergic reactions are common. At best, the reactions are embarrassing and uncomfortable. At worst, these reactions are fatal.

At the time of this writing, oral immunotherapy for food allergy is the main alternative to 'try to avoid the food'. This treatment raises the ToR of the patient. Since an allergic reaction is possible only if the ToR is reached, raising the patient's ToR to a high level makes it almost impossible to develop an allergic reaction through accidental exposure, and can allow the patient to eat a limited quantity of that food.

Thus, this treatment can transform the patient's situation from the tiresome 'I must always check and worry' to 'I do not have to check and worry'. This also removes a lot of the fear and restrictions for the rest of the family staying in the same household. After treatment of the patient with severe peanut allergy, the family members who like eating peanuts can start keeping and eating peanuts again in the home.

Though the benefits sound wonderful, as of the end of the year 2022, this treatment is not commonly available. It is widely considered the most difficult procedure in the Allergy speciality. Routine Allergy subspecialty training does not teach the effective and safe provision of this treatment. Patients seeking this treatment tend to be the patients who have frequent and severe reactions, which means the risk of anaphylaxis and death with a single misstep, is significant. Multiple visits (10 or more) for treatment are often necessary over the span of several months.

Some reliable centres offer this treatment, with the total cost often exceeding US$10,000 (potentially US$40,000 or more). The success rate is often quoted as 70 to 75%.

The success rate of this treatment at the Department of Paediatrics, National University Hospital of Singapore averages over 85% for most foods. The total cost of treatment is far less than US$10,000. The cost of living in Singapore is equal to or greater than living in affluent parts of the USA and Europe, so the far lower cost of this treatment is not due to the lower costs of everything in general.

Some patients fly in for each visit or migrate to Singapore to undergo this treatment, and then return to their home countries — including the USA and Europe — for follow-up.

You might ask, 'How are such success rates possible? And at dramatically lower costs?'

Some of the answers come from the concepts in this book. A full understanding of tests, treatments and their utility in a patient-centric fashion helps with success.

Understanding the patient and their family, and anticipating their needs in advance, contributes significantly to the high success rate and lower costs.

By taking the effort to understand the patient and their family, clarifying expectations, providing a short-term and long-term 'road map', and transparent do-not-rush-into-this-please discussions, the treatment team helps patients and their families understand the entirety of the treatment.

The patient can commence the treatment, confident that there are unlikely to be any surprises. The patient and their family are reassured by the treatment team's foresight, caution and effort to understand them. With this trust in the service and the team, there is a lower tendency to abandon the treatment. This also increases the uptake rate of patients who consider the treatment.

As the cost of living in Singapore is considerable, I worked with my colleagues to strike a balance between revenue (the service was not to operate at a financial loss) and affordability for the average patient. Thus, more patients can afford this treatment and can stay on if it takes longer than was initially expected.

Patients and their families are often anxious and scared about undertaking a treatment that can result in allergic reactions. The amount of information regarding the treatment and potential concerns of the patient, such as falling sick or forgetting a dose, is considerable. Thus, patients are given a thin file filled with concise answers to Frequently Asked Questions, so that they know what to do at any time. In addition, they are given the means to reach the treatment team any day of the week, through email and the telephone.

Capsule summary

- Getting the correct diagnosis and gathering additional information to understand the patient as a whole, facilitates making optimal decisions with and for the patient.

ANTICIPATORY CARE

Anticipatory care focuses on the maintenance of health. Anticipatory care can be divided into:

- Primary prevention: maintaining optimal health and preventing diseases from occurring
- Secondary prevention: detecting diseases at the earliest possible stage to maximise the chance of cure or control.

Anticipatory care is best addressed after the patient's primary concerns and current diagnosis are settled. The doctor who speeds through or dismisses the patient's concerns to tackle anticipatory care, appears unempathetic and foolish. The patient thinks: 'I came to you with a definite problem, but you ignore that to look for *potential* problems? Do you know how to prioritise? Do you even listen or care about my concerns?'

Since consultations are often time-limited, robust clinical reasoning allows efficient handling of the patient's primary concerns, thus freeing up time at the end of the consultation to tackle anticipatory care.

Primary prevention

Primary prevention involves health education and interventions.

Health education focuses on a healthy lifestyle:

1. Diet,
2. Exercise and
3. Other habits.

Interventions at the government level include sponsored vaccinations and fluoridation of water. People can opt out of some interventions, often to the detriment of their health and those around them. Misinformation (often deliberate, and accompanied by fear-mongering) on the Internet misleads many people into refusing vaccinations.

Diet

A healthy diet incorporates a mix of healthy food, including fruits and vegetables. A healthy diet reduces the risk of cancer and cardiovascular disease, and may also reduce the risk of atopic, autoimmune, and inflammatory disorders.

Grains are dietary staples in many countries. The consumption of fish has been shown to confer health benefits.

If ingested in small quantities, red meats and alcohol demonstrate mixed benefits. At much larger quantities, the risk of harm such as cancers and liver damage often overshadows any potential health benefit.

Raw food must be carefully sourced and stored.

If cooking is necessary, boiling and steaming are usually the healthiest methods. Some cooking methods, such as barbequing, grilling, frying and roasting are potentially dangerous, especially when dealing with starch-rich foods such as potatoes and bread, because carcinogenic substances such as acrylamide may be generated in the process.

Certain oils are healthier than others. As cooking oils degrade with each use and may be linked to the development of cancer, reusing cooking oil requires reading up on the limits and methods of safe reuse.

'Junk' food such as most processed snacks, fried food and soft drinks are unhealthy and should be avoided. Foods rich in nitrates and nitrites have been consistently linked to cancer; nitrates and nitrites can be metabolised in the human body into cancer-causing N-nitroso compounds.

The diet is affected by the patient's affluence, education level, and availability of food in the country. Patients with less education tend to know less about healthy diets than more educated patients. However, regardless of their educational status, people often knowingly eat unhealthy food. Teaching patients what to do is more useful than teaching them what not to do. Thus, an education on less desirable foods and cooking methods must be accompanied by a discussion on healthy foods and cooking methods. Affluence affects choices: poorer families cannot afford the more expensive foods and concomitantly may lack knowledge of the healthy diet. Free health education nationwide goes a long way.

Quality of life matters too. The mindful doctor recognises that telling people to totally avoid their favourite foods, is unempathetic and unfeasible; the patient is virtually certain to ignore such advice. Instead, the mindful doctor modifies their dietary advice to show respect for the patient's preferences. For example, instead of telling the patient to totally avoid junk food, the doctor recommends that the patient reduce their daily junk food intake to once every 1 to 2 weeks, and explains the reason for this recommendation.

Many studies provide conflicting conclusions on foods. Poorly designed and executed studies account for much of the conflict because of bias, dubious data-gathering, inadequate follow-up and inaccurate conclusions. Flawed studies uniformly fail to ask:

- 'Is the data reliable?'
- 'Would the data be the same if applied across a broader range of people?'
- 'Did I follow up with the participants well enough and long enough to detect the development of disease?'
- 'Is there another logical explanation for the same data?'

Some proponents of certain diets rely on anecdotes to try to substantiate their claims. If something is truly beneficial for many people, the results are so commonplace and obvious that you do not need anecdotes. When anecdotes are relied upon to support a fad, one should be careful. Furthermore, people have been bribed to make fictitious claims. Given these facts, a prudent reader would demand robust evidence that directly compares the outcomes of 1 diet to another.

Most potentially harmful fads do not have robust studies backing up their claims. Robust studies often are not conducted on these fads because:

- Grant providers usually fund studies that have some chance of being useful, instead of studies without a logical or scientific basis.
- Reputable researchers prefer not to waste their time on illogical flights of fancy.

Thus, the lack of robust studies should warn you away from a fad.

An example would be the 'Carnivore Diet', which is a meat-predominant diet and fad. This diet became popularised around the year 2018. Lennerz et al. (2021) conducted a study on this diet. The study participants were 2029 people who wanted to eat the food and were already doing so for at least 6 months. The researchers collected self-reported data online and did not report any follow-up. The participants' responses were unsurprising:

- They were satisfied and had few side effects. (Could anything else be expected from people who willingly ate this food for a long time?)
- They felt better about their health. (If they felt worse, would they have kept eating the food long enough to be eligible for this study?)
- Their LDL-cholesterol went up tremendously. (Increased LDL-cholesterol is bad for cardiovascular health.)

A minority of the participants reported having healthier body mass indices, slightly better indicators of glycemic control, and a reduction in the use of medication for diabetes mellitus.

The logical conclusions from this data are:

1. If you asked people who have voluntarily remained on a diet for a long time how they felt about their diet, do not expect surprises.

2. The diet dramatically raises LDL-cholesterol, which predisposes to devastating cardiovascular diseases such as heart attacks and strokes.

3. A minority of participants with diabetes mellitus claimed benefits from this diet, but these claims were not verified. Uncontrolled diabetes mellitus predisposes to devastating cardiovascular diseases. However, the tiny improvement in glycemic control that these participants claimed, would be overshadowed by the jump in LDL-cholesterol. Being on this diet would still increase the overall risk of devastating cardiovascular disease, regardless of whether the patient had diabetes mellitus.

I would not try this diet unless I wanted to be crippled or dead prematurely. It is unlikely that any ethics board or grant provider who realised the same, would approve any further study on this diet.

Exercise

Being physically active provides several benefits to health:

- Improvement in the strength of the heart, lungs, muscles, and bones
- Helping to maintain a healthy body mass index
- Reduction in levels of unhealthy stress.

Improved heart, lung and muscle strength increases one's functional capacity and ability to weather diseases and accidents later in life.

Bone strength diminishes over time, starting in young adulthood and decreasing faster in women than in men. This gradual weakening of the bones can lead to osteoporosis, which is a disease where the bones become so weak that they break easily. Fractures resulting from osteoporosis tend to occur in middle age and the elderly, more so in females, and can be crippling.

The body mass index (BMI), if too low or too high, is associated with various diseases. Low BMI is linked to osteoporosis, and high BMI is linked to diabetes mellitus and cardiovascular diseases. A healthy BMI is maintained through a healthy lifestyle: diet, exercise, sleep, and resilience to stress. Decreased sleep predisposes to higher BMI, and feelings of greater stress predispose to higher BMI.

Exercise helps to reduce unhealthy stress, partly because this time is spent on healthy activity and distracts the person from their source of stress. National guidelines can drive awareness of exercise among doctors and other healthcare professionals. In general, more exercise is healthier than less exercise.

Other habits

Harmful recreational substances

Cigarette smoking, recreational drug abuse, and some other hobbies are linked to diseases. For example, cigarette smoking predisposes to many types of cancer.

Though the doctor could tell the patients about the harm, this information often fails to convince patients to stop indulging in these hobbies.

The mindful doctor recognises that patients who use harmful substances often perceive some gain from this use, such as fitting in with their friends. This doctor explores the patient's perception of gain, suggests viable alternatives, and tries to lead them to take charge of their health and lifestyle. This doctor tells the patient about the harm from engaging in their hobby, but knows that it is more effective to come across as a caring human instead of a lecturer.

Screen time

Screen time is the time spent using a device with a screen such as a computer, television, handphone, or games console. More screen time (usually 2 hours or more in children and adults, every day) is linked to:

- Depression, mental illness, cardiovascular disease and obesity in adults, and

- Inattention, delayed development, poorer sleep and risk factors for cardiovascular disease in children.

Some of the consequences may come not from the direct effects of looking at a screen, but instead from opportunity cost: the person who is spending more time on the screen every day is spending less time on other, potentially healthier choices such as exercise, and therefore is giving up the benefits of healthier choices.

To assume that more screen time is automatically harmful regardless of how that time is used, is a mistake. Screen time can be useful for healthy, dedicated learning and communication. Conversely, prolonged entertainment on screens (including use of social media) is probably harmful. I suspect most of the adverse effects of prolonged screen time come from entertainment-type screen time.

Many parents resort to entertaining their young children with screens, which gives the parents more time to rest or relax. This scenario is common when parents are trying to get young children, especially picky eaters, to finish their food during mealtimes.

Violence on screens

Controversy exists over violence in entertainment, be it computer games, television shows or movies. It is often argued that watching violent behaviour in entertainment is linked to violent behaviour in the watcher: 'Those men fought because they often watch shows on fighting. Watching the shows made the men behave violently.' The evidence for this argument is weak and questionable.

Many adults who have seen 'violent' behaviour in computer games and shows, will not engage in such behaviour. The association between physical violence and screen violence in adults probably shares the same explanation as the feel-good data from the study on the Carnivore Diet. Specifically, people watch 'violent' shows and play 'violent' computer games because they find the violence exciting, sometimes gratifying.

Therefore, adults who enjoy 'violent' screen time and engage readily in violent behaviour, do both as a reflection of their preferences and values. Screen violence does not directly cause violent behaviour.

However, the causal link is clear in children. Studies in children demonstrate this link between exposure to violence in entertainment, with subsequent real-world aggression. This causal link is unsurprising once we consider the malleability of the brain in childhood.

Windows of vulnerability

A window of vulnerability is a crucial phase in the life of a human, where negative influences tend to exert amplified and long-lasting effects on their health.

Many windows of vulnerability occur in infancy and early childhood. Adverse influences, such as malnutrition, have a long-lasting impact on the health of these children, who will become adults.

These windows are opportunities to reduce the risk of many long-term problems.

One example is food allergy. Food allergies can be disabling or lethal chronic diseases; even in the best-case scenario, they are troublesome to the patient. Prevention of food allergies in children requires intervention during the window of vulnerability, which begins in early infancy. Young infants must regularly ingest potential 'food allergens' for several months, sometimes a few years. Delay or absence of this ingestion of many food types, especially in high-risk infants, can be disastrous. The parents who become aware of this retrospectively (they have at least 1 child with severe or multiple food allergies) often feel guilty; I advise them to be fair to themselves, because they are not experts in food allergy and should not blame themselves for not having this knowledge. Instead, they should focus on what they can do from now on for their child with food allergies, and especially if they intend to have more children. Some parents unhappily say that some guidelines and so-called 'experts' told them to avoid introducing feared foods such as peanut and egg. In response, I unhappily explain that 'experts' sometimes provide opinions based on bias, ignorance of biology, lack of logic and ignorance of the evidence, and write guidelines on the same basis.

The window of vulnerability for the brain is of particular interest. This window remains open for several years after birth.

Many studies have demonstrated the association between increased screen time in young children, with attention-deficit hyperactivity disorder (ADHD) and ADHD-like symptoms. Various theories put forth to explain this association, include:

1. The risk of developing ADHD is increased by more screen time

2. Having ADHD increases the risk of screen addiction

3. In children who already have ADHD, parents are predisposed to giving them more screen time

Combining our current understanding of neuroscience, brain development, and the research on screen time and its impact on mental health and ADHD-like behaviour, it is likely that all 3 theories are probably true, albeit to different degrees in different subgroups in the population. The most alarming is the first theory: that the risk of developing ADHD is increased by more screen time. The certainty of this alarming theory increases once the Bradford Hill's criteria for causality are considered. The same combination of knowledge, theory and evidence also strongly suggests that increased screen time, especially in boys, increases the risk of autism.

It is unlikely that any research study will ever be undertaken to directly prove that ADHD is caused by increased screen time. Such a study would require parents to willingly subject their young children to significant amounts of screen time daily. Even if an Ethics board could approve such a harmful study, the possibility of being left with a child with ADHD or autism after participating in the study, would scare parents away.

To argue that the first theory cannot be true because a study to prove it is neither ethical nor feasible, is like arguing that parachutes cannot save human lives when falling out of a plane at an altitude of 10,000 feet, because a study to prove that people cannot survive a fall of 10,000 feet without a parachute is neither ethical nor feasible.

The inability to conduct a study to directly prove that screen time increases the chance of ADHD, does not prove that screen time does cause ADHD. However, it is not difficult to predict the effects of exposing infants and toddlers at a time when their brains are vulnerable to external influences, to prolonged screen time where the content is unsuited to them. Research on prolonged screen time has demonstrated adverse effects on mental health and attention span in children, and worsening of ADHD symptoms in children known to have ADHD.

When multiple studies have been conducted on screen time and its effects on humans, the general absence of research findings (even after accounting for publication bias, where studies with 'negative' results tend not to be published) to show that increased screen time is not linked to inattention or ADHD, is telling. When the research on screen time and its relationship to autism is considered, where the pathogenesis of autism is likely related to the same windows of vulnerability, neuroscience and knowledge of brain development as ADHD, it becomes even harder to argue against the inevitable conclusion: increased screen time does predispose to developing ADHD.

Entertainment that does not stimulate the brain in a healthy way, is unlikely to improve the health and function of the neurons. Neurons get pared over time. Studies demonstrate that stimulating brain activities can stave off brain degeneration, preventing diseases such as dementia. Thus, a lack of healthy mental stimulation is likely to predispose to a more rapid decline in neuronal number and health.

Windows critical to pathways in brain development are open at a young age. During these windows, appropriate stimulation from the environment is critical to development. Failing to engage in mentally stimulating activity at a pace slow enough and in a form suitable enough for the young child to comprehend, is probably detrimental to the brain of the young child.

Frequently entertaining the infant or toddler with a screen instead of engaging them in slower-paced, stimulating and attentive social interactions, could explain the observations that children exposed to prolonged screen time tend to have delayed development and inattention, as if the neurons necessary for cognitive function and focus, are less developed or reduced in number.

Many adults, including paediatricians, underestimate the learning abilities of infants and toddlers. Investing time and energy daily to listen attentively to young children and infants, play with them, make eye contact with them, talk to them, and read children's books to them is crucial. At mealtimes, the adults at the table should role-model healthy behaviour in a social setting. These activities are more slow-paced than screen entertainment, allow the adults to adapt the activity to that child, and role model healthy social and attentive behaviour in front of these children.

Adding the dimension of empirical observation increases my certainty that increased entertainment-type screen time, increases the risk of autism and ADHD. Since 2010, I have noticed a massive surge in these behaviours in the clinics, the shopping malls, and so on. The surge is almost exclusively in young boys. Where possible, I have politely enquired or followed up on these children, and discovered virtually all were already diagnosed, or were soon afterwards diagnosed formally with autism or ADHD. The background (apparent intelligence, socioeconomic status, concern for their child, etc.) of the parents did not seem to correlate with these cases; however, the 1 striking consistency was the exposure to huge amounts of screen time, especially during the window of vulnerability I cited above, before the onset of these behaviours. Some of my students independently made insightful deductions in this area based on their own observations of the child's behaviour. They drew some of the abovementioned conclusions even though they did not know of the evidence on screen time, and I did not tell them my observations or suspicions.

Cognition and attention span in 'normal' children lie on a spectrum. If you subjected your young child to large amounts of entertainment-type screen time, and then thought that the absence of an official diagnosis of ADHD or autism automatically means they were not harmed by the large amounts of exposure, you are probably mistaken.

Entertainment-type screen time should be limited as much as possible, especially in young children. I have seen the various guidelines on screen time, issued by various countries as of the end of 2022. I feel that the cutoffs in many guidelines are too generous.

These are my recommendations on entertainment-type screen time:

1. Children below 2 years of age should not be subjected to entertainment-type screen time.

2. Entertainment-type screen time in children between 2 and 3 years of age, is probably dangerous and should be totally avoided. If such entertainment must be provided (I cannot think of a valid reason to thus endanger the child), it should be less than 2 hours a week.

3. Entertainment-type screen time in children between 3 and 6 years of age, should be strictly limited. At least 80% of the free time that these children have for entertainment, should be spent on imaginative play and social interaction with other children or adults. This suggestion of 'at least 80%...' is based on both the benefits of such imaginative or social activity, and my understanding of the effect of oppositional stimulation on developing neurons (like a see-saw in the playground, where 1 end represents the effect of entertainment-type screen time on the young brain, and the

other end represents the weight of healthier activity to counter that risk of harm).

4. Parents should watch the entertainment themselves and vet their suitability for their children. The parents should be vigilant for displays of violence or disrespectful behaviour towards other living beings. If the children see these displays, their parents should teach them about the problems that come with such behaviour.

5. Parents should be mindful of their use of screens in front of their children. Children tend to copy their parents, and may think that their parents' heavy use of screens may be ideal for themselves too.

6. Older children and adults should minimise entertainment-type screen time. The detrimental effects can be considerable, but tremendous self-awareness is needed to notice these effects on oneself. In addition, time spent on these screens means the loss of time that could have been better spent on healthy social interactions, hobbies, and exercise.

Windows of vulnerability: implications for national economics and health

The governments of countries faced with the burden of multiple chronic diseases and an ageing population, often focus on the chronic diseases and the elderly: opening more hospitals, providing more services for the disabled and the elderly, and so on. This is a short-term response.

The windows of vulnerability indicate that appropriate interventions at the population level, including family support and parental education, would delay or prevent the onset of various chronic diseases as children grow up. Optimising the health of these future adults benefits them and their productivity, helps the country's economy and harmony, and reduces the strain on the country's budget and infrastructure when they grow old.

Interventions

Checking the patient's vaccination status and recommending useful vaccines will help to protect the patient and the community:

- Many countries have national vaccination programs, the bulk of these vaccines being administered in infancy and pre-school age. Check the child's vaccination status regularly up until the end of the standard age for routine vaccinations.

- Patients with compromised function in vital organs such as the heart, lung or immune system are less able to weather infections than others. They should be encouraged to receive vaccinations for common diseases in their region.

Mandatory or sponsored vaccinations will encourage herd immunity. Herd immunity is the resistance to the spread of an infectious disease within a population that is based on pre-existing immunity of a high proportion of individuals, as a result of previous infection or vaccination. Thus, herd immunity helps to prevent and minimise outbreaks of infectious diseases. Lack of herd immunity often manifests as outbreaks of vaccine-preventable diseases.

Vaccine hesitancy contributes to these outbreaks. Vaccine hesitancy is more prevalent where 'freedom of speech' is promoted without requiring accountability for the predictable consequences of one's words. Words have power, and power must be linked to responsibility.

This 'freedom of speech with little or no responsibility' allows anti-vaccine activists to freely ply their trade, and facilitates the propagation of misinformation on the Internet. The initial years of the COVID-19 pandemic amply demonstrated the consequences of freedom without responsibility.

Some infectious diseases are so dangerous that vaccinations for these diseases should be mandatory *and* sponsored. Humans must accept that their freedom to interact with others, comes with the responsibility to those who interact with them. Even if someone was willing to contract measles and perish from it, others around them should not be unnecessarily put at risk of measles too. The joining of freedom with responsibility is the basis for criminal law, and is also the basis of governmental interventions for the benefit of everyone in the country.

Secondary prevention

Secondary prevention aims to detect diseases at the earliest possible stage to maximise the chance of cure or control.

These steps can be divided into clinical and testing steps.

Clinical screening for secondary prevention

Some patients have symptoms of the disease, but are unaware of the significance of the symptoms. Other patients are asymptomatic but have signs of the disease.

Clinical screening for signs is more accurate if the doctor has mastered Level 2 of the physical examination, as these doctors can notice subtle signs that others would miss. Examples include:

- **Noticing palmar crease or conjunctival pallor whilst glancing at the patient.** A 'Level 2 Master' of physical examination can detect the faintest shades of pallor, often at serum Haemoglobin levels just below 10 g/dL. In comparison, a doctor who has not mastered 'Level 2' may notice pallor only when the patient's serum Haemoglobin level has dropped to 8 g/dL or less. Pallor is commonly seen in nutritional disorders, some chronic diseases, and some cancers.

- **Poor eye contact, distinctive mannerisms or other unusual behaviour in the playing child.** These signs can be picked up by observant doctors and routine developmental screening. These signs may be present in children with developmental disorders, such as autistic spectrum disorder and attention-deficit hyperactive disorder.

- **Abnormal breathing pattern and facial colour whilst glancing at the patient.** This requires Level 2 mastery. When he was a junior consultant, Professor Lee Jiun could routinely recognise a sick baby in this manner.

Some measures for secondary prevention can be taught to patients. For example, breast self-examination is useful for detecting small lumps, which might be an early sign of breast cancer.

Testing for secondary prevention

Testing can be suggested by the doctor, and encouraged by government-sponsored population screening programs.

The doctor may recommend tests for the patient who belongs to a subgroup with risk factors for certain diseases. Risk factors include the patient's age, diet, lifestyle, and socioeconomic status. Examples include:

- Screening for anaemia in fully breastfed infants, some middle-aged folks, elderly folks, and vegetarians
- Vitamin D levels in people with little sun exposure.

Population screening detects many serious diseases before symptoms or signs appear. The doctor can educate patients on these screening programs, and encourage them to participate. Examples include:

- Colonoscopy for middle-aged and older adults, for rectal cancer
- Cancer markers in older adults
- Mammograms for breast cancer
- Papanicolaou smears for cervical cancer.

Capsule summary

- Doctors can provide guidance on anticipatory care to patients after addressing the patient's primary concern and current diagnosis. Robust clinical reasoning facilitates this process.

- Anticipatory care encompasses primary and secondary prevention. Having the necessary knowledge and physical examination skills facilitates this process.

Frequently asked questions

Q: What about opportunistic care?

A: Opportunistic care refers to addressing the patient's other chronic illnesses after the primary concern and diagnosis have been handled properly.

If following up with a patient with chronic disease, the doctor often 'cycles' between chronic diseases and anticipatory care, alternating between these for each consultation as necessary.

When handling chronic illnesses in this opportunistic fashion, robust reasoners use a focused assessment (this is discussed in the chapter 'Tackling the chronic disease').

QUIZ: CLINICAL APPROACH

Q1a: What is the basic diagnostic reasoning requirement?

Q1b: Explain how your answer to Q1a is important for diagnostic accuracy.

Q2 (scenario): A 20-year-old lady presents with vomiting water twice a day, diarrhoea 4 times a day with small to moderate amounts each episode, fever with a maximum ranging between 37.8 and 38 degrees Celsius daily, and severe episodic migratory abdominal pain. The pain occurs several times a day, lasting up to 1 hour per episode. The pain score is 6/10. The pain tends to occur around the umbilicus, but can travel to the left, right and lower parts of the abdomen. There is no pain between episodes.

These symptoms have been present for 3 days. There are no other symptoms. Her oral intake is decreased to about three-quarters of her usual.

She has no known chronic diseases and has never undergone any surgery. The rest of her family is well. Her last menstrual period was 1 week ago.

She has a temperature of 37.9 degrees Celsius initially. The other vital signs are normal. On examination, she has mild ascites. Her abdomen is non-tender. Bowel sounds are normal. The rest of the physical examination is normal.

Q2a: What are the top 2 to 4 differential diagnoses?

Q2b: What are the next steps to take?

Q3 (scenario): An 8-year-old girl presents with vomiting water 5 times and abdominal pain over the central and lower right portions of the abdomen. These symptoms began 1 day ago. The pain was initially episodic, with 3 episodes in the first 12 hours, each episode ranging from 30 minutes to 1 hour in length. The pain duration is now increasing with each episode, the latest lasting 4 hours. The pain score ranges from 6 to 8/10 per episode. There is no pain between episodes.

There are no other symptoms. Her oral intake is decreased to about three-quarters of her usual. She has no known chronic diseases and has never undergone any surgery. The rest of her family is well. Her pubertal development has not begun.

Her vital signs are normal. Her BMI is 16. She is complaining of pain as you begin your examination. Her abdomen is soft; there is mild tenderness over the right lower quadrant, without any guarding or rebound. No masses are palpable. Bowel sounds are normal. The rest of the physical examination is normal.

Q3a: What are the top 2 to 3 differential diagnoses?

Q3b: What are the next steps to take?

Q4: What is the proportion of consultation time you should spend on anticipatory care in every consultation?

SECTION 2

Decision Making: Tests

This section covers the considerations for testing and test result interpretation.

PATIENT-CENTRED TESTING

If tests are ordered, they should add value to that patient's care on top of the information and conclusions already drawn from the clinical evaluation.

All patient-centred tests fulfil at least one of 2 purposes:

1. Differentiate between the relevant differential diagnoses for that patient
2. Gather additional information to adjust treatment

Differentiate between the relevant differential diagnoses for that patient

Appropriately chosen diagnostic tests differentiate between the relevant differential diagnoses for that patient.

Diagnostic tests are indicated when the uncertainty of the most likely diagnosis or any differential that requires ruling out, is significant. The result of the test must differentiate between the differentials by:

- Ruling in the most likely clinical diagnosis, and/or
- Ruling out one or more of the less-likely differentials, if all 3 criteria to rule out that differential are fulfilled.

Other factors that contribute to a testing decision include the cost, discomfort and risks posed to the patient.

Consider the next 2 cases.

CASE #15: Tranh

Tranh is a 20-year-old man who limps into the Accident and Emergency Department with excruciating, progressive, unremitting pain in the right iliac fossa that began 1 day ago. This pain is associated with nausea and vomiting once, over the same period. There are no other symptoms. He has never had surgery.

He winces as he gets on the bed. He has a temperature of 37.8 degrees Celsius; the other vital signs appear normal. His abdomen is tender and guarded over the right iliac fossa. There is no rebound tenderness. Bowel sounds are normal. He can flex and extend his right leg at the hip, but winces at the extremes of the range of motion of the right hip.

--

You decide the relevant differential diagnoses are:

- Acute appendicitis (this diagnosis explains all the clinical features) — 97%

- Septic arthritis of the right hip (this diagnosis cannot explain most of the clinical features) — 2%

- Evolving viral gastroenteritis (this diagnosis cannot explain most of the clinical features) — 1%.

--

Given the 97% certainty of acute appendicitis, would the results of diagnostic tests to rule in appendicitis, be likely to change the management of this patient?

(Continued)

Is the likelihood of septic arthritis high enough (2%) to justify spending resources ruling it out, especially given that there is another more likely diagnosis?

At 1% probability, is it worthwhile to perform rule-out testing for evolving viral gastroenteritis? Even if you deemed the test worthwhile, gastroenteritis does not fulfil the 3 criteria for ruling out.

CASE #16: Rudra

Rudra is a 50-year-old Indian man who walks into the Accident and Emergency Department complaining of progressive pain in the right lower part of the abdomen that began 1 day ago. The pain initially began as brief episodes lasting several minutes, but has progressed until it has been non-stop for the last 4 hours. The pain score is 6/10. This pain is associated with other symptoms: nausea and vomiting once, and 1 episode of watery stools over the same period. There are no other symptoms.

He has never had any surgery.

On examination, he is overweight with a BMI of 30. His vital signs are normal. He winces on palpation of the right lower quadrant of the abdomen. There is no guarding or rebound tenderness. Bowel sounds are normal.

You decide the relevant differential diagnoses are:

- Early acute appendicitis (this diagnosis explains all the clinical features) — 60%

- Acute diverticulitis (this diagnosis can explain most of the clinical features. He is obese and middle-aged, which are supportive risk factors for this diagnosis) — 30%

(Continued)

(Continued)

- Viral gastroenteritis (this diagnosis cannot explain most of the clinical features) — 10%.

--

At a 60% certainty of appendicitis, do you need diagnostic tests to rule in appendicitis further?

Is the likelihood of acute diverticulitis high enough (30%) to justify spending resources to rule it out?

At 10% probability, is it worthwhile to perform rule-out testing for viral gastroenteritis? Even if you deemed the test worthwhile, gastroenteritis does not fulfil the 3 criteria for ruling out.

Cases #15 and #16 discuss the clinical certainty of the most likely diagnosis. By extension, the *un*certainty of that diagnosis, which is also the chance of being wrong, would affect decisions regarding diagnostic testing.

For Case #15, acute appendicitis is virtually certain. Delaying treatment to order diagnostic tests and wait several hours for the results, would probably waste resources and might endanger the patient. A prudent doctor would keep the patient nil-by-mouth in preparation for surgery, call the surgeons immediately and ask them if they required any pre-operative blood tests.

Viral gastroenteritis is very unlikely in both cases. Even if the probability of gastroenteritis was higher, at 40%, this diagnosis does not fulfil the criterion of 'dangerous' to warrant ruling it out.

For Case #16, the clinical features suggest acute appendicitis at the early stage. Given the demographics of the patient, many doctors would think of the differential of acute diverticulitis. However, the minor arguments against diverticulitis make it less likely than acute appendicitis.

Upon 'splitting up' the total of 100% certainty among the differentials, acute appendicitis might be assigned 60% certainty. Acute diverticulitis is assigned 30% because there is some clinical fit, with minor arguments against this diagnosis. That leaves the last 10% to the final differential of viral gastroenteritis, which has even less fit than acute diverticulitis.

A 60% certainty of acute appendicitis would mean a 40% chance of not having acute appendicitis and thus, a 40% chance of making poor decisions if the doctor insisted on treating for appendicitis.

A 30% chance of acute diverticulitis means a 30% chance of making poor decisions if the doctor ignores the possibility of acute diverticulitis.

The doctor then tries to differentiate between the differentials. The initial tests aim to rule in acute appendicitis because the highest-yield decisions usually target the most likely diagnosis. If the same tests to rule in appendicitis can simultaneously rule out acute diverticulitis, this is a bonus.

The reasoning steps in deciding test and treatment decisions will be explained further in subsequent chapters. Let us move on to the second purpose of all patient-centred testing.

Gather additional information to adjust treatment

Once the most likely disease has been decided with or without diagnostic testing, additional tests may be necessary to gather more information. This additional information helps to ensure that your treatment is optimal for that patient.

Ask yourself: 'What else must I know to provide adequate treatment?'

Three categories of information matter:

Information from Test	Importance
Assess disease activity/severity	Affects urgency and intensity of treatment
Detect treatment-related risks, due to the patient's co-morbid diseases or status conditions	Affects the safety of available options for treatment
Assess disease presence and activity, in diseases that can be present but are clinically occult	Monitoring of disease activity, since the absence of clinical symptoms and signs, may not mean full recovery

Assess disease activity/severity:

Tests may refine your initial clinical estimate of disease activity or severity, which in turn affects the intensity of your overall management. Examples include:

- Acute pancreatitis: serum calcium and other markers in Ranson's criteria
- Pneumothorax: chest X-ray to estimate its size.

Most tests provide information on disease activity, while some provide information on disease severity.

Is it important to distinguish between activity and severity? Yes.

When a disease has been 'masked' by treatment, disease activity is less than disease severity.

Disease activity comprises symptoms, signs, and most test results. Doctors often use this clinical and test-based information for diagnosis and subsequent decisions, with many textbooks and references recommending the same. Thus, many students and doctors assume disease activity is automatically equal to disease severity, which is untrue.

Disease severity carries almost all the weight for optimal decisions. Since disease activity is either equal to or less than the disease severity, conflating activity with severity predisposes to underestimating the severity of the patient's disease, which then predisposes to inadequate management and poor outcomes.

For example, the doctor who recognises the distinction between disease activity and disease severity, is not fooled by the patient who 'does not seem sick' when this patient's severe disease was partly masked by recent treatment. This doctor would commence optimal treatment immediately. Other doctors who are unaware of the distinction between activity and severity, tend to think that the same well-looking patient with partly masked disease does not have severe disease, and then erroneously under-treat the patient, with potentially tragic consequences.

The chapter 'Diagnosis: disease, severity and treatment' covers the distinction between activity and severity, and the implications of this distinction in far greater detail.

A clinical estimate of severity is important. Waiting for the results of tests can delay optimal decisions. Early recognition of the disease severity allows you to immediately match your treatment intensity to that patient. Examples include:

- If the doctor clinically recognises the patient has severe pancreatitis, they would promptly commence intensive treatment and send the patient to the Intensive Care Unit for the appropriate (intensive) management, before the test results are known.

- If a tension pneumothorax is recognised clinically, immediate needle decompression is warranted even if the chest X-ray has not been performed.

Detect treatment-related risks, due to the patient's co-morbid diseases or status conditions:

This information helps you ascertain if the treatment is safe to administer. Examples include:

- **Disease requiring major surgery, with the use of general anaesthesia and high risk of significant blood loss:** Pre-operative blood tests are often ordered. Abnormal results might increase the danger of surgery, and warn of another undetected disease. The robust reasoner reacts to abnormal results by figuring out the cause of these results, instead of merely 'optimising a number'.

- **Disease requiring drugs which are cleared by the liver or kidneys:** When the patient has impairment of the function of the organ, which is clearing the drug, the corresponding liver or renal panel is ordered. The test result affects the choice and dose of the drug used.

- **A Chinese patient with epilepsy, in whom you intend to commence Carbamazepine:** Genotype for the HLA-B*1502 allele, which increases the chance of Stevens-Johnson syndrome when Carbamazepine is used. If this allele is present, another anti-epileptic drug should be considered.

Assess disease presence and activity, in diseases that can be present but clinically occult:

Some diseases may be present but clinically undetectable in the consultation. They fall into 2 categories:

1. Diseases that required extended treatment to ensure a cure. The clinical features of these diseases are masked by treatment.

2. Diseases that do not require active treatment and may resolve spontaneously, but their continued presence affects the patient's risks and choices.

Examples include:

- **Leukaemia:** Initial treatment may mask the symptoms and signs of leukaemia. Tests for the minimal residual disease are performed to check for the presence and activity of tumour cells. Positive test results may suggest the patient needs additional treatment to maximise the chance of cure.

- **Osteomyelitis:** Antibiotic treatment can mask the symptoms and signs of deep-seated infections such as osteomyelitis. Even when the symptoms and signs are gone, inflammatory markers are tracked. If still significantly elevated at the intended end of treatment, extending the treatment is a consideration.

- **Food allergies in children:** Many food allergies resolve spontaneously in children. If the child has avoided all exposure to the allergen, it is clinically impossible to discern whether the food allergy is still present. In this situation, there are 2 ways to find out if the food allergies are still active as the child ages: either perform surrogate tests for the continued presence of an allergy, or perform food challenges (the child eats the food). As food challenges are resource-intensive and potentially dangerous, surrogate tests are often performed first.

Capsule summary

- All patient-centred tests must fulfil at least one of 2 purposes: differentiate between the relevant differentials in your patient, or gather additional information for adjusting treatment.

Frequently asked questions

Q: Is epidemiological testing part of patient-centred care?

A: Epidemiological testing is not part of patient-centred care. These are tests performed on cohorts of patients, which often track specific infections and pathogen strains. The data gathered can decide policy and coordinate healthcare efforts on a larger scale (such as regional or national level).

DIAGNOSTIC DIFFERENTIATION: LIKELIHOOD RATIOS

The first purpose for all patient-centred testing (if testing is indicated) is diagnostic: to differentiate between the differentials for each unique patient.

The result of the test must differentiate between the differentials by:

- Ruling in the most likely clinical diagnosis, or
- Ruling out one or more of the less-likely differentials, if all 3 criteria to rule out that differential are fulfilled

If your reasoning is robust, pursuing the most likely clinical diagnosis has the highest yield. Thus, ruling in the most likely diagnosis is the first step.

Ruling out is often unnecessary if the most likely diagnosis has been ruled in with a near-100% certainty. This was explained in the earlier chapter 'Ruling out: when, why and how'. The probability-based thresholds for diagnostic testing are discussed in the next chapter 'Decision thresholds for diagnostic testing and treatment'.

If your reasoning is deficient, it may not matter which diagnosis you pursue, because you are unlikely to make the right decisions.

Since it is not always clear if your reasoning is robust enough for each unique patient's disease, you may as well pursue the most likely clinical diagnosis.

Let us start with the common statistical terms.

Sensitivity and specificity

Sensitivity refers to the number of people in a group with the test result being negative, who truly do not have the disease.

Test result negative: sensitivity	Of every 100 patients with a negative test result, the sensitivity means…
100%	All do not have the disease.
90%	90 do not have the disease, and 10 do. The 10 who do have the disease, have a False Negative result.
50%	50 do not have the disease, and 50 do. The 50 who do have the disease, have a False Negative result.

Specificity refers to the number of people in a group with the test result being positive, who truly have the disease.

Test result positive: specificity	Of every 100 patients with a positive test result, the specificity means…
100%	All have the disease.
90%	90 have the disease, and 10 do not. The 10 who do not have the disease, have a False Positive result.
50%	50 have the disease, and 50 do not. The 50 who do not have the disease, have a False Positive result.

It is tempting to assume that if a test is 90% sensitive, where only 10% of the people with that result have the disease, the negative result in your patient means the chance of disease is 10% in your patient.

Likewise, it is tempting to assume that if a test is 90% specific, where 90% of the people with a positive result have the disease, the positive result in your patient means the chance of disease is 90% in your patient.

Such assumptions would be incorrect. The chance (if neither 0% nor 100%) of disease at the cohort level is not equal to the chance of disease at the individual level. For this (neither 0% nor 100%) chance of disease at the cohort level to be equal to the chance of disease at the individual level, the individual patients must be clones of each other, with identical clinical presentations.

Your patients are not clones of each other, with identical clinical presentations.

The actual probability of the disease in your patient is determined by 2 major factors:

- The pre-test probability of having the disease, modified by
- The likelihood ratio of the diagnostic test result.

The likelihood ratio is based on combining sensitivity and specificity, which allows an accurate application of the test result to the individual patient's pre-test probability.

If your clinical reasoning has been robust, the pre-test probability of the disease will be similar to your certainty of that clinical diagnosis. Robust reasoning enables you to apply the likelihood ratio of the diagnostic test to your clinical estimation, to obtain an accurate post-test probability.

Likelihood ratios

Likelihood ratios are numbers that increase or decrease the existing probability of an outcome.

As with sensitivity and specificity, each type of likelihood ratio is associated with a particular test result: positive versus negative.

If the test result is positive, you use the positive likelihood ratio for that test. The equation to calculate the positive likelihood ratio is:

> ### POSITIVE LIKELIHOOD RATIO
> **(For positive test results):**
>
> $$\frac{\% \, \text{Sensitivity}}{(100 - \% \, \text{Specificity})}$$

If the test result is negative, you use the negative likelihood ratio for that test. The equation to calculate the negative likelihood ratio is:

> ### NEGATIVE LIKELIHOOD RATIO
> **(For negative test results):**
>
> $$\frac{(100 - \% \, \text{Sensitivity})}{\% \, \text{Specificity}}$$

Combining the pre-test probability (% certainty of your clinical diagnosis) with likelihood ratios

Likelihood ratios are not directly equal to probability, and thus cannot be directly applied by multiplying the pre-test probability by the likelihood ratio to get the post-test probability.

There are 2 methods to combine the pre-test probability with the test result's likelihood ratio to obtain the post-test probability.

1. Fagan nomogram
2. Mathematical calculation

Fagan nomogram

To use the nomogram, mark the pre-test probability on the leftmost vertical axis, then mark the corresponding likelihood ratio on the middle axis. Using a straight edge (such as a ruler), draw a straight line connecting your 2 marks and extend that line to the rightmost vertical axis. The intersection of that line with the rightmost axis provides your post-test probability.

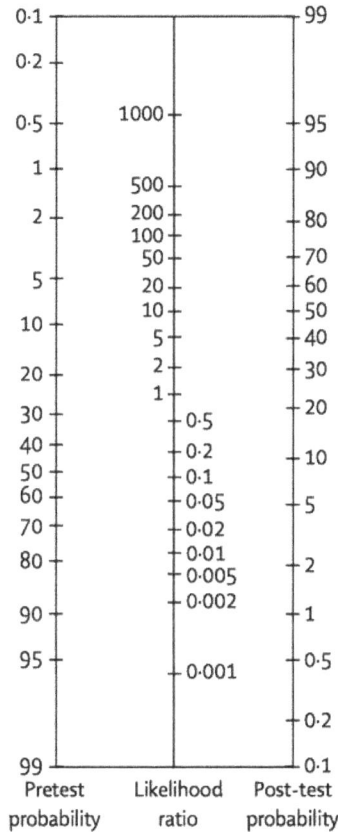

The figure on the next page shows the Fagan nomogram applied to a patient with a 60% pre-test probability of disease (leftmost vertical axis), with a positive test result and thus, application of a positive likelihood ratio of 4 (middle vertical axis). Drawing a straight line through both points gives a post-test probability of about 83% (rightmost vertical axis, arrowhead).

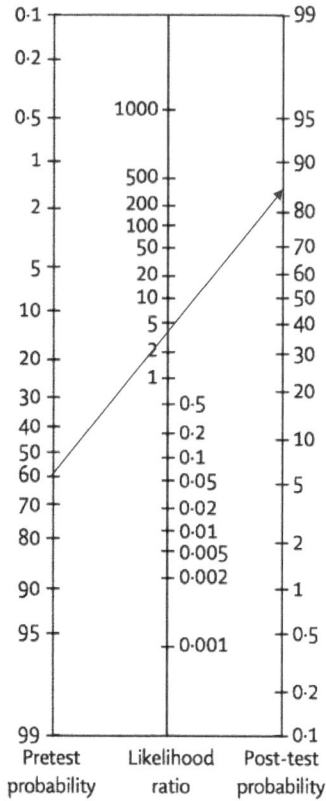

Pretest probability	Likelihood ratio	Post-test probability

Mathematical calculation:

Calculating the patient's post-test probability requires 3 steps:

1. Converting pre-test probability into pre-test odds, then
2. Multiplying your pre-test odds of having that disease with the corresponding likelihood ratio to obtain the post-test odds, then
3. Converting the post-test odds back to the post-test probability

Odds are the ratio of the chance of having an outcome, to the chance of not having that outcome. For example, if you threw a six-sided die, the odds of getting the number '6' on a throw, would be (chance of getting a '6': chance of not getting a '6') = 1:5.

If the pre-test probability of having acute appendicitis was 60%, the chance of not having acute appendicitis would be (100-60) = 40%.

Thus, expressing this pre-test probability as odds, becomes a chance of 60% 'has acute appendicitis' to a chance of 40% 'does not have acute appendicitis'.

The odds are expressed as 60:40, which can be simplified to 3:2.

You have 2 numbers, one to the left and one to the right of the colon.

Then, you multiply the number on the side that corresponds to your outcome of interest — this will usually be the number to the left — with the likelihood ratio of the diagnostic test result. This is the post-test odds.

In the last step, you convert the modified ratio back to probability, using the equation below:

$$POST\text{-}TEST\ PROBABILITY\ (expressed\ as\ \%):$$
$$\frac{Post\text{-}test\ Odds\ of\ Having\ Disease}{Combined\ Odds\ of\ Having\ Disease\ plus\ Not\ Having\ Disease} \times 100$$

Let us demonstrate mathematical calculation with an example: Rudra (Case #16 in the previous chapter).

Rudra had a pre-test probability estimate of acute appendicitis, at 60%.

The pre-test odds are 60:40 (60% chance of appendicitis to 40% chance of not having appendicitis), or 3:2.

He undergoes an ultrasound scan of the abdomen, which has an 80% sensitivity and 80% specificity for acute appendicitis.

You calculate the likelihood ratios of the results of the ultrasound scan for acute appendicitis. The positive likelihood ratio of the ultrasound scan is 4; the negative likelihood ratio is 0.25.

If the ultrasound scan is:

- Positive (the images suggest the patient has acute appendicitis): you apply the positive likelihood ratio to the pre-test probability estimate of acute appendicitis. The pre-test probability was the '3' to the left of the colon, so $(4 \times 3){:}2 = (12{:}2)$. Converting this into post-test probability with the formula above, this becomes $[12/(12+2)] \times 100 = 83\%$. The plotted Fagan nomogram earlier in this chapter mirrors this result. This post-test probability is high enough for most doctors to call the surgeons immediately.

- Negative (the images suggest the patient is unlikely to have acute appendicitis): you apply the negative likelihood ratio to the pre-test probability estimate of acute appendicitis. The pre-test probability was the '3' to the left of the colon, so $(0.25 \times 3){:}2 = (0.75{:}2) = (3{:}8)$. Converting this into post-test probability gives you $[3/(3+8)] \times 100 = 27\%$. This chance is too high for most doctors to dismiss the likelihood of acute appendicitis. This result would come as a surprise because you initially thought the most likely diagnosis was acute appendicitis.

If the ultrasound scan result was negative, this would be a surprising result. When a diagnostic test result is surprising, it is tempting to perform another test immediately. To rush into more tests or treatments, is usually a mistake.

Any surprise suggests that your initial clinical assumptions about the patient could be mistaken. The disastrous chain of dominoes suggests that making more decisions based on mistaken clinical reasoning would be imprudent.

Since your clinical assumptions were based on your clinical evaluation, you must revisit the patient's clinical evaluation and re-analyse the clinical information. If you recheck your clinical assumptions and there truly seems to be nothing wrong about them, the next step is to ask yourself if you have interpreted the test result correctly. The inability to explain the surprise should warn you to proceed with caution; it may be prudent to ask a robust reasoner for assistance.

No clinical diagnosis or inaccurate clinical estimate of the probability of the diagnosis

An accurate post-test probability for the diagnosis, requires an accurate estimate of the pre-test probability.

Thus, diagnostic tests are virtually impossible to use accurately if you have no clinical diagnosis, or your clinical estimate of the probability of the diagnosis is inaccurate.

Without any clinical diagnosis, you have no pre-test probability to use. If you tried to use the Fagan nomogram, there is no starting point on the left vertical axis. How are you going to draw the straight line using the test result, to reach the right vertical axis? If you tried to use mathematical calculation, your pre-test probability is '?', which makes accurate mathematical calculation impossible.

When doctors have no clinical diagnosis, they have 2 options:

1. Use the test result's sensitivity and specificity directly on the patient. Though this is not correct, this is better than wildly guessing.

2. Wildly guess the meaning of the test result.

Under these circumstances, most doctors seem to employ option 2; they wildly guess. I and my students have noticed that the doctors who do not make clinical diagnoses, also do not know the sensitivity and specificity of the test. The interpretation of the test result is 'if I see this result, I guess this is the diagnosis'. Sometimes the diagnosis that is guessed, has no relationship to the test result.

If your clinical estimation of the probability of the diagnosis is inaccurate, your final post-test estimate of disease likelihood will often be inaccurate too. Using the wrong starting point on the left axis on the Fagan nomogram leaves you with the wrong finishing point on the right axis. Using the wrong pre-test probability when attempting mathematical calculation, will leave you with an inaccurate post-test probability.

All of this demonstrates the chains of dominoes: accurate clinical diagnosis often accompanies accurate test result interpretation, whilst poor clinical reasoning predisposes to inaccurate (or no) clinical diagnosis and erroneous interpretation of test results.

Clinical information: clinical features and risk factors have maths too

By this point, your head may be swimming at all the numbers. Even more so when you realise that if you are going to perform more than 1 diagnostic test, there is more maths.

Clinical features and risk factors have their likelihood ratios too. If you tried to apply all the likelihood ratios of every symptom, sign and risk factor for each patient you saw, either using the Fagan nomogram or mathematical calculation, you would be overwhelmed even before considering the use of diagnostic tests.

I have seen senior educators debate this concern of the learners being overwhelmed. Some rightly say that learners must know the concept of likelihood ratios. Others contend that memorising all the numbers is impossible, then recommend that the teaching of likelihood ratios be avoided, thereby avoiding any concern about overwhelming the learner.

I agree with the educators who say that learners must know the concept of likelihood ratios. However, the maths *is* overwhelming. Teaching must be usable and practical for the learners, and not overwhelm them. I disagree with the suggestion that refusing to teach important concepts is justified because this avoids the chance of overwhelming learners. Perceived limitations about oneself or others regarding teaching ability, cannot justify a failure to seek help.

You may not have realised that the preceding chapters in this book had simplified all of that maths into patient-centred concepts. I have held off explicitly telling you about this simplification, until now. The diagnostic information categories and the 3 rules of clinical reasoning are the practical manifestations of this simplification of the likelihood ratios, for the clinical evaluation:

1. **The categorical priority of clinical features over risk factors:** These categories come from recognising that most Clinical Features have stronger positive and negative likelihood ratios than Risk Factors for the current diagnosis. In addition, most patients have more information about Clinical Features than Risk Factors, that can be used for their clinical diagnosis.

2. **Rule #1 of clinical reasoning:** Since Clinical Features have stronger positive likelihood ratios than Risk Factors, the Clinical Features are the focus for ruling in the most likely diagnosis. The more of the patient's Clinical Features and the details of those Features that you explain, the more positive likelihood ratios you are applying cumulatively to your most likely diagnosis. Thus, Rule #1 compels you to use all of these positive likelihood ratios to nail the most likely diagnosis.

3. **Rule #2 of clinical reasoning:** Universal clinical features of a disease have strong negative likelihood ratios. Thus, their absence strongly rules out that disease.

4. **Rule #3 of clinical reasoning:** Secondary specific clinical features of a disease have strong positive likelihood ratios. Thus, their presence strongly rules in that disease.

The clinical application of the odds ratios, done properly over years or not at all, explains the differences in behaviour and outcomes between robust reasoners and poor reasoners.

By trying to meet the basic diagnostic reasoning requirement, robust reasoners apply multiple likelihood ratios to their differentials during the clinical evaluation.

The robust reasoner's great certainty in the most likely diagnosis, makes diagnostic tests unnecessary in most patients and allows them to make confident, swift and effective decisions. These reasoners usually use tests to adjust treatment.

The most powerful reasoners use Rules #2 and #3 to apply the strongest likelihood ratios during the clinical evaluation. The intuitive application of these likelihood ratios leads to dramatic differences in certainty between the most likely diagnosis and every other relevant differential. Thus, reasoners who employ all 3 Rules, need diagnostic tests far less often than those who only employ Rule #1.

On the rare occasion the robust reasoner needs a diagnostic test, their intuitive understanding of the use of likelihood ratios in clinical evaluation, leads them to choose the most appropriate test. The choice of this diagnostic test may seem bizarre to everyone else who lacks the same reasoning and intuitive grasp of likelihood ratios. The robust reasoner usually interprets the results of diagnostic tests accurately. The correct conclusions are usually made, which then predispose to optimal decisions. This is the optimal chain of dominoes.

In contrast, poor reasoners tend to skimp on the proper clinical evaluation. Either there is a scant clinical evaluation, which leaves little useful information and thus few likelihood ratios to apply clinically, or the clinical evaluation is encyclopaedic, which reveals ignorance of the most useful diagnostic information. Regardless of how much clinical information the poor reasoner obtains, their poor reasoning predisposes them to cherry-picking information that is 'easier' to use, such as Risk Factors. However, Risk Factors have weak likelihood ratios. The poor reasoner then ignores most or all of the other information obtained from the clinical evaluation.

With no (or few) useful likelihood ratios applied to the differentials, the poor reasoner then relies on diagnostic tests. However, their neglect of the proper clinical evaluation and general inattentiveness towards information, returns to plague the poor reasoner. Without an accurate sense of the relevant differentials, diagnostic tests are often chosen erroneously. The lack of intuitive understanding of likelihood ratios during the clinical evaluation, predisposes to the misinterpretation of diagnostic test results. Mistaken conclusions are usually made, which then predispose to erroneous decisions. This is the disastrous chain of dominoes.

Capsule summary

- If diagnostic tests are required, the final probability of the disease is the pre-test probability modified by the likelihood ratio of the diagnostic test result.

- Surprising test results warrant a recheck of your clinical assumptions.

- The diagnostic information categories and 3 rules of clinical reasoning are the simplified and practical manifestations of the likelihood ratios, applied to the clinical evaluation.

DECISION THRESHOLDS FOR DIAGNOSTIC TESTING AND TREATMENT

Excellent decisions in personal and professional life are reliant on 2 universal factors:

1. Accuracy of gauging the current situation
2. Logical probability thresholds for each option

Translated into healthcare decisions for your patient, the same 2 universal factors become:

1. Accuracy of the current (clinical) diagnosis
2. Logical probability thresholds for each option in diagnostic testing and treatment

Section 1 has covered the 1st factor. This chapter will discuss the 2nd factor.

Each model is dedicated to 1 disease.

The x-axis indicates the probability of the disease. This axis spans from 0% (left side) to 100% (right side).

The Decision Threshold model

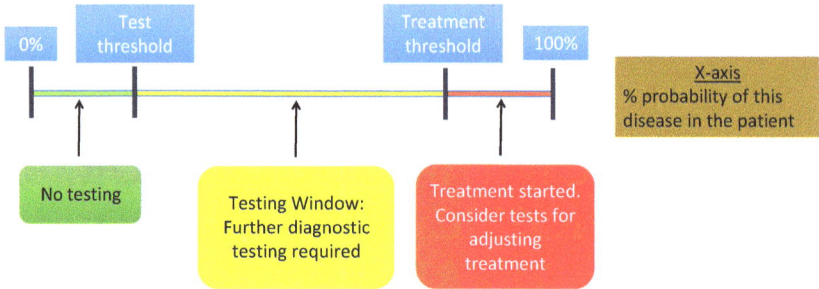

Each of the 2 decision thresholds is represented by a large blue box above the x-axis:

1. **Test threshold:** The minimum probability of this disease being present in the patient, to consider any testing.

2. **Treatment threshold:** The minimum probability of this disease being present in the patient, to consider commencing treatment.

The test threshold will lie to the left of the treatment threshold.

For each disease, the doctor decides the decision thresholds. These are pre-generated before meeting the patient, often from the sum total of the doctor's experience, knowledge and reasoning.

Each disease has its own model in the doctor's head. Thus, if the doctor has 100 diseases in their head, they have 100 models, 1 model per disease.

The 2 large blue boxes that represent these decision thresholds, occupy positions that can differ from 1 disease to another. The doctor with 100 such models would have the large blue boxes occupying 2 positions in the model for disease #1, 2 positions in the model for disease #2, and so on.

The x-axis is broken up into 3 coloured zones. The decision thresholds represent the border joining 2 adjacent coloured zones.

All probabilities of the disease below the test threshold lie to the left of the test threshold. This zone is coloured green. In any patient, should the probability of this disease lie below the test threshold (i.e. in the green zone), the probability is so low that diagnostic tests are not indicated.

All probabilities of the disease above the treatment threshold lie to the right of the treatment threshold. This zone is coloured red. In any patient where the probability of this disease lies above the treatment threshold (i.e. in the red zone), the probability is so high that commencing treatment should be considered. In this red zone, diagnostic tests are unlikely to add value to the patient's care. Sometimes, more information is needed before optimal treatment can begin. Any tests performed would be for adjusting treatment.

The yellow zone represents the window of diagnostic testing. Within this zone, the disease has a sufficiently high probability to warrant thinking about diagnostic testing. The probability is neither low enough to 'discard' the possibility of the disease, nor high enough to sensibly consider commencing treatment. Thus, diagnostic testing is performed to move the probability of that disease out of the yellow zone, into either the red or green zone.

Choosing diagnostic tests

If the most likely diagnosis is in the diagnostic testing window, rule-in tests should be performed. These are tests with strong positive likelihood ratios.

For all other differentials in the diagnostic testing window, which fulfil the 3 criteria to rule out, rule-out tests can be performed. These are tests with strong negative likelihood ratios.

The best tests for ruling in a disease may be different from the tests for ruling out that disease.

If diagnostic testing is warranted, ruling in the most likely diagnosis should be the first step, and often the only step, in most patients:

- If your reasoning is robust enough for the patient's disease, this is the highest-yield step.

- If your reasoning is inadequate for the patient's disease, then it is difficult to predict if anything you do would help much. Thus, you might as well go for the most likely diagnosis.

If the most likely diagnosis ever reaches the probability of 97% or more, the chance of any other disease is 3% or less. Thus, a very high probability of the most likely diagnosis effectively 'excludes' all other differentials automatically. At such high probability, the most likely diagnosis is usually in the 'red zone', which is enough to consider commencing treatment.

If the most likely diagnosis cannot be ruled in with near-100% certainty, and if a differential that lies in the yellow zone also fulfils the 3 criteria for ruling out, then the rule-out test for the differential should be employed.

There is 1 exception to this recommended sequence. In emergencies where:

- There is a differential that fulfils the 3 criteria to rule out,
- Major harm or death would occur if the dangerous-but-less-likely-diagnosis was correct but the doctor did not act promptly,
- There is no clinical information that can 'rule in' the most likely diagnosis with near-100% certainty, and
- The rule-in test for the most likely diagnosis would take more time than is prudent whilst
- The rule-out test for the dangerous differential would provide results in time to avoid major harm or death,

then performing an immediate rule-out test is required.

Let us illustrate using acute appendicitis.

We assign an 80% treatment threshold for acute appendicitis and a 30% test threshold for acute appendicitis. The next figure shows this threshold model for acute appendicitis.

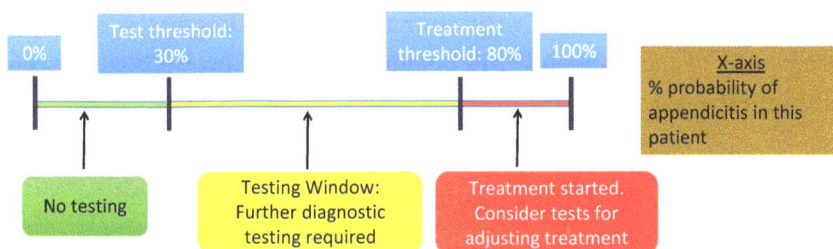

Let us go back to Case #15, which was described in the chapter 'Patient-centred testing'.

Case #15, Tranh, was a young adult with an overwhelmingly convincing picture of acute appendicitis. The relevant differentials and their certainty, were:

- Acute appendicitis — 97%
- Septic arthritis of the right hip — 2%
- Evolving viral gastroenteritis — 1%

What do you do?

Patient's diagnoses (probability): Appendicitis (97%), Everything else (3%)

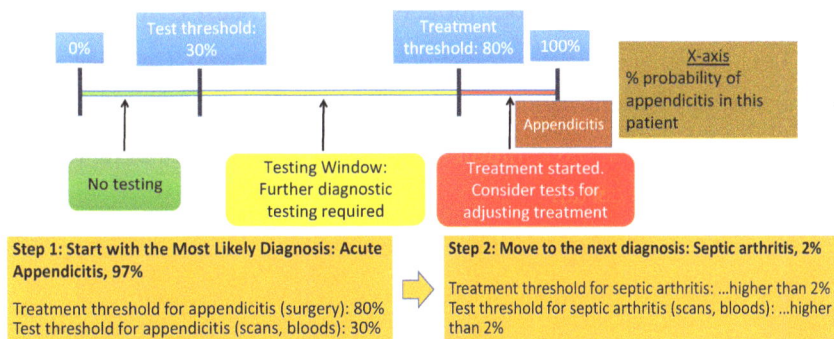

Above the model are your differentials for the patient. Below the model are the orange boxes depicting the thought process.

The first step begins with your most likely diagnosis. The 97% probability of acute appendicitis, is shown as a small brown box. The box falls into the red zone.

You are sure enough of the diagnosis of acute appendicitis that you consider commencing treatment. You call the surgeons, and keep the patient nil-by-mouth. The certainty of acute appendicitis (97%) is so high that the risks of delayed treatment outweigh the slim chance that diagnostic tests would suggest another diagnosis instead. The certainty of the other differentials is so low, that diagnostic testing or treatment for those would be inappropriate.

If you perform tests, they are aimed at adjusting treatment: can Tranh undergo surgery safely?

Translating your reasoning and actions into decision probability thresholds becomes: the probability of acute appendicitis exceeded your threshold for treatment. You commence treatment when the time is right, avoid delays, and ensure treatment is safe and adequate.

Considering any other differential becomes unnecessary. You could go through the same steps for septic arthritis and viral gastroenteritis, but no action would be warranted for those because their probabilities will fall into the green zone of your models for those diseases.

Let us apply the decision thresholds to Case #16, which was described in the chapter 'Patient-centred testing'.

Case #16, Rudra, was a middle-aged man where the most likely clinical diagnosis is not as certain:

- Early acute appendicitis — 60%
- Acute diverticulitis — 30%
- Viral gastroenteritis — 10%

The next figure shows the model for acute appendicitis with the same decision thresholds: 80% treatment threshold, and 30% test threshold.

The differentials for the patient are stated above the model. Below the model are the orange boxes depicting the thought process.

What do you do?

Patient's diagnoses (probability): Appendicitis (60%), Diverticulitis (30%)

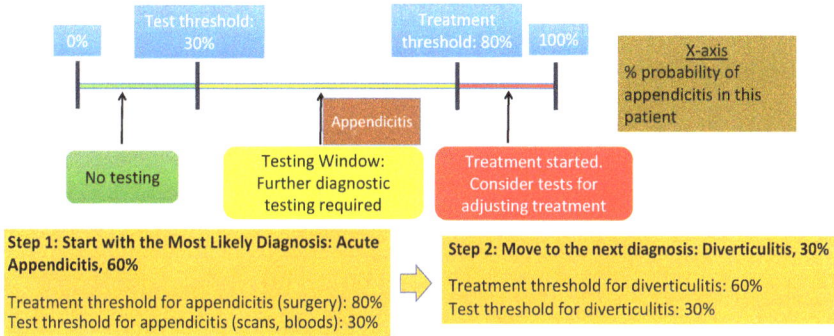

The first step begins with your most likely clinical diagnosis. The 60% probability of acute appendicitis in this patient is shown as a small brown box. The box falls into the yellow zone. You order rule-in tests for the most likely diagnosis, which is appendicitis.

You aim to rule in acute appendicitis until you reach the red zone of 80% probability or more, which is enough to consider commencing treatment. Thus, your rule-in test must have a strong positive likelihood ratio.

Translating your reasoning and actions into decision thresholds becomes: the probability of acute appendicitis sits in the diagnostic testing window. You require rule-in tests for this diagnosis.

You go to Step 2. You consider the next differential with the next-lower probability: diverticulitis.

The next figure depicts your thresholds for acute diverticulitis: 60% treatment threshold, and 30% test threshold.

What do you do?

Patient's diagnoses (probability): Appendicitis (60%), Diverticulitis (30%)

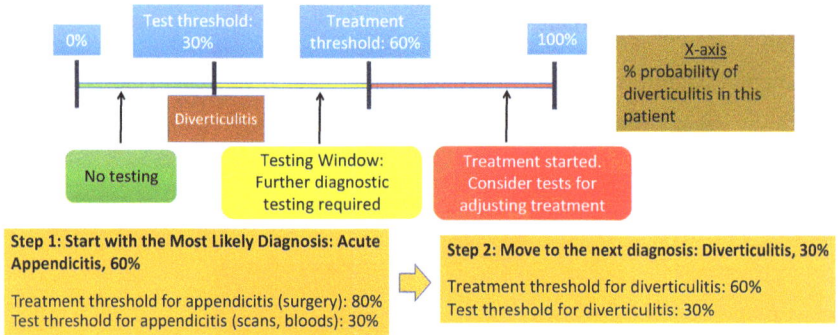

You put the 30% probability of diverticulitis on your mental model, as shown by the small brown box. This small brown box lies exactly on your test threshold of 30%. Most doctors would consider a probability sitting on the test threshold, to be in the yellow zone. You consider rule-out tests for diverticulitis.

Though you think the patient has acute appendicitis, you feel uncomfortable because there is a 30% chance of acute diverticulitis instead. Acute diverticulitis requires different management from appendicitis.

Since diverticulitis is not your most likely diagnosis, your ideal first step would not be to rule out diverticulitis. You aim to rule in acute appendicitis, first. If possible, you would like your rule-in diagnostic testing for acute appendicitis to simultaneously rule out acute diverticulitis. Some diagnostic tests can address both differentials, such as a CT scan of the abdomen.

You move on to your 3rd differential. Viral gastroenteritis is so unlikely (10% probability) that it falls into your green zone for your model for this disease. Even if the probability of viral gastroenteritis was high enough to be in your yellow zone, viral gastroenteritis does not fulfil the 3 criteria for ruling out anyway.

Considering your intent to 'rule in' appendicitis and 'rule out' diverticulitis, and the constraints of this patient (an ultrasound scan may be inaccurate in an obese patient like Rudra), you order a CT scan of the abdomen. You know your CT scan should be accurate enough to discern between appendicitis and diverticulitis.

If you want to order blood tests simultaneously, you must ask yourself: are the results of the blood tests going to add value to the diagnostic utility of the CT scan, or are needed for adjusting treatment once the CT scan result is available? If the blood tests do not add diagnostic value in this situation and are not needed for adjusting treatment, then performing these blood tests is, at best, a waste of resources.

Wait and see: watchful waiting

'Wait and see' is a viable option when facing diagnostic uncertainty. To undertake watchful waiting without performing any diagnostic tests, there must not be a dangerous diagnosis that falls into the yellow zone.

For example, if you had a patient with an 80% probability of viral gastroenteritis and a 20% probability of acute appendicitis and you decided this patient's 20% likelihood of acute appendicitis is below your testing threshold of 30%, diagnostic testing would not be indicated. However, a 20% chance of missing acute appendicitis would worry most doctors. Though you would not order diagnostic tests, you feel uncomfortable.

Thus, you recommend an extended observation period of 4–6 hours for watchful waiting and serial abdominal examinations.

How test thresholds are decided for each disease

How do doctors formulate their decision thresholds?

Part of the formulation is theoretical; the remainder of the formulation is often based on painful experiences.

The factors affecting test thresholds are:

1. Danger if this disease is not diagnosed promptly

2. Risks of the test, especially for patients who did not have this disease

3. Cost of the test, especially for patients who did not have this disease

If the delay or missing of a disease is likely to cause significant harm, the test threshold becomes lower. In the decision threshold model, this threshold moves to the left, widening the yellow zone for diagnostic testing. You are more willing to perform tests for patients who may not have this disease, because the consequences of delayed or missed diagnosis are worse than for common, benign diseases. The lower threshold means more patients who do not have the diagnosis will also undergo testing.

There is an intuitive limit to how low the threshold should go. The lower the threshold, the more often patients without that disease are tested. For example, you could set a test threshold of 1% for appendicitis and other dangerous diseases. This means any dangerous diagnosis with at least a 1% pre-test probability would require diagnostic testing. You will perform diagnostic tests on almost every patient, which will annoy many patients. Though some patients might seem willing to pay for batteries of tests initially, even these patients often stop coming to see you because they find other doctors who can get better outcomes without so much testing. Some patients will complain about you and warn other potential patients away from you.

If the test is risky (e.g. an invasive test or involves significant radiation such as a CT scan) or expensive, the test threshold becomes higher. In the decision threshold model, this threshold moves to the right. The yellow zone for diagnostic testing is narrower. Raising the threshold reduces the number of patients without this disease, who suffer the unnecessary risks and costs of the test:

- Invasive procedures carry risks such as bleeding and unexpected damage to other structures.

- CT scans slightly increase the chance of various types of cancer in the future.

For most of the common and dangerous illnesses with basic, safe and affordable tests, the test threshold might lie around 10% to 20%.

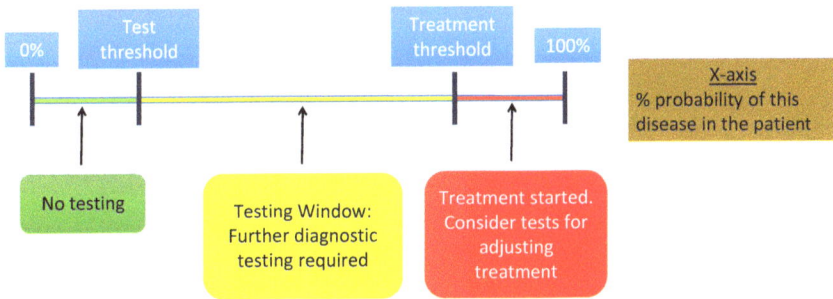

The changes in test thresholds will be illustrated by discussing diagnostic tests for leukaemia.

When considering a peripheral blood film (PBF) for a patient with leukaemia, the test threshold for this cheap, safe and noninvasive test would decrease because leukaemia can easily be fatal. In the threshold model, the test threshold for the PBF would move to the left. The yellow zone becomes wider. See the next figure.

Test threshold moves to the left

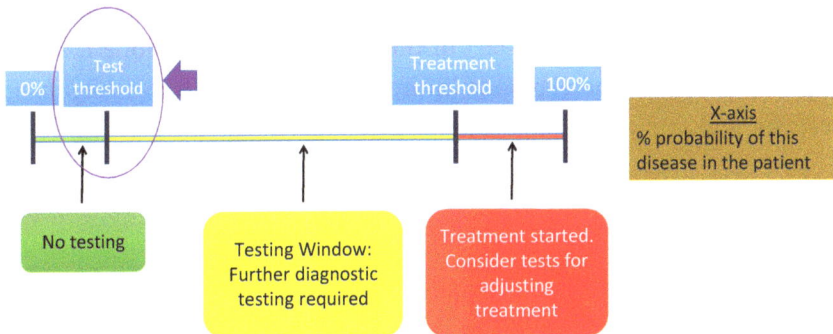

There are other diagnostic tests for leukaemia, such as a bone marrow aspiration (BMA). As the BMA is invasive and expensive, the decision threshold for the BMA increases. You want to reduce the number of patients without leukaemia, undergoing the BMA unnecessarily. In the threshold model, the test threshold for the BMA would move to the right. The yellow zone becomes narrower. See the next figure.

Test threshold moves to the right

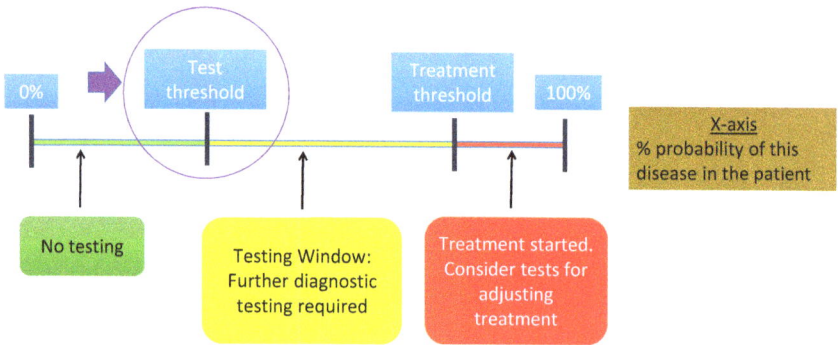

Multiple diagnostic tests, which means multiple test thresholds for a disease

Different diagnostic tests can exist for each disease. The threshold differs between basic tests and discussion-type tests for that disease. Basic tests are usually safe and relatively cheap, and thus have a lower threshold whereas discussion-type tests tend to be more expensive or risky, and thus have a higher threshold. The distinction between basic and discussion-type tests is further explained at the start of the next chapter. The bone marrow aspiration and peripheral blood film are examples of 2 different diagnostic tests for leukaemia.

Consider the next 2 cases.

CASE #17: Ria

Ria is a 16-month-old girl who received the measles-mumps-rubella vaccine 1 month ago. She presents with petechiae over her trunk for the past 1 week. There are no other symptoms. Her vital signs are normal. The only sign on examination is petechiae over her trunk.

Your differentials for her are:

- Idiopathic thrombocytopenic purpura — 90%
- Leukaemia — 10%

Assume that our decision threshold model for idiopathic thrombocytopenic purpura (ITP) has a 10% test threshold for a full blood count and a treatment threshold of 90%.

Ria has a pre-test probability of 90% for ITP. You are unable to rule in this diagnosis any further. Though she meets the treatment threshold of 90%, you need more information to decide on optimal treatment. Tests for adjusting treatment, such as a full blood count, can assist you.

You move to your next differential: leukaemia.

Assume that our decision threshold model for leukaemia has a 5% test threshold for a peripheral blood film (PBF) and a 30% test threshold for a bone marrow aspiration (BMA). The treatment threshold is 90%. Her pre-test probability of 10% for leukaemia, falls into the diagnostic testing window for the PBF (5 to 90%), but not the BMA (30 to 90%).

Thus, to rule out leukaemia in Ria, you would perform a PBF but not a BMA.

Given the low chance of leukaemia, which is just above the test threshold, a weak 'rule out' test like a PBF, if negative, will suffice to move the probability into the green zone. Once in the green zone, no further testing is necessary.

Ruling Out:

Diagnosis is Less Likely than the most likely diagnosis, but still in the Testing Window

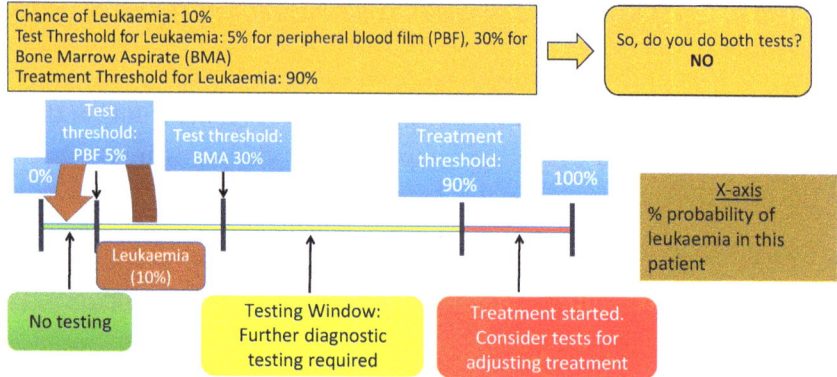

Since the most likely diagnosis is not leukaemia, instead of ruling out leukaemia, could you treat for ITP in such a way that leukaemia would not respond but ITP would? The treatment should not mask any disease activity from leukaemia. Thus, one could administer intravenous immunoglobulin (IVIG) but not steroids. Though both IVIG and steroids can be used for treatment of ITP, steroids can mask some of the activity of leukaemia.

If the patient responded to this treatment, the response has ruled in ITP. There would be no need for rule-out tests for leukaemia.

This 'rule-in-the-diagnosis trial of treatment' option is valid in scenarios where:

1. Treatment for the most likely diagnosis is warranted,

2. The treatment would work quickly if the most likely diagnosis was correct,

3. Waiting for the treatment to work would not significantly endanger the patient more in the event the correct diagnosis was the dangerous differential, and

4. The treatment would not mask the dangerous differential.

If this treatment worked, the treatment rules in the most likely diagnosis and simultaneously rules out the dangerous differential.

However, as IVIG is often expensive, Ria's scenario thus far does not warrant such treatment, and a PBF is cheap and safe, the more prudent next move in this scenario would be to perform the full blood count and a PBF.

CASE #18: Zoe

Zoe is a 16-month-old girl who received the measles-mumps-rubella vaccine 1 month ago. She presents with petechiae over her trunk for the past 1 week. There are no other symptoms. Zoe's appetite has also decreased in the last 3 days. Her vital signs are normal. On examination, there is petechiae over her trunk. There is hepatomegaly, the soft liver being palpable 4 cm below the right costal margin. She seems happy and playful.

Your differentials for her are:

- Idiopathic thrombocytopenic purpura — 60%
- Leukaemia — 40%

Zoe's clinical picture is concerning. Though you think she has ITP, why does she have decreased appetite and hepatomegaly, which cannot be explained by this disease? You eventually decide on a probability of 60% for ITP and 40% for leukaemia.

Assume that we use the same decision threshold model for ITP: a 10% test threshold for a full blood count and a treatment threshold of 90%.

You are unable to rule in ITP any further, and she does not meet the threshold for treating ITP.

You move to your next differential: leukaemia.

Using the same decision threshold model for leukaemia with a 5% test threshold for a PBF and a 30% test threshold for a BMA, her pre-test probability of 40% for leukaemia lies in the diagnostic testing window for both tests. You would perform a PBF and a BMA to rule out leukaemia. If you performed a PBF alone, even a negative PBF result would not suffice to move her post-PBF probability into the green zone.

Ruling Out:

Diagnosis is Less Likely than the most likely diagnosis, but still in the Testing Window

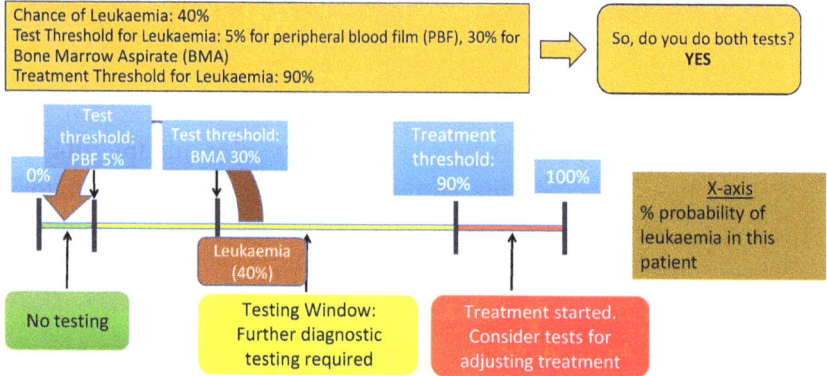

Chance of Leukaemia: 40%
Test Threshold for Leukaemia: 5% for peripheral blood film (PBF), 30% for Bone Marrow Aspirate (BMA)
Treatment Threshold for Leukaemia: 90%

So, do you do both tests?
YES

Test threshold: PBF 5%

Test threshold: BMA 30%

Treatment threshold: 90%

0%

100%

X-axis
% probability of leukaemia in this patient

Leukaemia (40%)

No testing

Testing Window: Further diagnostic testing required

Treatment started. Consider tests for adjusting treatment

This case demonstrates the need for a stronger rule-out test when there is a higher pre-test probability of a dangerous disease. Moving a higher pre-test probability of disease into the green zone often requires 'discussion-type' tests, because these tests tend to have the strongest negative likelihood ratios.

How treatment thresholds are decided for each disease

The factors affecting treatment thresholds are:

1. Danger if this disease is not treated promptly

2. Risks of the treatment, if administered to a patient who did not have this disease

3. Cost of the treatment, if administered to a patient who did not have this disease

If a disease causes significant harm in the event of no or delayed treatment, the treatment threshold becomes lower. In the decision threshold model, this threshold moves to the left. The yellow zone narrows and the red zone widens. You are more willing to commence treatment for patients who may have this disease and less willing to wait for the results of diagnostic tests, because the consequences of delayed or missed treatment are worse than for common, benign diseases.

If the treatment is risky (e.g. chemotherapy for cancer) or expensive, the treatment threshold becomes higher. In the decision threshold model, this threshold moves to the right. The red zone narrows and the yellow zone widens. The increased risks or costs require you to be more certain before you give this treatment to a patient. Without raising the threshold, these risks and costs would be imposed on more patients who did not have this disease.

For many common illnesses with cheap and safe treatment, the treatment threshold might lie around 60%.

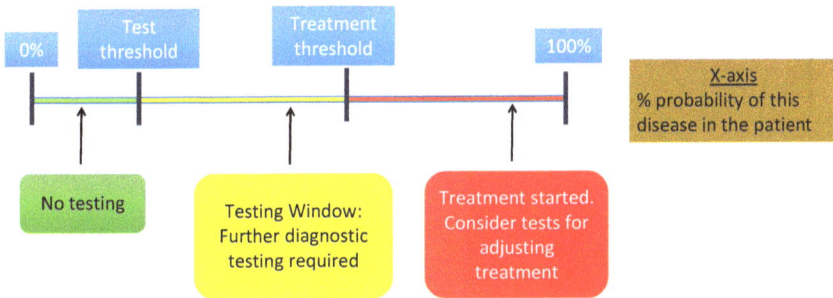

If the disease had a significant chance of causing permanent harm or death, the treatment threshold would become lower. In the decision threshold model, this threshold moves to the left. The red zone widens. An example would be bacterial meningitis; at 50% probability, many doctors would commence treatment. See the next figure.

Treatment threshold moves to the left

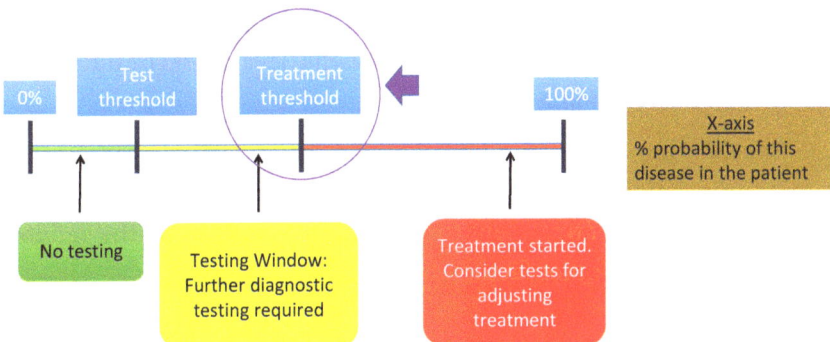

Conversely, if the treatment for the disease is risky or expensive, the threshold to treat is higher. In the decision threshold model, this threshold moves to the right. The red zone becomes narrower. An example would be chemotherapy for leukaemia. Even though leukaemia is dangerous, chemotherapy has significant costs and side effects. You want as few patients as possible to erroneously receive chemotherapy. See the next figure.

Treatment threshold moves to the right

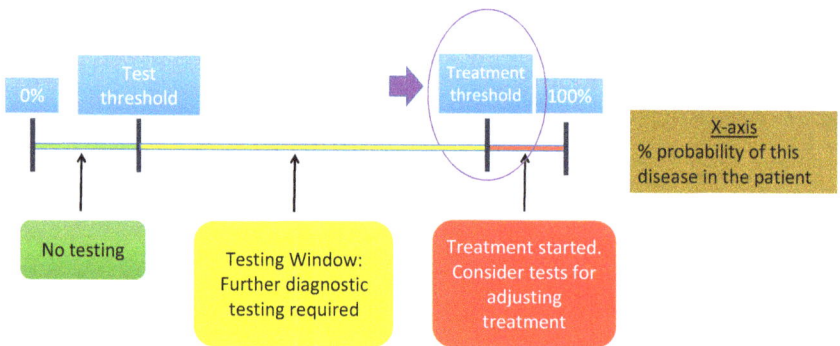

Multiple treatment thresholds for disease?

In theory, there are multiple treatment options for some diseases, so you could use decision thresholds to choose between these options.

In practice, this is illogical. Though different treatment options do exist for each disease, the fundamental principle of effective treatment is: treatment intensity must at least match disease severity. The choice among different treatment options is secondarily affected by the balance of acceptability, costs and risks of each treatment. Treatment considerations are discussed in Section 3 of this book.

The decision threshold model is useful for providing a gauge of the minimum certainty to consider commencing treatment for that disease. The specific choice of treatment (or treatments) depends on the patient's disease severity and other factors instead of probability.

Must we always perform the tests and treatment immediately, if indicated by the decision threshold model?

The answer: No.

The threshold model provides a logical way of deciding whether diagnostic tests and treatment are indicated. The red zone suggests starting treatment, but it is sometimes necessary to gather more information to decide the optimal treatment.

As Case #17 (Ria) showed, the clinical information and disease severity did not mandate immediate treatment. More information might be needed to estimate the activity of the disease, hence the suggestion of performing a full blood count. Another treatment option for ITP is wait-and-see, which does not have the side effects and high costs associated with administering IVIG. Wait-and-see in ITP, is often a viable option.

For Case #18 (Zoe), the rule-out tests include performing both a PBF and BMA. In theory, a BMA alone would suffice. However, many doctors often perform both because the PBF is cheap and on very rare occasions, the BMA can report a false negative result. If the PBF shows lymphoblasts before the BMA has been scheduled, the most likely diagnosis becomes leukaemia instead and changes the management plan, even before the BMA has been performed. The BMA is still necessary if Zoe is deemed to have leukaemia clinically, because samples from the BMA can provide important information for adjusting her treatment.

Not using these thresholds: how decisions are made illogically

There are 2 common ways decisions can be made without using thresholds:

1. Not assigning an estimated probability/certainty to your diagnosis and differentials

2. Having no diagnosis and differentials

When the doctor has differentials but decides not to use probability, the decisions can be entirely whimsical. Even if these decisions can seem relevant to one or more differentials, a robustly reasoning observer (or patient) will realise that the doctor is prioritising other factors to make decisions, such as the inconvenience of ordering a test being the basis of the doctor refusing to order a test, or the prospect of profit, which drives the doctor to order expensive treatments.

When the doctor has no diagnosis or differentials, the doctor makes decisions based on either wild guesses, or ulterior motives, or both.

Capsule summary

- Decision thresholds are useful for making decisions about diagnostic tests and treatment.

- Ruling in the most likely clinical diagnosis should be attempted first.

- Rule-out tests are a consideration only if a disease fulfils the 3 criteria for ruling out.

- The tests chosen depend on the probability of that disease in that patient.

- Decision thresholds are not useful for deciding between different treatment options for a patient.

- Without using decision thresholds, indiscriminate ordering of tests and treatment becomes easy.

Frequently asked questions

Q: Which test (which carries significant risks, especially if repeatedly performed on the same patient) is most often ordered unnecessarily, without regard to logical decision thresholds?

A: CT scans. CT scans are useful and convenient because they can be performed quickly, and they can pick up signs of many diseases. These factors make them tempting for doctors who wish to rule out OAF.

A robust reasoner often can make the diagnosis clinically, thereby making the CT scan unnecessary. Robust reasoners order CT scans only when necessary.

In contrast, poor reasoners blithely order CT scans to rule out OAF. Since misinterpretation of test results is more common in poor reasoners, this indiscriminate ordering of CT scans predisposes to missing the diagnosis in 3 common ways:

1. A CT scan is ordered even though the scan is not accurate for detecting or differentiating between the patient's relevant differentials. The poor reasoner readily misinterprets the subsequent negative CT scan result as 'there is no dangerous problem'.

2. A CT scan is ordered for relevant differentials where the CT scan is usually accurate. 'Usually accurate' is not 'always accurate'; a CT scan is neither 100% sensitive nor specific for most diseases. Poor reasoners readily assume that the CT scan has 100% accuracy. When the CT scan comes back negative for Disease X despite the clinical features pointing to Disease X, the poor reasoner insists Disease X cannot be present 'because the CT scan was negative'. The unspoken, additional fallacy in their insistence is 'clinical features are unimportant compared to the tests'.

3. Even when the CT scan shows signs that point to another disease, the poor reasoner who is fixated only upon their list of diseases, can readily ignore the warning information on the radiologist's report of another (sometimes dangerous!) disease.

Each CT scan slightly increases the risk of cancer in the patient. Doctors who rule out OAF often demonstrate a callous disregard for this risk to patients. They can order multiple CT scans in the same patient over the course of a few weeks, significantly increasing the chance of future cancer in that patient whilst finding nothing on the scans.

Thus, the misuse of CT scans and the harm inflicted on patients by poor reasoners who indiscriminately order these scans, demonstrate the universal truth: tools are often useless, and sometimes dangerous, in the hands of the unskilled.

Furthermore, over-ordering of unnecessary CT scans can result in many patients being sent for these CT scans. The demand for CT scans places a huge strain on the CT scanners and staff (radiologists, radiographers, hospital porters, and so on). As a result, truly urgent and important CT scans are often delayed for the patients who needed them.

When a leader in education told me about the increased demand for scans and radiologists in his country, I replied: 'You can spend more money on training and paying radiologists, and buy more imaging machines. However, that does not solve the problem: the reasoning of the doctors ordering the scans. Thus, the patient outcomes will not get better.'

COUNSELLING: TESTS

Tests can be divided into basic tests, and discussion-type tests.

Basic tests fulfil 3 criteria:

1. Non-invasive

2. Safe

3. Cheap

Examples include most of the commonly used blood tests, urine tests, stool tests, and X-rays.

Discussion-type tests will not fulfil all 3 criteria. Thus, these tests require strong justification and a discussion with the patient:

1. Invasive tests have small risks of significant harm and often cause pain, frequently prompting the use of drugs to mitigate this pain.

2. Tests that have small risks of significant harm, such as a higher chance of cancer after a CT scan, must have those risks weighed against the expected value that the tests add to the patient's care.

3. Open, prompt communication requires the cost of expensive tests to be explained to the patient.

Examples of discussion-type tests include:

- Blood tests: tumour markers, functional stimulation tests (endocrine, immunological), genetic, serological testing
- Invasive: endoscopies, biopsies
- Imaging other than X-rays: ultrasound scans, CT, MRI, PET scans.

Counselling

Informed consent is a requirement for all patient-centred healthcare (not just in surgeries and procedures).

I define informed consent as a discussion that adequately informs the unique patient of the viable options, and explores that patient's concerns to the best of the doctor's ability.

Informed consent for treatment purposes is slightly different than for testing purposes. In addition, counselling can encompass discussions on tests and treatment in tandem, contingency plans, and require additional customisation beyond what is discussed in this chapter. All of this is explained in more detail in the chapter 'Treatment decisions'.

When counselling on tests, explain these 4 points in sequence:

1. The nature of the test
2. The change in the management plan that is expected after seeing the test results
3. The approximate cost of the test, or combined cost of all tests if performing more than one
4. The approximate time on the same day, or the approximate date that the results become available

Basic tests often do not require much discussion. Many patients are familiar with these tests. Even when they are not familiar with the tests, patients who trust their doctor usually go along with the doctor's recommendation of basic tests. Thus, counselling on all 4 points for basic tests is often unnecessary. However, if the patient is seeing you for the first time or seems unconvinced by your diagnosis or management, do explain the 4 points.

Discussion-type tests require an explanation of all 4 points. Given the more specialised nature of these tests, this explanation helps to reassure the patient.

In an emergency, such as a CT scan of the head for an unconscious patient with suspected intracranial haemorrhage, it may not be feasible to talk to the patient or a representative of the patient, to cover all 4 points.

1. The nature of the test: The purpose of the test and how it is performed. Patients want to know the risks and the implications of abnormal results.

2. The change in the management plan that is expected after seeing the test results: The test should dramatically change the certainty of the diagnosis or a differential, or provide crucial information for optimal treatment.

3. The approximate cost of the test: Expensive tests are not affordable to some patients. Common mistakes include assuming the patient will always pay for all tests regardless of cost, or that wealthy patients will not mind paying huge bills. Some wealthy patients are wealthy because they are financially prudent, and thus dislike being treated as rich, unthinking clients who have money to throw away.

4. The approximate time (or day) the results become available: Patients dislike waiting for results. Patients dislike it even more when the doctor does not tell them when the results become available. In an age where results can be obtained electronically, knowing when to look out for these results, and when to realise something is amiss when the results do not appear, does matter. Some countries such as Singapore have individual-linked online portals for each person's health results.

Discussing alternative plans for diagnostic tests

In some situations where diagnostic uncertainty is present, there are up to 3 viable options:

1. Wait and see
2. Perform the most accurate single diagnostic test

3. Perform other tests initially, instead of the most accurate single test

Wait and see is safe only if all relevant differential diagnoses have been considered, and the doctor remains vigilant for any changes in the patient. This option is usually not exercised when a diagnostic test is warranted, unless the patient has refused the test.

Perform the most accurate single diagnostic test is ideal, provided this test is available. However, sometimes this single test may be expensive or carry significant risks, especially if it is an invasive test such as an angiogram or biopsy.

Perform other tests initially, instead of the most accurate single test is an alternative when the most accurate single test is unavailable, is far more expensive or carries much more risk than the other tests. If the most accurate single test does exist, the combined accuracy of the alternative tests is often less than the accuracy of the most accurate single test.

See the following case:

CASE #19: Daphne

Daphne is a 3-year-old girl who was clinically diagnosed with chicken egg allergy at the age of 1 year. She had presented with perioral urticaria, 30 minutes after ingesting one-quarter of a hard-boiled chicken egg at first exposure. The skin prick test at that time showed a 4-millimetre (mm) wheal (positive result) to egg white and yolk. Since then, she has been taking baked egg products without reaction, and avoided all other foods that contain egg. At her previous follow-up visit a year ago, her skin prick test result to egg white and yolk was a 3-mm wheal (still positive). These tests indicated the allergy was probably still active.

She visits the allergy specialist's clinic today for a follow-up. Her parents report that she had eaten half a hardboiled egg 1 week ago, without their knowledge at that time. They were told of the ingestion afterwards. She did not develop any allergic reaction.

(Continued)

Her parents have reported a clinical picture consistent with a rising Threshold of Reactivity (ToR) (described in the example at the end of the chapter 'Gathering additional information to manage patients'). Their account suggests she is outgrowing her egg allergy. It is unknown if she would react upon eating larger quantities of egg protein, or egg protein that is less cooked. The specialist concludes she is outgrowing her egg allergy.

The viable options are:

1. Wait and see: let her eat more eggs at home, slowly and carefully?

2. Perform the most accurate single diagnostic test: a supervised egg challenge in the allergist's office or hospital.

3. Perform other tests initially, instead of the most accurate single test: a repeat skin prick test.

Wait and see: The allergist can discuss the option of letting her eat a fully cooked egg at home in slowly increasing amounts, watching carefully for reactions each time, with antihistamines on standby. With proper advice and caution, and given her initial presentation, severe allergic reactions would not be expected. The allergist can recommend avoiding half-cooked and raw eggs until the next clinic visit 1–2 months later. This avoids the time and money spent on diagnostic tests. If attempting this option, the allergist must be accurate in their prediction and advice.

Perform the most accurate single diagnostic test: The allergist offers a supervised challenge to egg in a healthcare facility. This is the safest and potentially fastest way of verifying her outgrowing of the allergy. Allergists recommend this when they sense the child's parents are scared of letting the child eat egg in any form, even if it is certain the child can tolerate egg. If she reacts, the challenge also allows direct estimation of her new ToR. Half-cooked or raw egg can be considered for the challenge.

(Continued)

(Continued)

Perform other tests initially instead of the most accurate single test: The allergist performs a skin prick test to the egg. If the skin prick test result remains positive to both egg white and yolk, this puzzles the allergist because the history from the parents clashes with this result. The allergist should recheck the history and consider another indirect marker of the presence of egg allergy, such as a specific Immunoglobulin E test. Conversely, if the skin prick test wheal is negative, which correlates with the clinical diagnosis, the allergist is more confident about recommending either of the first 2 options.

The viable options are dependent on the patient's diagnosis.

If Daphne had presented with anaphylaxis (a severe allergic reaction) upon exposure to a small amount of egg, the diagnosis would be a severe egg allergy because she has a low ToR. Without overwhelming proof that the egg allergy is gone, a careful allergist would hesitate to recommend that her parents try giving her significant amounts of egg at home.

Informing patients of test results

In many settings, patients have gone home when the results become available.

Calling the patient for a brief update and discussion instead of demanding they return to the doctor's office, helps everyone: the patient saves time and money because they do not have to return to see the doctor, and the doctor can give the consultation slot that this patient would have filled, to another patient.

Physically recalling the patient to the office/hospital may be necessary if the doctor deems the results warrant a significant change in plans (and hence, a discussion) or a careful explanation of the significance of those results.

Capsule summary

- Counselling for tests should cover the nature and cost of the test, the anticipated change in plans after seeing the test result, and the approximate date/time of availability of the result.

INTERPRETING TEST RESULTS

The results of tests usually reflect the underlying pathophysiology of the patient's disease. Pathophysiology explains the test results being abnormal or normal.

All test results must be interpreted in the clinical context of that patient: their clinical features and the most likely clinical diagnosis. Interpretation of diagnostic test results also requires consideration of the differential diagnoses.

Without this clinical context, misinterpretation is common.

Clinical context: how it helps the doctor and the patient

The clinical context helps you ascertain the accuracy and significance of the test result. Textbooks and references list the multiple possible causes of each abnormal test result. The clinical context of the patient with that result instantly narrows the list down to one or a few causes for that patient.

Without the clinical context, the 'possible interpretations' of each test result multiply severalfold, which leads to a higher chance of misinterpreting the result. Common examples include the 'patch on the chest X-ray', anaemia and electrolyte abnormalities:

- A patch on the chest X-ray is not always caused by pneumonia.

- Anaemia has multiple textbook possibilities, but the reasonable possibilities (often, only one) in that patient are based on the patient's clinical context.

- Electrolyte abnormalities are often mismanaged because poor reasoners 'treat the numbers' and make wild guesses, instead of paying attention to the clinical context.

Radiological reports can end off with a reminder: 'Please correlate clinically'. To a robust reasoner, this reminder is unnecessary because it is the same as saying 'the sky looks blue'. All test result interpretation, radiological or otherwise, requires clinical correlation.

Though this reminder may be intended to remind poor reasoners of the importance of clinical context, poor reasoners tend to fixate selectively upon parts of the radiological report, and ignore the reminder too.

For example, a doctor who is fixated on ruling out appendicitis can order a CT scan of the abdomen, and then pay attention only to the part of the report that mentions the appendix. If the report says 'the appendix is normal' and simultaneously mentions abnormalities in other structures that point to the correct diagnosis, the poor reasoner either:

- Does not read the rest of the report, or

- Reads the report and deliberately ignores the other abnormalities, or

- Jumps to the wrong conclusion about the abnormalities.

Recall Conversation #5 in the chapter 'Common mistakes in the clinical approach': Dora encountered experienced doctors who kept ignoring her clinical context to fixate on 'scary' diseases.

Thus, the accuracy of the doctor in interpreting test results is dependent on their clinical reasoning.

Robust reasoners recognise that deducing the most likely clinical diagnosis enables the appropriate choice of tests and interpretation of the test results. Thus, they undertake the interpretation of results within the clinical context of the patient. Any struggle with the clinical diagnosis warns them to tread carefully when interpreting the test results. Rather than order batteries of tests when a patient's diagnosis is unclear, they are more likely to seek help first. The optimal chain of dominoes shows itself.

Poor reasoners skim through or ignore the patient's clinical scenario, tend to order irrelevant tests, and tend to misinterpret the results of these tests. Ironically, poor reasoners often assume their choice of tests and their interpretation of test results is accurate — 'It is a number, just treat the number!' and 'The cause can only be this (insert wild guess)!' The disastrous chain of dominoes shows itself.

Poor reasoners can insist on clinging to their beliefs and defending their decisions even when their decisions consistently lead to suboptimal outcomes for the patient.

In contrast, robust reasoners who mistakenly ignored even a fraction of the patient's clinical context to prioritise test results, tend to notice when they have gone astray. Robust reasoners are likely to realise and thus, avoid repeating their errors.

Surprising test results

If the doctor is on the right track for the patient, there should be no surprises most of the time.

Thus, any surprise, be it a test result or lack of expected improvement in the patient's condition, is a warning sign that the doctor's clinical approach, diagnosis, and subsequent decisions may be in error.

There are 2 reasons for any surprise:

1. Flawed clinical reasoning (the most common)

2. Lack of knowledge

Poor reasoning and ignorance tend to coexist in poor reasoners. Even when poor reasoners are knowledgeable, their indiscriminate inattention to almost everything (sometimes, even to their own knowledge) effectively leaves them ignorant. Having knowledge is often pointless if you do not know how to prioritise or adapt it to each patient.

Poor reasoners habitually ignore inconvenient information. Unfortunately for them and their patients, 'surprises' also fall under the category of inconvenient information. Thus, the poor reasoner often ignores surprises and continues blithely on their disastrous course.

Robust reasoners use surprises as warning signs to themselves, often rechecking their clinical evaluation and assumptions. This is how robust reasoners promptly detect their mistakes, change course, and rescue the situation.

False positive and false negative results

False positives are interpretations of test results that suggest the disease is present, even though the disease is absent.

False negatives are interpretations of test results that suggest the disease is absent, even though the disease is present.

There are 2 consistent ways that doctors discover false positive and false negative results:

1. Retrospective. They managed the patient as per their interpretation of the test result but the patient did not respond as expected. Eventually, the final diagnosis and truth of the false positive/negative test result become clear.

2. Prospective. They recognise the false positive/negative result there and then for what it is, and are not misled. This requires robust reasoning.

The retrospective way is unpleasant and potentially dangerous.

The prospective way usually occurs after a decent reasoner is prompted by the surprising result to recheck their clinical assumptions. If the doctor realises there was truly no error in their clinical approach and diagnosis, they then realise the surprising test result is likely to be a false positive or false negative result.

The most powerful reasoners are rarely surprised by test results, partly because they choose the most appropriate tests and partly because their interpretation of the test results has 'shifted' away from the commonplace norms to match the patient's clinical context. These reasoners can look at a test result that everyone else has interpreted using common population-level norms, and instantly recognise that the correct interpretation for that patient is different from everyone else's interpretation. Their instant recognition of the truth is based on a combination of attentiveness to the patient's clinical context, an intimate understanding of pathophysiology, encyclopaedic knowledge, and proficiency in the universal equation (this equation is discussed in the chapter 'Diagnosis: disease, severity and treatment'). The subsequent outcome of the patient inevitably proves that this reasoner was correct, whilst everyone else who interpreted the test result conventionally was wrong. Most tests, including laboratory tests and imaging tests, can be interpreted in this patient-centred way.

For example, the unwell patient with an unknown diagnosis may have a full blood count result that seems totally normal. Everyone else looks at the result and thinks the full blood count does not show anything significant. The powerful reasoner who is walking by is asked to look at the same result. This reasoner asks for the patient's clinical context and ongoing treatment while looking at the result, and then clinically diagnoses the patient with a dangerous illness that no one else thought of. This reasoner proceeds to explain why the full blood count result looks normal, points out the seemingly normal cell parameter which is a clue to the correct diagnosis, and then suggests the definitive test for that diagnosis. The definitive test result comes back positive.

Consider Conversations #8 and #9.

Conversation #8

Doctor T, a junior doctor of the ward, presents the patient to his consultant: 'This 30-year-old lady has been admitted for acute myocardial infarction. She presents with episodic chest pain lasting several minutes each episode, on the right side of the chest, associated with difficulty breathing and palpitations. The symptoms began yesterday.'

Consultant: 'Are there pain-free intervals between the episodes of pain?'

Doctor T: 'Yes.'

Consultant: 'Is her heart on the right side?'

Doctor T: 'Uh…I think it's on the left. I did not check.'

Consultant: 'Your diagnosis does not make sense. Why did you say "myocardial infarction"?'

Doctor T: 'The cardiac enzymes were elevated!'

Consultant: 'That would not be surprising. In episodic tachycardias. Especially for the duration of the episodes you described. At a sufficiently high heart rate for a sufficiently long time, perfusion of the myocardium can be compromised enough to injure the myocytes. How high was the heart rate during the episodes?'

Doctor T: 'It went as high as 190 beats per minute in the Emergency Department, which was also captured on the ECG.'

Consultant: 'The cardiac enzymes would have been mildly elevated, then.'

Doctor T: 'Er, yes. They were. We referred to Cardiology overnight, and they also disagreed with the diagnosis of acute myocardial infarction. They…said what you said.'

Consultant: 'Sure. More importantly, what did the cardiologist say about the diagnosis and plans?'

Conversation #9

Doctor E is confused about an 80-year-old lady who was hospitalised. The patient has been lying in bed for the past 3 weeks. She is bedbound and not communicative verbally. She was admitted for a generalised tonic-clonic seizure, attributed to scar epilepsy. New symptoms and signs appeared soon after admission, the diagnosis being unknown. Multiple specialities were consulted, with no answer.

Doctor E asks me: 'Hey, I have a patient. I cannot explain her hyponatremia. The SIADH results were puzzling. We do not know the diagnosis either. Can you help?'

Doctor E shows me the test results. There are a few hundred test results, accumulated over this admission and the past few months from other admissions to the hospital.

By the 30th result, I have a headache.

Me: 'Stop. I am getting a headache. I cannot figure out the patient's diagnosis based on these, and I have no idea why she has hyponatremia.'

Doctor E: 'Why not?'

Me: 'Let us assume we are in a city. A stranger drops their wallet on the ground. This wallet contains money, and nothing else. Could you pick up this wallet, look at the money inside, and then guess the exact occupation of this stranger?'

Doctor E: 'Of course not!'

Me: 'Trying to figure the occupation out from the money alone, is the same as guessing a puzzling diagnosis using test results alone. Let us do it my way. Go clinically.'

Doctor E: 'Okay.'

Me: 'What are the patient's symptoms and signs?'

Doctor E: 'She was admitted for a seizure, likely due to scar epilepsy. Soon after admission, she gradually developed ascites. We noticed pedal oedema.'

Me: 'Was the ascites ascertained clinically?'

Doctor E: 'No, the other doctors just ordered a CT scan to "find the cause of abdominal distension". They don't examine patients as we were taught in medical school. I did find the ascites clinically.'

Me: 'If tests are ordered so indiscriminately, no wonder there are so many test results. Clinical skills that are not used, will fade away. Can I at least assume you clinically checked for the symptoms and signs of the causes of ascites? Since you did not mention signs of congestive cardiac failure, liver failure or kidney failure, can I assume there were no signs of these?'

Doctor E: 'Yes, and yes.'

Me: 'And there were no other symptoms?'

Doctor E: 'Correct.'

Me: 'Then she probably has nephrotic syndrome. This often causes distension and pedal oedema with a paucity of other symptoms or signs. Was a urine test for protein quantity, performed?'

Doctor E looks through the pages of results. 'Hey, yeah! She has nephrotic-range proteinuria. Oops, we missed seeing this result. It was there 2 months ago, at the previous admission! That also explains the low serum albumin we have been seeing for the past 6 months. She has been admitted more than once and we have been rechecking the albumin intermittently.'

Me: 'Missing test results, often happens when many tests are ordered indiscriminately. Some results get missed in the flood of test results. Or the doctor who ordered the test, ignored the test result. Now, let us think for a bit. We are dealing with a disease that can result in nephrotic syndrome, especially in an elderly person, with no other overt symptoms. What is the most common chronic disease in our population that does not cause overt symptoms and affects the kidneys like this?'

Doctor E thinks through the diseases of affluence, then says: 'Diabetes mellitus. Oh. The high sugar levels! And HbA1c!'

Me: 'They were high?'

Doctor E: 'Yes. The HbA1c was 10%. Endocrine was called in to titrate the insulin.'

Me: 'So it is uncontrolled diabetes mellitus with diabetic nephropathy, resulting in nephrotic syndrome. Would that explain her clinical picture?'

Doctor E: 'It does not explain her hyponatremia.'

Me: 'It would, if she had chronic hypovolemia. You said her serum albumin had been low for months.'

Doctor E: 'Yes. She has been bedbound. Thus, we assumed she did not get enough nutrition because we assumed her family might have been neglecting her. I don't think we checked her nutrition or diet. Okay, we should not have assumed so much. Er, we also did not see the nephrotic-range proteinuria result ever since it came out 2 months ago.'

Me: 'How long was the pedal oedema present?'

Doctor E: 'Not sure. Someone just documented it when the ascites appeared. We probably were not looking for it. Might have been there before admission, even.'

Me: 'I suspect so. Inadequate clinical evaluation and excessive testing often coexist. Bear with me, we are almost done. If she had nephrotic-range proteinuria and was chronically hypovolemic in the intravascular space, what would her body do?'

Doctor E: 'Produce antidiuretic hormone.'

Me: 'And if the body must keep producing antidiuretic hormone for a long time to preserve volume, what does that do to the serum sodium eventually?'

Doctor E: 'Oh! Water is conserved preferentially, so the serum sodium goes down! That would explain the hyponatremia! And the puzzling results of our "SIADH workup", which looked like appropriate ADH secretion instead of SIADH. Gosh, you have explained all the test results! Now we know what is going on, and what to do!'

Me: 'You are welcome. Remember: go clinically. First. And always. And please do not copy the behaviour of these doctors. I taught you to be better.'

--

Both conversations demonstrate the folly of prioritising test results over the clinical context.

To use test results as the mainstay of reaching the correct diagnosis, is inefficient and sometimes impossible. Using the test results to guess the diagnosis, is to indulge in wild guessing.

Always go clinically, first.

If you can explain the patient's entire clinical picture with your clinical diagnosis, the test results are often unsurprising and easy to understand. Case #14 in the chapter 'Pathophysiology in reasoning' illustrates this too.

The next case illustrates the common fixation on testing, accompanied by the usual inability to interpret the results accurately.

CASE #20: Kim

Kim is a 12-year-old boy who presented to the Children's Emergency with the presenting complaint of a headache and fever.

He had 5 days of fever. The fever reached a maximum of 39 degrees Celsius.

The headache was in the frontal region and radiated to the back of his head every day. The headache was worse with coughing. The headache did not wake him from sleep. No other information was obtained about the headache.

He had a mild cough with rhinorrhea in the first 4 days of the illness. The cough and rhinorrhea resolved spontaneously after the 4th day.

His father had a headache and fever about 4 days before the onset of Kim's symptoms. His father recovered within 2 days.

The physical examination was unremarkable. An ovoid erythematous area over his forehead was explained as a birthmark by his parents; other members of the family had marks like that too.

The doctor diagnosed Kim with a viral upper respiratory tract infection because his father had rhinorrhea and cough recently.

The full blood count was performed to 'confirm' this diagnosis. Acetaminophen and Ibuprofen were administered for symptomatic relief. The full blood count returned normal. His parents were told that Kim had a viral infection 'because the full blood count shows a viral picture'. Kim was discharged from the Children's Emergency Department.

Six days later, Kim returned to the Children's Emergency at night. The fever and headache were unchanged. The headache improved slightly and transiently with each dose of Ibuprofen. Additional questioning revealed that the headache was unremitting. Kim's appetite and energy levels had worsened since the last visit. There were no other symptoms.

On examination, his vital signs were normal. The previously noticed 'birthmark' on his forehead was tender. The rest of the examination, including a neurological examination, was normal.

Kim was labelled with 'prolonged fever for investigation', and hospitalised.

The on-call team — the doctors handling all admissions — assessed him. Additional history from Kim's parents suggested uncontrolled perennial allergic rhinitis: years of daily rhinorrhea, nasal itch and congestion.

The label remained the same: 'Prolonged fever for investigation'. The doctors decided to perform blood tests to determine if this unknown illness was dangerous.

The full blood count returned with mild leukocytosis (13×10^9 cells/litre) and neutrophilia (9×10^9 cells/litre). C-reactive protein was elevated (90 mg/L). Procalcitonin was unremarkable, at 0.11 micrograms/litre.

The doctors decided this patient probably had a prolonged viral infection with headache because:

- There were no 'red flags' of raised intracranial pressure.
- The neurological examination was normal.
- Procalcitonin was normal.

- The abnormal full blood count and C-reactive protein results could be seen in viral infections.

When the ward consultant arrived for the morning rounds, Kim's information and the abovementioned arguments for viral infection with headache were presented to him. He glanced at Kim, then pointed to the birthmark.

Consultant: 'How do you explain this tender swelling over the forehead?'

The consultant then told Kim's family that there was probably a serious bacterial infection in the frontal sinus that invaded the bone: Pott's puffy tumour. An urgent MRI scan revealed frontal sinusitis, osteomyelitis of the frontal bone, a small subdural collection, and signs suggestive of frontal lobe meningitis. Kim received high-dose intravenous Ceftriaxone. Multiple specialities became involved in his care.

He received 6 weeks of intravenous Ceftriaxone. He was cured.

One week after discharge, he was readmitted for episodic severe abdominal pain lasting 2 days, mainly in the epigastric region, which caused him to curl up in pain. There was 1 episode of vomiting. This was his 6th such episode, with previous episodes occurring during his 6-week stay for intravenous Ceftriaxone. No other history was taken about the presenting symptoms. On examination, he was screaming in pain. The doctors were unsure if he had mild tenderness over the epigastrium and right hypochondrium.

He was diagnosed with gastritis, because 'this is the most common cause of abdominal pain in children and this was the diagnosis made for the previous 5 episodes'. Given the presence of tenderness involving the right hypochondrium, an immediate referral to the paediatric surgeon was made to rule out a liver abscess. A battery of tests — full blood count, C-reactive protein, liver panel, amylase and procalcitonin — was performed. Only the liver panel returned abnormal: the aspartate aminotransferase (AST) and alanine transaminase (ALT) were both elevated. The AST was 480 units/litre and the ALT was 600 units/litre. A bedside ultrasound scan did not show a liver abscess.

Kim was labelled as having 'acute liver injury'. He was hospitalised and remained in pain overnight.

The following morning, the junior doctors of the ward brought the ward consultant (a paediatric subspecialty consultant who had pitched in to help Kim in the previous admission) to see Kim.

Doctor Z told the consultant: 'You have seen this child before.' The scant clinical history was presented. Before Doctor Z could present the test results, the ward consultant stopped her.

Consultant: 'You say this pain happened multiple times during the 6-week-long stay recently?'

Doctor Z: 'Yes.'

Consultant: 'The diagnosis back then was…?'

Doctor Z: 'Gastritis.'

Consultant: 'Did the treatment for every episode of presumed gastritis, work?'

Doctor Z: 'Uh, no. He remained in severe pain for hours, every time. The pain eventually stopped within 12 hours each time, so we assumed it was gastritis.'

Consultant: 'If you do the same thing over and over again, it is insanity to expect a different result. This is universal wisdom. In healthcare, if the treatment fails even once, the diagnosis should have been questioned! Never mind presuming the diagnosis was correct despite treatment failure for 5 episodes! Well, the pain is clearly the biggest concern. Tell me more about the pain.'

Doctor Z: 'Uh, we did not take any more history.'

Consultant: 'Okay. Then I will take the history myself.'

The consultant walks up to Kim, who is sitting in bed. The pain is temporarily better; he is not screaming. The consultant asks a few questions. He listens to the answers and quickly palpates Kim's abdomen. Two minutes later, he turns around.

Consultant: 'The pain is over the epigastrium and sometimes the right hypochondriac region. It occurs an hour or so after meals, especially fatty meals. I did not find any signs on examination. This is biliary colic!'

Doctor Z: 'Wow. That would explain the funny liver panel results. Uh, do you want the liver panel results? And the other test results?'

Consultant: 'This is a clinical diagnosis. I doubt the other test results change the diagnosis. It is unsafe to ignore test results, so I will look at them later. For now, we must focus on his diagnosis and relevant management.'

Doctor Z: 'Biliary colic is rare in children! Kim is not fat or female!'

Consultant: 'Yes. What was the antibiotic he received?'

Doctor Z: 'Ceftriaxone.'

The consultant waits impassively. After about 10 seconds, Doctor Z then realises aloud: 'Oh, Ceftriaxone predisposes to gallstones!'

Consultant: 'See? You have the knowledge. However, knowledge alone is not enough. Kim's diagnosis is clear just from taking a proper history of the symptoms, and then thinking about the relevant differentials. Please do not assume the most common diagnosis you see in everyone else, is the diagnosis for every patient forever. Patients are not clones of each other.'

'Please call the paediatric surgeons. Keep Kim nil-by-mouth for the operation. Obtain a hepatobiliary ultrasound to assess the gallstones, as the surgeons will want that before surgery. He has suffered long enough.'

The ultrasound scan came back demonstrating gallstones. Kim underwent surgery successfully, with no further episodes of biliary colic over the next 3 years.

--

Case #20 demonstrates the difference between robust and poor reasoning. In both admissions, the answer was always clinical: thinking of the relevant disease, and then performing the targeted evaluation that nails the correct diagnosis.

Poor reasoners readily believe fallacies such as 'the tests are always accurate' or 'we only need to focus on ruling out a checklist of dangerous diseases'. Thus, they often skimp on the clinical evaluation.

Tests are tools. Tools require skill to use well. Poor reasoners lack skill. Thus, tests are often misused by poor reasoners.

If you did not think of the correct diagnosis, you would not look for it. In history, in physical examination, and in testing.

Even if the poor reasoner 'gets lucky' by accidentally choosing the appropriate test as part of the battery of tests, their poor reasoning and disregard of the clinical context predispose to the ignoring or misinterpretation of the results.

Implications of a colleague who asks about or interprets tests without interest in the clinical context or existing clinical diagnosis

Given the abundance of testing in high-tech healthcare, there is ample opportunity to realise that tests must be interpreted whilst considering each patient's clinical context. Failure to undertake this patient-centred interpretation is inexcusable for many reasons. The existence of this book is one such reason.

A colleague who shows little or no interest in the patient's clinical context even as they discuss test results, is often a poor reasoner.

Four common manifestations of poor reasoning when discussing test result interpretation, include:

1. The senior doctor asks the junior to interpret a test result for a patient, whilst withholding the clinical context and the clinical diagnosis. This senior only seems interested in the junior's recitation of the textbook list of 'all possible causes of the result' (i.e. knowledge) instead of the ability to interpret the result to help that unique patient (i.e. clinical reasoning)

2. The colleague who makes a referral based on 'an abnormal test result' whilst omitting most of the clinical information and diagnosis.

3. The junior doctor or medical student who, when asked to interpret a test result, does so without referring to the clinical context.

4. The colleague who knows both the result and clinical context, but only reports the test result without mention of the clinical context. If asked about the clinical context or clinical diagnosis, they often hesitate or fail to answer.

Poor reasoners are often not interested in the clinical context, even though that clinical context is necessary to interpret the test result correctly and recommend appropriate action.

Thus, all their actions are automatically dubious. Even if the poor reasoner is a 'messenger' for another doctor who evaluated the patient, a poorly reasoning messenger can readily mislead and misinform you. Poor reasoners tend to misunderstand or ignore the information they were instructed to pass on, and sometimes change the message to suit their beliefs.

The 4th manifestation is sometimes accompanied by intentional deceit. This is especially so when the poor reasoner is asked about the clinical context. Poor reasoners are often surprised by such questions, thinking: 'I did not think the clinical context is important. Why should you care about it?'

Rather than admit their inattention to the patient's clinical context, they fabricate answers on the spot. What these poor reasoners fail to realise is that a robust reasoner who notices their surprise, instantly realises that the poor reasoner cannot be trusted. Any attempt at deception confirms the poor reasoner cannot be trusted *and* readily deceives their colleague, regardless of the risk of tragedy for the patient and that colleague.

Though most of these manifestations take place over teaching encounters or routine work without obvious tragedy, the same cannot be said when a handover of patients occurs in this fashion.

Implications of a handover focused on tests, without interest in the clinical context

Doctors take over the care of patients when they rotate to new locations, and change shifts during the day (also known as going on-call). 'Handover' refers to the process of conveying information to the next team of doctors taking over the care of the patients.

The strongest of my former students often complain about poor handovers by doctors, junior and senior. These handovers focus on tests and test results, whilst omitting the patient's clinical context.

There are 2 patterns:

1. The test-obsessed doctor asks the next doctor to trace a pending test result and then take action on the result, but cannot give the clinical context or a proper diagnosis, either of which is needed to choose the optimal action.

2. The test-obsessed doctor tells the next doctor about an abnormal test result, then suggests often irrelevant (and sometimes, dangerous) actions to execute over the next few hours to days. The clinical context which is needed to predict the consequences of such actions is inaccurate or absent.

When the first pattern is seen, the test-obsessed doctor can be vague about the test result and the decisions too. The classic example is: 'If the patient has a fever, send off the CRP and ESR. If the inflammatory markers are high, start antibiotics.' No other information is provided. The receiving doctor does not know what the primary team is thinking about the cause of the anticipated fever, does not know the cutoffs for the C-reactive protein (CRP) and erythrocyte sedimentation rate (ESR) that the team had in mind, and does not know the primary team's preference for the specific antibiotic(s). If the receiving doctor is a robust reasoner, this doctor realises that the absence of specific information during the handover is not a coincidence. The primary team is unsure of the diagnosis, unsure if the patient will have a fever, unsure of the interpretation of the inflammatory markers, and probably does not even know that the inflammatory markers are less important than reviewing the patient clinically.

Handovers are often at pre-arranged times with an unspoken time limit. The receiving doctor is supposed to focus purely on understanding and crystallising the information. However, if the doctor who is handing over cannot be trusted in anything they say, a decent reasoner must find someone else who can perform a proper handover, or go and check the patient themselves. This situation puts the recipient in a difficult spot, because other doctors want to hand over their patients and then go home instead of waiting for the recipient to check every poorly handed-over patient.

The consequences of poor handovers are common and painful for the next team of doctors. At best, poor handovers occur because the messenger is a poor reasoner. More often, poor handovers occur because the entire team of doctors is reasoning poorly; the patient is already being mismanaged, which increases the chance of unpleasant developments. The team of poor reasoners then sends one of their team members to hand over their patients.

If the next team of doctors does not go to check these patients for themselves, they can expect nasty surprises such as sudden deteriorations, collapses, and explosive outbursts by angry patients whose concerns were repeatedly brushed aside by the previous doctors.

Here is 1 example.

Doctor R goes on-call. Going on-call means that she is on duty from 5 p.m. to 8 a.m. the next morning, whilst the other doctors taking care of various patients in the hospital go home. These doctors hand over their patients to Doctor R at 5 p.m.

Though a decent reasoner, Doctor R just graduated from medical school 1 month ago. She has not yet experienced the terrible shocks that can take place after a poor handover.

An elderly man is handed over as 'trace the result of the renal panel that was performed at 4 p.m.', with no other information.

In this hospital, registrars are mid-rank specialist trainees who are often the most senior doctors staying in the hospital overnight. The same handover is given by the registrar of the day team to the registrar of the on-call team, with an additional reassurance: 'Nothing will go wrong. This patient is stable.'

The renal panel results return at 6 p.m. and are normal, so Doctor R thinks her job is done for that patient.

At 7 p.m., Doctor R is called by an alarmed ward nurse. She is told that the patient for whom she had seen the normal results on the renal panel, is 'still breathless despite being on 15 litres of oxygen via a non-rebreather mask'.

Doctor R is horrified. Doctor R realises the implications of the word 'still' in the nurse's panicked words: the day team knew about the patient's breathlessness and put the patient on intensive oxygen therapy, yet did not hand over this critical information to the on-call team.

Doctor R knows this patient is on the verge of collapse; this exact scenario was taught in medical school. Doctor R wonders how the entire day team, which includes experienced doctors, could lack such basic knowledge. The other unpleasant and most likely possibility is that the day team had this knowledge, but ignored it: 'Anything is possible. Maybe the patient will miraculously get better on their own and the problem will go away. If the patient collapses during your shift, that is your problem to handle. Not mine.'

Doctor R rushes over to see the patient and checks the medical notes of the day team. Doctor R gets more shocks. The patient had been hospitalised, sick and bedbound for over a month. The patient had been having pain in the left calf for the past few days, which was labelled as 'leg pain for investigation'. The patient was breathless since 2 p.m. and was placed on increasing amounts of oxygen in the ward, but remained breathless. The impression in the medical note since the onset of breathlessness was 'fluid overload' (which is not a proper diagnosis), based on the patient having a positive fluid balance of +300 mL per day.

A 300 mL positive fluid balance is not a valid reason to label 'fluid overload' in an adult. Look up 'daily insensible fluid loss'.

There was no record of any history to back up the label of fluid overload. The physical examination stated 'the lungs are clear', with no other mention of significant positives or negatives expected in 'fluid overload'. A chest X-ray earlier that day was normal.

In summary, Doctor R realises there is no diagnosis and no evidence to back up the label of fluid overload. Furthermore, the patient was placed on oxygen support 'for symptomatic treatment', starting at 5 litres per minute. When the patient did not feel better, the day team increased the oxygen flow to 15 litres per minute. Pulse oximetry readings ranged from 94 to 96% whilst on oxygen supplementation. The patient was given intravenous diuretics, which brought the fluid balance on paper down to -100 mL by 5 p.m. but did not help with the breathlessness. The label of fluid overload was casually made for the sake of writing something, anything. The 'leg pain for investigation' was to be investigated with an ultrasound scan of the calf 2 days after Doctor R's current shift.

No one challenged the senior doctors' impression or decisions. None of this crucial information, known to the day team, was handed over to Doctor R or anyone else in the on-call team.

Doctor R thinks through the scant information in the day team's notes and performs a rapid, focused clinical evaluation. Doctor R makes the clinical diagnosis of a pulmonary embolism due to a deep vein thrombosis of the left calf. A passing doctor tells Doctor R that he just saw the day registrar in the hospital, and this registrar is probably still in the hospital for reasons unknown.

Expecting the day registrar to be more familiar with the patient's condition than the on-duty registrar, Doctor R calls the day registrar to convey her diagnosis and plans.

The day registrar:

- Scolds Doctor R for 'not doing an electrocardiogram because the patient is tachycardic at 110 beats per minute, and you must always rule out an arrhythmia in a patient with tachycardia'. (Following this advice is illogical and wastes precious time.)

- Scoffs at Doctor R's suggestion that the patient has a pulmonary embolism. He says a pulmonary embolism is impossible because the coagulation times were elevated a few days ago. (This assertion is nonsensical.)

- Tells Doctor R that the pulse oximetry levels are above 93%, therefore there cannot be anything seriously wrong with the patient. (The intensive oxygen supplementation was 'masking' the patient's true severity of the disease. Even with this supplementation, oximetry readings of 94–96% are not normal. Doctor R knows this, but her far-more-experienced senior does not.)

- Disagrees with everything Doctor R suggests. Instead, the day registrar suggests a broad array of non-specific lab tests, and then orders Doctor R to talk to the on-call registrar.

Realising that talking to the day registrar is futile, Doctor R calls the registrar-on-call in the hospital to convey her diagnosis and plans. This registrar angrily tells Doctor R: 'You must be talking rubbish. The day registrar said nothing will go wrong and the patient is stable. The renal panel was normal too, right? So there cannot be any danger, right?'

Doctor R realises the day registrar intentionally misled the registrar-on-call with a false reassurance about the patient's condition. Is the day registrar fixated on appearing in control and confident, to the point of being inattentive to the patient and the consequences of deception?

Doctor R realises her seniors are not reasoning, cannot interpret basic tests accurately, and do not want to hear bad news. Doctor R pleads with the on-duty registrar to come to see this patient for himself. He does so. When he sees the patient, he is worried about the patient's vital signs but cannot figure out the diagnosis. Even though he is baffled and panicking, he does not believe Doctor R's diagnosis. This registrar calls the specialist consultant in charge of the patient to ask for advice.

Meanwhile, Doctor R executes her plans. Doctor R ignores the day registrar's suggestions because she has realised that this senior doctor cannot be trusted. The on-duty registrar does not stop her because he does not know what to do anyway.

The consultant-in-charge takes the call from the registrar, is alarmed and orders the patient to be immediately intubated and transferred to the Intensive Care Unit (ICU). The ICU consultant rushes over to see the patient. The ICU consultant becomes annoyed when he realises the patient has been deteriorating since mid-afternoon without any effective assessment or management.

In patients with dangerous diseases, the delay in appropriate care often leads to catastrophic deterioration, which then creates more work for the doctors.

The ICU consultant tries to speak to the senior doctors who were supposed to be taking care of the patient. Unsurprisingly, none of them knows what is going on. Finally, Doctor R briefly stops what she is doing for the patient, walks up to the ICU consultant and hands over the patient properly.

The patient is near to collapse when he arrives in the ICU. Had Doctor R not intervened, the patient would have collapsed soon afterwards in the general ward.

The results of the urgent tests that Doctor R ordered return, which back up the result of the subsequent urgent CT pulmonary angiogram (also ordered by Doctor R). The patient has pulmonary embolism.

These results greatly help the ICU team. Delays in requesting the appropriate tests and by extension, obtaining their results, would have impaired the care of this patient.

All this while, Doctor R was tied down with the necessary work to help this patient and the ICU team. Hence, the other less-sick patients who were entrusted to Doctor R had to wait whilst she took care of this patient.

Doctor R goes home the next day, exhausted. She is silently satisfied with herself, but is annoyed and disappointed in her seniors. Doctor R says nothing to her seniors about her feelings.

When Doctor R returns to work the day after, she is taken aside and scolded by the day team for 'not responding on time to the nurses on-call'.

The nurses on-call had called Doctor R that night for non-urgent requests about other patients. Doctor R had been unable to contact another doctor on-call who could promptly help with the nurses' requests. Thus, Doctor R told the nurses to wait because she had to prioritise the patient who was about to collapse. The nurses complained to the day team about having to wait for Doctor R.

The day team knew that:

- They had failed to assess and manage the patient appropriately.
- They had failed to hand over this sick patient properly, and intentionally misled the on-call team.
- Doctor R did the work they were supposed to do, which they did not do.
- The nurses were complaining because Doctor R had been held up doing the work the day team should have done.

Instead of admitting their responsibility to the nurses, they told the nurses that they would reprimand Doctor R. When speaking to Doctor R, the day team did not acknowledge their responsibility for the mess. The day registrar did not apologise for their behaviour towards her during the call. No word of thanks is uttered to Doctor R.

Doctor R stoically weathers the unprofessional and ungrateful behaviour of her seniors. She realises they are pretending they did nothing wrong. She realises they are like this because they have chosen to behave like this for years: never admitting their mistakes and thus never learning to be better.

She resolves never to become like these seniors. She realises the sloppy medical notes, the illogical impression and the poor handover are all due to poor reasoning and apathy. She resolves to always check for the clinical context, especially when a handover is poor.

Several less-accurate tests are performed instead of the single most accurate test: interpretation of results

'Perform other tests initially, instead of the most accurate single test' may be an alternative when the most accurate single test is unavailable, is far more expensive or carries much more risk than the other tests. If the most accurate single test does exist, the combined accuracy of the alternative tests is often less than the accuracy of the most accurate single test.

When the clinical context clashes with the interpretation of the alternative tests' results, be careful. Surprises often mean your clinical reasoning was insufficient or flawed for that patient. Recheck your clinical evaluation and assumptions. If you remain certain the clinical diagnosis was indeed correct, proceed with the single, most accurate test.

For example, a minority of patients with acute myocardial infarction have normal ECGs and cardiac enzymes. The doctor who obeys Rule #1 of clinical reasoning and clinically recognises a myocardial infarction, would not be fooled by these normal results. This doctor would order a more accurate test for these patients, such as the myocardial perfusion scan (called a 'cardiac MIBI scan'). If the reasoning was robust, the MIBI scan result will match their clinical diagnosis.

One such case was presented by a student during a universal clinical reasoning lesson in 2021. The ECG and cardiac enzymes were normal. However, the universal clinical reasoning template pointed to myocardial infarction as the only likely clinical diagnosis, which the MIBI scan subsequently affirmed.

Capsule summary

- Interpretation of all test results for a patient must be in the clinical context of that patient.
- If the test result appears to clash with your clinical diagnosis, recheck your assumptions about the patient and the test result.
- Tests are tools. Their proper use and interpretation are dependent on your reasoning.
- A surprise should always prompt a recheck of your clinical assumptions.

Frequently asked questions

Q: Conventional teaching around test results often ignores the clinical context. How is this ignorance of the clinical context, harmful?

A: Teaching that does not mirror effective clinical practice, is misleading and can be worse than no teaching at all.

If clinical reasoning is ignored, any hypothetical approach is easy to concoct and justify because it is detached from reality.

Teaching and educational resources can mimic local practice, instead of striving to improve local practice. Such teaching derives from common human instincts: familiarity is appealing.

Prioritising familiarity is ideal when relaxing, but problematic when trying to improve the competence of learners.

By showing learners what they usually see anyway and are comfortable copying, instead of teaching them what they need for improvement, the teacher puts the learners in an echo chamber that may improve the teacher's popularity but fails to improve healthcare.

Many American education resources, including commercial platforms, demonstrate a test-heavy, devoid-of-clinical-context format.

When teaching is test-heavy and devoid of the clinical context, clinical reasoning is nonexistent.

When this teaching is widespread, the poor healthcare outcomes in some countries are unsurprising.

When this teaching also creates an echo chamber for the learners, the *continued* poor healthcare outcomes in these countries are unsurprising.

Common examples of test-heavy, devoid-of-clinical-context teaching include approaches to:

- Hypokalemia
- Hyponatremia

- Liver transaminitis
- Type 1 respiratory failure
- Type 2 respiratory failure

…and so on.

Examples of the test-heavy, devoid-of-clinical-context scenario, either on a platform or in face-to-face teaching, include:

- 'What is your approach to Type 1 respiratory failure? By the way, you do not know anything about the patient. You know nothing about the symptoms or signs, and you cannot see the patient.'
- 'Read this X-ray and tell me what the patient has. You do not know anything about the patient's symptoms or signs and you cannot see them.'

Trying to guess the patient's diagnosis based on lab results alone (either with a single result or a few hundred results) is like using the currency in a random wallet found in a city, to try to guess the owner's job: absurd and often impossible.

The robustly reasoning students complain about such absurdities in teaching. They also stay away from all such teachers and commercial platforms. I applaud their reasoning and wisdom. A patient is not a lab test or X-ray result. Illogical teaching can be worse than no teaching at all.

Even the argument 'What if the patient was found unconscious? So you cannot take a history?' ignores the fact that the patient *was found,* period. Otherwise, there is no patient to perform tests upon, to give you a result to interpret.

The description of the patient when he/she was found, the vital signs or even the physical examination will clinically narrow the differentials, decide the appropriate tests, and help to explain the test results.

How do these detached-from-real-world lessons and platforms affect their learners' reasoning?

These lessons and platforms discourage reasoning. By ignoring clinical reasoning whilst purporting to teach the proper approach or interpretation of test results, they indirectly tell users that reasoning is not required for accurate interpretation of test results. Ignoring reasoning is bad enough, but discouraging it is even worse.

As of the end of 2022, lucrative education markets are not held accountable for their advertising and teaching. Thus, commercial platforms can have hundreds of questions and hypothetical approaches focused on test results, with zero clinical reasoning.

Platforms that provide knowledge instead of reasoning should not make false claims. However, misleading advertising is common worldwide. Profit-driven education is no different.

If these platforms claim to improve clinical reasoning, then they are being doubly deceitful. They are doing the exact opposite of what they claim. It would be like charging a customer for a health supplement that you claim helps hair growth, but the supplement does not improve hair growth and even causes the remaining hair on the customer's head to fall out.

Does the inclusion of clinical context in the products of commercial platforms, automatically equate to teaching clinical reasoning?

The answer is 'No'. Many commercial platforms provide knowledge of a hypothetical scenario and teach more knowledge on how to approach those scenarios and make decisions. Some teach knowledge about individual symptoms, signs, tests and treatments, but all of this teaching is still knowledge. If real-world performance is any indication, many users can go through hundreds of cases in tutorials and on platforms that provide a clinical context, be taught the knowledge about those cases and diseases, and still learn nothing about reasoning.

Poor reasoners are most tempted by such platforms because the questions and lessons (regardless of any advertised claims about reasoning) imply that only theoretical knowledge is needed for healthcare. Even semi-competent reasoners may be tempted to use the platforms because many humans feel more comfortable when others are doing the same: 'Hey, lots of people are using these platforms. Surely they can't all be wrong?'

Robust reasoners automatically stay away from such platforms because they know it is more important to learn the right thing than the common thing. Especially if the common thing is more harmful than helpful.

When learners are taught that reasoning is unnecessary, they tend to order tests indiscriminately. Without clinical context, the results of the initial tests are confusing and easily misinterpreted. Since the constant message to these learners is 'tests are accurate and important', they react to their confusion by ordering more tests. The vicious cycle continues.

I hear doctors — medical specialities, surgical specialities, you name it — discussing the lab results of patients in the hospital corridor from time to time. They are always puzzled, and they then suggest performing more tests. There is no mention of the clinical context. They have no idea what is going on and no idea of the best way to solve their predicament. Some even declare this loudly: 'The test results are weird. Maybe more tests are needed.' They should listen to themselves; they do not know how to interpret simple test results. They are inadvertently proclaiming the root cause of their dilemma. If they were more attentive to themselves and their patients, it is unlikely that discussion would ever have taken place.

Should future doctors be taught, even indirectly, to ignore the most useful information they need to be competent?

To match teaching to effective care in the real world, the clinical context should be mentioned before any test results. For example, an 'approach to respiratory failure on blood gas' can present a few variations in the clinical presentation of such patients, each belonging to 1 relevant disease, and *then* present the blood gas results for each presentation. To make such teaching even more effective, clinical reasoning must be woven into the lesson and taught explicitly.

Teaching to match the context of effective healthcare, helps to produce competent doctors.

Teaching to match the behaviour of ineffective healthcare, helps to produce incompetent doctors.

UNDERSTANDING COMMON LABORATORY TESTS

This chapter summarises the patient-centred uses of some common laboratory tests.

Each entry will cover:

- Name of the test, including common alternative names
- Components of the test, if more than 1 component is present
- Indications
- Common fallacies
- Common consequences of fallacies

--

Full blood count/complete blood count

Components: Total white cell count, breakdown of white cell types (neutrophils, lymphocytes, eosinophils, etc.); serum haemoglobin, mean corpuscular volume, mean corpuscular haemoglobin, mean corpuscular haemoglobin concentration, haematocrit, red cell distribution width; platelet count, mean platelet volume (additional components vary with different labs)

Indications:

- Diagnosis of haematological diseases

- Anticipatory care: secondary prevention by screening for anaemia

- Early detection of adrenal insufficiency in patients in shock (inappropriately normal eosinophil counts)

- Diagnostic support for specific infections, if there is diagnostic uncertainty

- Adjustment of treatment:

    o Assessing disease activity

    o Before major procedures where significant bleeding is anticipated

    o When treatment (e.g. some drugs, chemotherapy) may lead to dangerous drops in certain parameters in white cell count, haemoglobin or platelet counts.

Common fallacies:

These involve variations of 'the full blood count screens for infection':

1. A high total white cell count or neutrophil count means there must be a bacterial infection.

    Truth: there are multiple causes of high total white cell counts and high neutrophil counts, including marked physiological stress, some viral infections and systemic steroid use. Extremely elevated levels are usually caused by clinically obvious diseases or situations, rendering a full blood count unnecessary for diagnosis or treatment (unless the doctor is ignoring the clinical context, which is needed for the correct diagnosis and treatment no matter what the full blood count shows anyway).

2. A normal white cell count or normal neutrophil count means there is no serious problem.

   Truth: many serious diseases, including bacterial infections, have a normal white cell and neutrophil count. A normal result gives false reassurance.

3. Every patient who has a fever for 3 to 5 days, must have a full blood count. A normal result means the patient is fine.

   Truth: see point number 2.

Common consequences of fallacies:

If a doctor believes a high total white cell count or neutrophil count automatically equates to bacterial infection, this is often accompanied by further tests, indiscriminate prescription of antibiotics, and complacency. This becomes dangerous when the patient has another dangerous disease that is not a bacterial infection.

If the doctor believes a normal white cell or neutrophil count means there is no serious problem, they tend to stop thinking, tell the patient that there is no danger, and then send the patient home.

Insisting on performing a full blood count on days 3 to 5 of the illness irrespective of the clinical picture, often tempts doctors to skimp on the clinical evaluation.

--

Renal panel/serum urea and electrolytes/chemistry panel

Components: Urea, creatinine, sodium, potassium, chloride and bicarbonate

Indications:

- Significant fluid losses or extensive skin barrier compromise (e.g. burns, severe uncontrolled eczema): checking for electrolyte levels

- Kidney disease: diagnostic as well as adjusting-treatment purposes

- Other diseases causing large disturbances in the renin-angiotensin-aldosterone axis, such as pituitary and adrenal disorders

- Determining the type of anion-gap metabolic acidosis

- Adjustment of treatment:

  o Assessing disease activity, such as estimating the degree of chronic kidney disease before initiation of dialysis

  o Dose adjustment of drugs that are cleared by the kidneys, in patients with suspected kidney injury

  o When treatment (e.g. some drugs, chemotherapy) has a significant chance of causing kidney injury.

Common fallacies:

A normal electrolyte result means everything will be okay for at least 24 hours.

Truth: the frequency of checks depends on the doctor's prediction of the dynamics of the electrolyte changes.

Common consequences of fallacies:

When any of the components of this panel can change rapidly and catastrophically (such as in patients with extensive burns), failing to anticipate and check accordingly can be dangerous.

--

Liver panel

Components: Serum albumin, total bilirubin, conjugated bilirubin, unconjugated bilirubin, aspartate aminotransferase (AST), alanine transaminase (ALT), lactate dehydrogenase (LDH), alkaline phosphatase (ALP), gamma-glutaryl transferase (GGT). Some laboratories add a coagulation profile (PT, PTT) to this panel.

Indications:

- Liver disease
- Neonatal jaundice (various causes)
- Diseases causing haemolysis
- Diseases causing hypoalbuminemia
- Adjustment of treatment:
  - Assessing disease activity, such as the degree of transaminitis in drug-induced hepatitis
  - Dose adjustment of drugs that are metabolised by the liver, in patients with impaired liver function
  - When treatment (e.g. some drugs, chemotherapy) has a significant chance of causing liver injury.

Common fallacies:

For AST and ALT, where hepatic inflammation was previously severe (with these numbers extremely elevated), decreasing numbers mean that the patient is recovering.

Truth: if liver damage is so extensive that most of the hepatocytes are dead or dying, the AST and ALT eventually do trend downwards because there is very little of the viable liver remaining, not because the patient is recovering.

Common consequences of fallacies:

When AST and ALT trend downwards in a patient with liver failure, the doctor assumes the patient is recovering and decides to cut down on supportive treatment. This can be dangerous when the patient's clinical status and other markers of liver function (e.g. coagulation, serum ammonia levels) are ignored.

Coagulation panel

Components: Prothrombin time (PT), partial thromboplastin time (PTT)

Indications:

- Diseases causing disturbed coagulation, which can manifest as increased bleeding or thromboses
- Adjustment of treatment:
  - Titration of anticoagulant regime
  - Before any procedure where significant bleeding is anticipated.

Common fallacies:

If the PT or PTT is high, the patient has a disease or is more likely to bleed. If the PT/PTT is normal-to-low, there is no problem.

Truth: interpretation of these results must be within the clinical context. For example, in asymptomatic children, an elevated PTT is often due to a transient, harmless lupus-type anticoagulant. As another example, thrombotic thrombocytopenic purpura can have normal PT and PTT.

Common consequences of fallacies:

Healthy children may be over-investigated for an abnormal PTT.

It can be lethal to miss the diagnosis of a coagulopathic disease.

--

C-reactive protein

Indications:

- Increase suspicion of serious illness in a neonate.
- Adjustment of treatment: titration of antibiotics for infectious diseases, which may be present but clinically occult.

Common fallacies:

The C-reactive protein (CRP) is accurate in diagnosing dangerous illnesses. A high CRP means there is a dangerous illness. A low CRP means there cannot be any dangerous illness such as a bacterial infection.

Truth: many factors affect CRP. Lung infections and diseases involving the gastrointestinal tract tend to elevate the CRP; these diseases are not always bacterial or dangerous.

Common consequences of fallacies:

The doctor orders inflammatory markers (like the CRP and ESR) for anyone with a fever, a fever of more than X days, a new fever whilst in hospital, and so on. They assume the test screens for dangerous diseases.

When the CRP is high, the doctor may fixate on a label of 'sepsis' and treat the patient with antibiotics inappropriately.

If the CRP is high in a patient who has abdominal pain, the doctor may fixate on appendicitis or another random intestinal disease that they think will cause a high CRP. This fixation can lead to missing the patient's true disease.

If the doctor relies on a low CRP to assume the patient cannot have a dangerous disease, the doctor tends to miss these diseases. For example, a significant minority of patients with brain abscesses have normal CRP. A doctor who assumes a normal CRP excludes dangerous diseases, tends to miss brain abscesses and other dangerous diseases where the CRP can be normal.

Erythrocyte sedimentation rate

Indications:

- Increase diagnostic certainty when paired with CRP, for certain systemic diseases such as systemic lupus erythematosus.
- Assessing chronic disease activity, if symptoms and signs cannot be relied on.

- Adjustment of treatment: titration of antibiotics for infectious diseases, which may be present but clinically occult.

Common fallacies:

1. A high erythrocyte sedimentation rate (ESR) means the patient has a dangerous disease. A low ESR means the patient cannot have a dangerous disease.

   Truth: many benign diseases, such as self-limited influenza infection, can result in elevated ESR levels several days after the onset of illness. Conversely, ESR can be normal in patients with dangerous diseases.

2. ESR is useful for ruling out inflammation. Low ESR means the patient cannot have an inflammatory disease. If the patient has a known chronic inflammatory disease, a low ESR means the disease is not active.

   Truth: ESR can be normal in a minority of patients with active inflammatory disease. This includes diseases like Kawasaki disease and inflammatory bowel disease.

Common consequences of fallacies:

The doctor orders inflammatory markers (like the CRP and ESR) for anyone with a fever, fever of more than (insert arbitrary number) days, a new fever whilst in hospital, and so on. They assume that the test screens for dangerous diseases.

Patients with high ESR may be unnecessarily hospitalised and over-investigated.

Patients with low ESR can have dangerous diagnoses that are missed because the doctor believes that the low ESR excludes those diseases. Patients with an active chronic inflammatory disease are misdiagnosed because the doctor believes the low ESR excludes the possibility of active disease.

COMMON MISTAKES IN TESTING

Mistakes in testing can be divided into 2 categories:

1. Choosing tests wrongly
2. Interpreting test results wrongly

The disastrous chain of dominoes often shows itself when doctors make these mistakes. Mistakes in both choice and interpretation of the test results, usually coexist. This coexistence can lead to a vicious cycle of demanding even more inappropriate tests, which are then misinterpreted, which leads to more confusion and requests for yet more inappropriate tests which are again misinterpreted, and so on.

Choosing tests wrongly can be further subdivided into:

- Testing without a diagnosis (assuming patients are pieces, not whole patients; because the patient asks for the test; because the patient will not object)

- Tests that do not differentiate between the relevant differentials for that patient.

Interpreting test results wrongly can be further subdivided into:

- Ignoring clinical context (chasing unrealistic possibilities; failing to consider other diagnoses when the results are surprising; interpreting test results without knowing how to)

- 'The test is 100% accurate'.

Categories of Mistakes

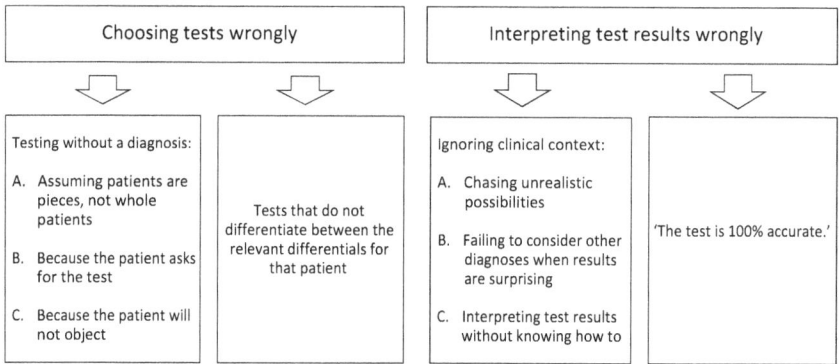

Choosing tests wrongly		Interpreting test results wrongly	
Testing without a diagnosis: A. Assuming patients are pieces, not whole patients B. Because the patient asks for the test C. Because the patient will not object	Tests that do not differentiate between the relevant differentials for that patient	Ignoring clinical context: A. Chasing unrealistic possibilities B. Failing to consider other diagnoses when results are surprising C. Interpreting test results without knowing how to	'The test is 100% accurate.'

1. Choosing tests wrongly

Choosing tests wrongly often leads to inappropriate and excessive testing for the patient.

Tests require machines, manpower and time to perform. The number of technicians in the biochemical laboratory is finite, as is the number of machines that can run a full blood count or renal panel. Likewise, there is a finite number of Computed Tomography (CT) and Magnetic Resonance Imaging (MRI) machines available in the Department of Radiology in each hospital, along with a limited number of radiographers and radiologists.

If several doctors in a hospital are indiscriminately ordering tests, this can strain the hospital's testing capacity. Other patients who truly require these tests may suffer delays in testing and appropriate care.

Testing without a diagnosis:

Deciding the most likely disease and relevant differentials in the patient allows specific and high-yield decisions. Conversely, having nothing in mind or a vague descriptor such as 'sepsis', leads to vague and often-irrelevant decisions.

A. *Assuming patients are pieces, not whole patients*

The doctor assumes every 'piece' (symptom, sign or test result) of information in the patient can occur coincidentally, without any relationship to other symptoms, signs and test results in the same patient.

The next assumption is that arbitrarily choosing tests based on that isolated piece, removes the need to reason clinically. This test is usually the most common test the doctor has seen being performed by other doctors for patients with this symptom or sign, regardless of diagnosis.

For example, the doctor decides that if the patient has pain in the arm, X-ray the arm. If the patient has pain in the leg, X-ray the leg. If the patient has a fever, perform a full blood count. And so on.

Since X-rays only pick up some diseases that cause pain, performing X-rays on a painful area and then deciding that a normal X-ray means there is no disease at all, predisposes the doctor to miss every other disease that causes the same pain. If the X-ray looks normal, this doctor often thinks 'there is no serious problem', reassures the patient, prescribes analgesia, and then sends the patient home.

As poor reasoning often coexists with inattention, this doctor may arbitrarily ignore any other piece of information. Sometimes, this doctor goes through all of the patient's pieces in this manner, picking one or more tests for each piece whilst pretending the other pieces are unrelated. A long list of tests is ordered and often misinterpreted.

B. *Because the patient asks for the test*

Patients may consult the doctor, asking for one or more tests. Some of these suggestions come from reading articles on the Internet; others from friends or family whose sources are unknown.

Some doctors ignore their fundamental jobs and readily perform these tests. When questioned, these doctors often use the flimsy rationalisation: 'If I do not do what the patient wants, another doctor will do it anyway.' This is similar to the rationalisation used by some criminals: 'If I did not steal the jewels, someone else would have done it anyway.'

The correct clinical diagnosis is required for all healthcare decisions to be excellent.

Do not unthinkingly perform the test requested by the patient. Obtain and analyse the symptoms and signs first, make the most likely diagnosis, and then recommend the appropriate management to the patient. This management plan will simultaneously decide the necessity of the requested test.

Sometimes, patients will not be convinced and just want the test anyway to 'rule out' their concern. Before you agree, remember that you share responsibility for anything that subsequently happens. Thus, you can acquiesce if the test is not risky and you are proficient in the interpretation of the results.

For example, a patient with eczema may request tests for food allergies. You take a history from the patient about their symptoms. You check for symptoms of food allergy, and there are none. You may have a diagnosis in mind; if there is no disease, say so. Regardless of your words, the patient insists on the test. If you are not fully proficient in interpreting allergy tests, you should refer the patient to a reliable specialist. If you are proficient, you can perform the allergy tests, because you can inform the patient accurately about the overall conclusion based on your clinical evaluation and the test results.

You cannot acquiesce if the test is risky (such as an invasive test) and not clinically warranted. Should something go wrong, you would be unable to defend yourself against accusations of incompetence because a reasonable or competent doctor would not have ordered that test. Making the argument 'the patient wanted the test and knew the risks and consented!' does not change your culpability and makes you look even worse; not only are you incompetent, but you are also deliberately irresponsible.

Do not perform a test whose result you cannot interpret accurately, unless you can get help interpreting that result. It is indefensible to give patients wrong information based on gross ignorance and overstepping your professional limits.

C. *Because the patient will not object*

The lack of objection from the patient sounds good. Which doctor wants patients who will (reasonably) object to their suggestions?

The answer: the robust reasoner. A patient who objects to a logical proposal is a surprise. Surprises warn the robust reasoner that something is wrong, be it a lack of clear communication, ignorance of the patient's perspective or anything else that must be addressed.

Doctors who perform tests because their main reason is a lack of patient objection instead of clinical indication, often fail to explain their thoughts to the patient. There is no explanation because there are no thoughts to explain, or the thoughts are so bizarre that merely admitting them would scare off many patients.

This behaviour is further fuelled by assumptions that the patient's opinion does not matter ('I am the doctor. You must listen to me'), and that the patient should be so grateful that they must pay any bill and bear any consequences without complaint.

Hence, by failing to explain to and understand the patient, these doctors create a situation that prevents objection.

Patients who mistakenly assume that doctors always act in their best interests and always reason properly, and therefore should not voice their opinion or objections, often painfully discover the consequences of their assumptions.

At best, such treatment of patients is self-serving and disrespectful. Too often, doctors omit explanations, intentionally order lots of unnecessary tests and treatments, and then over-charge the patient.

My former students have complained about some seniors ignoring clinical context and ordering lots of unnecessary tests. When these junior doctors object, the senior tells them: 'It does not cost you anything, so just order!' That single sentence is terrifying for 2 reasons:

1. It reveals the ignoble intentions of that doctor.

2. Some seniors encourage their juniors to make self-serving decisions at the expense of the patient.

Tests that do not differentiate between the relevant differentials for that patient

Recall the analogy of being the welcoming driver/official tasked with identifying 1 specific person out of the crowd of people leaving the airport terminal. You were given an information sheet with many details about your target.

Instead of using all the details on the sheet, you decide to use only 1 detail: 'This person is wearing shoes'.

You then randomly fixate on 1 person out of the many people wearing shoes, grab that person and drag him/her along with you. If they resist, you knock them unconscious, carry them to your vehicle and drive off.

Sounds like kidnapping, right?

Sounds like the kidnapper failed to use a detail that would differentiate between the potential targets, right?

The mistake of choosing tests that fail to differentiate between the differentials for the unique patient, is often preceded by target fixation. The doctor fixates on a single disease. This doctor then cherry-picks a test that he/she believes confirms that disease, whilst ignoring the differentials. Unfortunately, this test often does not distinguish between two or more clinically relevant differentials.

The result of the test returns and the doctor declares 'this test result supports my suspicion'. The doctor is 'kidnapping' 1 possibility on the textbook list and carries on stubbornly, through to the final disastrous outcome.

Having fixated on the single disease, this doctor fixates on their pre-decided treatment plan. Though they might not knock the protesting patient unconscious, the doctor aggressively tries to persuade the patient to follow their plan.

The classic example is a fixation on the label of 'bacterial infection'. A full blood count is ordered even though it cannot differentiate between the relevant differentials. This doctor insists any leukocytosis or neutrophilia must point to bacterial infection, and then insists on the patient taking a course of antibiotics.

Another example is a patient whose differentials are infectious mononucleosis, (hepatotropic) viral hepatitis, and adenovirus infection. The doctor is fixated on infectious mononucleosis. The liver panel reveals mild transaminitis. Such transaminitis can be seen in all of the differentials, not just infectious mononucleosis. However, the doctor declares the transaminitis proves the patient must have infectious mononucleosis.

2. Interpreting test results wrongly

Ignoring clinical context:

A. *Chasing unrealistic possibilities*

The doctor is fixated upon and chases diseases without regard to clinical context or probability.

The classic example was demonstrated by Dora, the female medical student who had dengue fever in Conversation #5, in the chapter 'Common mistakes in the clinical approach'. The fixation by her first doctor on systemic lupus erythematosus was not borne out by testing. The next doctor then fixated on leukaemia while ignoring her clinical context.

As another example, a teenage patient presents with an intentional drug overdose. There is mild transaminitis on the liver panel: AST and ALT are mildly elevated at 40 U/L and 50 U/L, respectively. This transaminitis is explained by the drug overdose. Even though the patient volunteered a history of drug overdose, which matched the physical examination and test results, the doctor decided to rule out every cause of transaminitis they could think of! This teenage patient then undergoes tests for Wilson's Disease, hepatotropic viruses, liver cancer, and so on.

Patients with artefacts or 'odd' findings on tests can undergo more expensive and risky tests because of this mistake. Some of these patients are started on treatment for dangerous diseases such as cancers. Many of the patients and their families are devastated by the fixated doctor telling them they have a dangerous disease, such as leukaemia.

When a sensible doctor comes by, provides the correct diagnosis and result interpretation and then stops the nonsensical management, the patient often expresses mixed feelings: relief that they do not have the dangerous disease, and anger at the target-fixated doctor who misled them.

B. *Failing to consider other diagnoses when results are surprising*

When the test results are surprising, the doctor should always return to the clinical context and review their assumptions.

However, poor reasoners often ignore surprises. They usually insist on their mistaken diagnosis and dismiss the surprising test result with a wild guess, such as 'sepsis can cause anything, including this test result'.

Sometimes, the poor reasoner cannot explain the surprising test result, does not recheck their assumptions, and still insists on their diagnosis or label for the patient. The worried patient replies: 'But you have just said the test result does not fit the disease!' Poor reasoners tend to reply: 'The test must be wrong! I am sure I am right!'

If the patient is wise, they will realise this doctor is delusional, and consult another doctor.

Test results can be false positives or false negatives. A surprising test result does not always mean the doctor's diagnosis is wrong. This is where a robust reasoner differs from a poor reasoner. A robust reasoner will be diligent and recheck their clinical assumptions and clinical diagnosis.

They will be able to explain the surprising test result, instead of dismissing it. They will also be more careful afterwards, as they realise it would be embarrassing and potentially dangerous if it turned out the test result was indeed accurate and their diagnosis was wrong!

C. *Interpreting test results without knowing how to*

If a doctor does not know how to accurately interpret the results of a test in a patient-centred fashion, they should not order the test.

Poor reasoners often make these mistakes as part of the disastrous chain of dominoes: ordering a test without knowing how to interpret its results properly, then misinterpreting the results, and then using that misinterpretation to make poor decisions.

Sometimes, the test that was ordered is irrelevant. The poor reasoner lacks the reasoning to realise their mistake, then misinterprets the test result, and then draws the wrong conclusions.

This is especially common in healthcare cultures that facilitate or encourage batteries of tests, creating a dual problem: the culture often gives the impression that tests are necessary whilst failing to ensure that the tests are used appropriately.

Interpretation of tests without knowing how to, occurs in 2 situations:

- The doctor has no idea how to interpret the test result at all.
- The doctor has some theoretical knowledge but struggles to interpret the test result within the patient's clinical context.

The classic example is 'all patients with fever must have a full blood count', followed by the doctor misinterpreting the test result as 'all neutrophilia on the full blood count is equal to bacterial infection, regardless of the patient's clinical context'.

Another example is C-reactive protein (CRP). Doctors may order this test with the erroneous intent of 'confirming' or 'excluding' their diagnosis. Many poor reasoners do not know the literature about CRP, order the test anyway. Even the poor reasoner who has read the literature on CRP can readily misinterpret the test result. For example, if the test is reported to have a 90% sensitivity, the doctor wrongly assumes a negative result automatically means the patient's chance of having the disease is $(100-90) = 10\%$.

Robust reasoners and experts in evidence-based medicine know that CRP adds little or no value in the diagnosis of pneumonia and most other diseases, in the setting of a proper clinical evaluation.

Specialised tests are likewise mis-ordered and misinterpreted. For example, the specific Immunoglobulin E (IgE) tests using ImmunoCap for allergies, require interpretation in the context of an allergic reaction. In addition, the cutoffs for 'positive' vary from substance to substance, instead of the usual Class 0 to Class 6 at the bottom of the standard printout (as of the end of 2022). Furthermore, there is an individual variation based on that patient's total IgE production; accounting accurately for this variation is unknown to many doctors and specialists.

Some doctors order panels of IgE tests for multiple foods. They then tell patients to avoid anything whose result returns at Class 1 or above. When one or more of the results return 'positive' in this manner, this erroneous interpretation unnecessarily scares the patient, restricts the patient's lifestyle, and impairs their quality of life.

Sometimes, a patient who was misled by a doctor will consult another doctor. They ask the next doctor for their interpretation of the existing test results. If this doctor is accurate in their interpretation and is thus compelled to disagree with their predecessor, their predecessor's mistakes are impossible to conceal. The most diplomatic response is: 'I cannot comment on what the previous doctor told you, because I was not there.'

A robust reasoner cannot agree with their predecessors' inappropriate decisions or advice, without harming the patient. In addition, the robust reasoner deduces the patient already suspected the truth.

Trying to lie to the patient is often futile because reality eventually asserts itself. A patient who suspected the previous doctor was wrong, would not be easily fooled.

'The test is 100% accurate'

Most tests are not 100% accurate.

The doctor who assumes the test is perfect, often skimps on the proper clinical evaluation: 'Since the test is 100% accurate, why should I bother to evaluate or think clinically?'

Without a clinical diagnosis and likely differentials, tests are often performed as a vague 'screen' for equally vague labels such as 'sepsis', 'infection', and so on. A negative result is assumed to mean no disease; a positive result is assumed to mean the disease is present. Even if the result is positive, the doctor still has no specific diagnosis, instead sticking to their vague label.

Common variations of this fallacy include:

- For anyone with a fever, perform a full blood count. If the blood count is normal, there is nothing dangerous.
- For anyone with pain, perform an X-ray of the painful area. If the X-ray is normal, there is nothing dangerous.
- For someone whose inflammatory markers (CRP and/or ESR) are normal or only slightly elevated, there is no dangerous infection or inflammatory disease.
- For someone with normal serum Procalcitonin, there is no bacterial infection.
- For someone whose CT scan of the painful area seems normal, there must be no disease in that area.

An example is the infant whose serious bacterial infection (such as osteomyelitis or septic arthritis) was missed. The doctors often argue that the baby 'looks clinically well', and then ignore the rest of the clinical picture. They then order inflammatory markers and insist that if these inflammatory markers are not elevated, there cannot be a dangerous disease.

However, infants with these diseases may not show much pain or mount a marked inflammatory response on testing.

For another example, see Case #21.

CASE #21: Adela

Adela is a 17-year-old girl who presents to the Emergency Department with severe, unremitting neck pain for 1 day. There are no other symptoms. Her vital signs are normal. On examination, she is looking forward and dares not move her neck. There is no apparent swelling, warmth, skin changes or tenderness over the neck. The rest of the examination is normal.

The doctor orders an X-ray of the neck. The X-ray looks normal. The doctor tells Adela there is nothing wrong with the bones. Adela is prescribed Ibuprofen for symptomatic relief of the pain. She is then sent home, with an appointment in the clinic.

Three days later, Adela is reviewed by Doctor Y in the Medicine clinic. The pain improved transiently with each dose of Ibuprofen. However, the pain is still severe, leaving her unable to move her neck or sleep comfortably. There are no other symptoms.

Doctor Y has a strong grasp of pathophysiology and clinical reasoning. Given the pattern of pain and absence of other symptoms and signs, he concludes that Adela has a subtle vertebral subluxation; invasion by a cancer into a tissue with pain fibres is a differential. He reasons that subtle subluxation is often not detectable on X-ray.

He requests a direct admission into the hospital ward, requests an urgent CT scan of the neck and simultaneously makes an urgent referral to Orthopaedic surgery (spine) to advise on the CT scan.

(*Continued*)

The Orthopaedic spine surgeon agrees with the plan and suggests the CT scan to include rotation of the head. The CT scan is performed.

The CT scan reports the diagnosis of rotatory atlantoaxial cervical subluxation. Adela undergoes treatment in the hospital for the next few days, and recovers.

In addition to demonstrating the danger of assuming a test is 100% accurate, Case #21 also demonstrates the synergy of pathophysiological understanding and clinical reasoning for unfamiliar diagnoses.

Capsule summary

- Mistakes occur commonly in the choice and/or interpretation of tests.
- Poor reasoners often make multiple mistakes in each patient.
- Mistakes in testing are usually preceded by mistakes in clinical approach and diagnosis.

QUIZ: TESTS

Q1: When are diagnostic tests necessary?

Q2: What are the pros and cons of performing a single most accurate diagnostic and invasive test, versus several, non-invasive, less-accurate diagnostic tests?

Q3: What are the 3 categories of information that tests help with, for adjusting treatment?

SECTION 3

Decision-making: Treatment

This section covers the principles of effective treatment, interpretation of response to treatment, and counselling.

TREATMENT DECISIONS

Treatment should help to cure the patient. If a cure is not possible, then control of the chronic disease is often the aim. Sometimes, neither cure nor control is viable, such as a self-limited common cold or incurable cancer.

Cure and control must be accomplished safely and quickly.

If the costs and risks of treatment are significant to the patient, these decisions must be balanced against the expected benefits of treatment. 'Significant' from the doctor's perspective is not always 'significant' from the patient's perspective. Thus, doctors should never unilaterally decide this balance.

The most skilful and empathetic doctors never force their expectations upon patients. They know excellent healthcare comes from partnership, not dictatorship.

What is 'treatment'?

Treatment includes all measures that will cure or control the disease. These measures include pharmacotherapy (drugs) in any form, procedures, and lifestyle changes. Counselling is part of the potential treatment for mental and mood-related illnesses.

All formal decisions for treatment, including referrals, must have the patient's informed consent.

Informed consent

'Informed consent' is a phrase that is widely debated. The debate centres around accountability versus feasible clinical practice.

Accountability for possible consequences implies having to discuss in full, all possible consequences and their management and the contingency plans for these consequences, regardless of their probability, time constraints, and the impact on the listener.

Feasible clinical practice recognises that mentioning all ultra-rare consequences tends to overload and scare many patients, requires a lot of time and esoteric knowledge that is probably beyond the capabilities of most doctors, and runs the risk of scaring off patients who needed the treatment.

Since decisions are adapted to the unique patient, informed consent must be adapted to that patient. Thus, the discussion must adequately inform the unique patient of the viable options and explore their concerns to the best of the doctor's ability.

Informed consent is relevant to all decisions, not just for treatments or procedures. This principle guides all shared decision-making.

For each option, the doctor must cover, in this order:

1. What the option is
2. The expected benefit (for tests, this is the usefulness of the test result for the diagnosis and decision-making. For treatment, this is the aim and the likely time-to-effect of treatment)
3. The safety risks and common side effects

Since the discussion must be customised, the extra elements can include:

- Costs, especially for non-basic tests, for treatment using non-basic everyday drugs, and for patients with financial difficulties.

- The rarest and worst side effects, especially when patients appear anxious or demand to know the worst side effects.

- Contingency plans, especially if the test results are surprising or the treatment did not achieve its goal within the stated period. Some patients like to think ahead.

- The scenario if no tests or no treatment is performed, especially for patients who seem reluctant to undergo tests or treatment.

All discussions, especially for uncommon tests and treatments, should be documented succinctly. A fellow doctor reading the entry should be able to understand:

- The essence of the counselling

- The patient's main concerns

- The essence of the patient's response.

During the discussion, the mindful doctor will:

- Check in with the patient every few minutes: Do they understand? Do they have any questions? If the patient has not understood the information thus far, going on will leave the patient even more lost than before and often wastes the doctor's time.

- Avoid the use of medical jargon. Patients do not readily understand medical abbreviations and terms.

- If the doctor does not know something, honestly admitting 'I don't know, but I will find out and get back to you' is preferable to fabricating information.

- Limit the total discussion time to 20, at most 30 minutes. Humans have a finite attention span. Schedule a second session for further discussion, if necessary.

Cases #22 and #23 demonstrate counselling with the elements of informed consent.

CASE #22: Dave

Dave is a 60-year-old man who presents to the Emergency Department with fever, productive cough and worsening breathlessness for 2 days. His temperature is 38 degrees Celsius. There are no other symptoms. He has no chronic illnesses. He is hypoxic with an oxygen saturation of 90% on room air.

On examination, he is tachypneic. There are crepitations and bronchial breath sounds on auscultation over the right lung field. There is dullness to percussion over the right hemithorax.

You diagnose him with bacterial pneumonia.

You plan to hospitalise him for antibiotic treatment, supportive therapy, and close monitoring. Though this plan seems obvious to you, Dave does not know what to expect.

You must tell him:

- The tests and their purpose: the chest X-ray may provide more information that guides the management
- The treatment, then proceed to explain the benefits of each:
  - o The aim of using the antibiotic to cure him, with the expected time to improvement
  - o Supportive therapy such as oxygen may help to reduce his work of breathing
- The need for monitoring, in case he worsens unexpectedly
- The common side effects of the antibiotic.

If Dave seems reluctant to agree to the tests, explain the contingency plan for this no-tests scenario: treatment proceeds, but if he does not improve rapidly, he needs another evaluation and potentially more tests.

If he refuses treatment, you discuss the scenario of no-treatment: he would be in danger, as he is deteriorating rapidly.

CASE #23: Edith

Edith is a 2-year-old girl with uncontrolled persistent asthma, as evidenced by 3 hospitalisations for moderate asthma exacerbations in the past 6 months, 4 other consultations with her family doctor for milder exacerbations during that period, and dry nocturnal cough twice a week for the same 6 months.

You have reviewed her home setting: there are no triggers to address.

She has not been on any controller therapy.

You decide Edith requires moderate-intensity controller therapy: inhaled Fluticasone propionate at 100 micrograms (mcg) twice a day. This treatment should be administered daily by her parents via a spacer and facemask. She has a Salbutamol inhaler on standby at home.

Edith's parents want to know the plans.

You need to discuss:

- The inhaled corticosteroids and their aim: prevent all attacks and clear all the nocturnal symptoms
- The expected time-to-effect, and the contingency plan if such a response is not seen
- The side effects of the inhaled corticosteroids.

If Edith's parents cite their fears of dangerous side effects from the steroids, you counter with facts: the moderate dose of inhaled corticosteroids does not cause those side effects. Those side effects have a small chance of occurring with significant doses of systemic steroids given for several months or longer. You explain the continued symptoms and risks to her if they refuse controller therapy.

If her parents decide not to proceed with controlling her asthma, and you are unable to change their mind, suggest that they seek a 2nd opinion and write the referral letter. You must respect your patient's wishes, but should not abandon them because they (or in this case, their parents) disagreed with you.

Styles of decision-making

There are 3 overall styles of decision-making:

1. Shared responsibility (partnership)
2. Top-down (dictatorial)
3. Abandonment of responsibility (apathetic)

Shared responsibility

The doctor is the health expert but cannot fully empathise with the patient, whereas the patient understands themselves best but lacks the doctor's expertise.

The shared responsibility style recognises this combination of strengths and weaknesses in the doctor–patient dynamic. Thus, in this style, the doctor provides the expertise, and the patient provides their understanding of themselves. The doctor must spend time and energy listening and explaining to the patient, but the benefits are often worth the doctor's effort: more satisfaction for the patient, better chances of patient compliance and an excellent outcome, and more safety for the doctor should things go awry.

Responsibility for decisions is shared. The patient has the final say. A holistic treatment plan that is acceptable to the patient, is mutually agreed upon. The doctor shows they respect the patient.

Should anything go wrong, the final decision-maker was the patient. If the doctor did a proper job of reasoning, assessment and explanation, the patient has virtually no grounds to find fault. The chance of a formal complaint or lawsuit is much lower than in the top-down style, partly because poor outcomes are less likely if the doctor has done a proper job, and partly because the patient knows that the final decision was made by themselves, not the doctor.

Top-down style

The top-down style involves the doctor making all the decisions and dictating to the patient. The patient has almost no say in the options, and can only agree or disagree. This style is often self-serving because there is no requirement to explain or listen to the patient. The doctor who uses this style is tempted to skimp on the counselling: since the patient has no say, why should I bother to explain the rationale, costs, risks, and so on about the decisions?

However, many patients dislike being dismissed, ignored, and left in the dark. Compliance with the management plan may be compromised because unhappy patients can obey the classic rule of human behaviour: 'If you do not listen to me, I do not have to listen to you.' If anything goes wrong, most or all of the blame lies with the doctor, increasing the risk of formal complaints and lawsuits.

Patients who seem harmless and submissive can still lodge a formal complaint or lawsuit against the doctor who failed to counsel them adequately. Even if the patient directly tells you: 'Doctor, do not explain. Just tell me what to do. I will obey you,' you should think twice about using this top-down style.

Abandonment of responsibility

A minority of doctors push all responsibility for decision-making to the patient. This is 1 manifestation of the 'apathetic' tier of performance (discussed in the chapter 'Tiers of performance'). The doctor skimps on the clinical evaluation and then offers treatment options based on:

- The most common disease they think they see, or
- The most common request they get from their patients, or
- Any treatment the patients request.

The classic example is the doctor who asks patients, 'do you want antibiotics?' regardless of whether antibiotics are indicated.

If the patient says 'yes', the doctor prescribes an antibiotic.

In addition, this doctor often prescribes everything the patient requests, without any regard for costs or side effects. This is how some doctors prescribe addictive medications to patients whilst ignoring the warning signs that point to the patient being a drug addict.

Such indiscriminate prescription can be fuelled by the flimsy rationalisation: 'If I do not give the patient antibiotics and whatever else they want, another doctor will do it anyway'. This is similar to the rationalisation used by some criminals: 'If I did not steal the jewels, someone else would have stolen them anyway'.

This practice of abandoning responsibility can stem from the mindset that 'if anything goes wrong, it is the patient's fault. They wanted the medicines. I did not make any recommendation; I just asked'.

The doctor does not care about the consequences to anyone else: to the patient, to other doctors, or to society. This is the abandonment of duty and responsibility to everyone else.

Indiscriminate prescribing makes some patients happy because they are being given what they want, with no need to think or listen to explanations from the doctor. However, the problems are manifold.

Indiscriminate prescription of medicines increases the frequency of patients developing adverse drug reactions. Indiscriminate use of antibiotics increases microbial resistance to antibiotics in the community. This practice also feeds a culture of misinformation and drives unreasonable patient expectations.

Misled by doctors who prescribe indiscriminately, some of these patients will routinely demand antibiotics from other doctors regardless of the disease. The other doctors are mystified by the demand, and even more mystified when the patient gets angry at them for refusing to prescribe antibiotics. The doctor who explains 'the antibiotics will not treat this disease and may cause even more problems instead!' often finds their explanation falling upon deaf ears. The patient is angry that this doctor is not like the previous doctor who freely gave them what they wanted.

Such practice proliferates when there is no auditing or obvious consequence to the apathetic doctor.

Specificity in counselling

The more specific and patient-centred you are in your counselling to the patient, the more useful the discussion is to the patient. Patients can tell the difference between patient-centred counselling and non-patient-centred counselling.

The specificity of the doctor's counselling has some correlation with their style of decision-making (see table below).

Style of decision-making	Shared responsibility	Top-down	Abandonment of responsibility
Categories of counselling	• Patient-centred • Averages	• Averages • Nothing useful	• Averages • Nothing useful

There are 3 categories, or manners, of counselling. Each category varies in its specificity towards the patient:

1. Patient-centred

2. Averages

3. Nothing useful

1. Patient-centred: The doctor uses their knowledge about the patient to customise the discussion. This knowledge includes disease severity, co-morbid conditions, patient's perspective and potential caregivers, and was covered in detail in an earlier chapter 'Gathering additional information to manage patients'.

Patient-centred counselling requires mindfulness and considerable knowledge about the medical aspects of the patient. Doctors who meet these requirements will usually engage in the decision-making style of shared responsibility.

Patients with more severe disease that is uncontrolled for long enough, have a higher chance of complications. Explaining the risk of complications can serve as a huge motivator for compliance with the treatment plan. The doctor does not engage in scaremongering or exaggeration; for example, they will not tell the patient with a mild disease that non-compliance will increase their risk of getting complications attributed only to patients with uncontrolled moderate or severe disease.

Where co-morbid conditions, status effects and medications can cause additional problems for the management of the patient's current disease, the doctor discusses these with the patient and works out a mutually agreed plan to handle these problems.

Understanding the patient's perspective and potential caregivers, facilitates a patient-centred management plan.

The classic example of a lack of patient-centred counselling, is life expectancy in the patient with terminal cancer. Laypeople (and mindful medical students) complain that the doctors cite averages and cannot seem to provide the patient with more patient-centred information. If the doctors could give the patient a more accurate estimate of their life expectancy, this would help the patient in planning how to use their remaining lifespan.

To be fair to oncologists, giving an accurate prediction about lifespan is difficult. Giving this prediction under such unhappy circumstances is even more difficult; when stressed, humans tend to want certainty. Here is where the dilemma arises: the patient wants more certainty about their remaining lifespan, but the oncologist wants more certainty about the prediction they are going to give the patient.

There is a huge difference between trying to be patient-centred whilst respecting uncertainty, versus not trying at all. Consider the next 2 statements, either of which could be applied to the same patient with cancer.

- 'You are going to live for 1 year. This is the average quoted in the research.' Though the oncologist may be factually accurate, this average will not apply to many patients.

- 'Your cancer is progressing quickly. You have told me about the things you want to do before you pass away. I think you have about 6 months left. We can discuss the treatment visits and side effects, and see if we can accommodate your plans. Tell me more about your plans.'

When the discussion focuses on the unique patient instead of the hypothetical 'average patient', the doctor can give more relevant advice to that unique patient.

2. Averages: The doctor relies on their theoretical knowledge and experience to provide common information and averages. For example, the doctor tells the patient to use an average dose of the medication regardless of the disease severity, or only mentions the most common side effects of the antibiotics without paying attention to the patient's other concerns about the antibiotics. Predictions on the duration of recovery or life expectancy likewise use averages in the population or textbooks.

Factually speaking, the doctor is accurate. In comparison to the patient-centred manner of counselling, less mindfulness and knowledge are required. For example, if the doctor is not going to discuss the effects of the patient's co-morbid conditions, status effects and other medications on the current treatment, the doctor does not need the knowledge of these effects. The trade-off is the inability to fully customise the discussion to suit the patient's needs.

Doctors using any style of decision-making can engage in this manner of counselling.

If using the style of abandonment of responsibility, the doctor may indiscriminately prescribe antibiotics to patients and tell them about the common side effects of the antibiotics. Though the doctor seems to be providing useful information, providing this information changes neither the intentional abandonment of proper healthcare nor the consequences of indiscriminate prescription to the patient, one's colleagues or society.

3. Nothing useful: When the doctor lacks either knowledge or reasoning (or both), the doctor often lacks accuracy and genuine confidence. It is difficult to counsel accurately or confidently if you lack accuracy and confidence. In addition, the doctor may be consumed by the fear of being held accountable for mistaken predictions.

This doctor may decide it is safer not to provide useful information to the patient: 'If I tell them nothing specific, they cannot use my words against me. If something goes wrong because of my vague advice, I can claim that they misunderstood me. If I tell them nothing unless they ask for the information, I minimise the words that can be used against me.'

This manner of counselling is usually seen in the decision-making styles of top-down and abandonment of responsibility. 'Nothing useful' often means nothing was said, or nothing specific in what was said.

When used in the top-down style, the doctor is not being vague. Instead, the doctor simply tells the patient nothing.

When used in the style of abandonment of responsibility, the doctor deliberately provides vague information. Similar self-deceptions are used in everyday life when someone is trying to evade responsibility for their abandonment.

Consider this example.

Ken is a sports trainer. Ken's mother tells him that she wants to start exercising. Ken asks her about the exercises that she wants to do. Ken knows that his mother knows his occupation. Even though Ken knows that many people injure themselves inadvertently when they undertake the same exercises she describes, and knows how to teach her to avoid these mistakes, he only says: 'Exercise can be healthy.'

Ken's mother starts exercising and then suffers an injury.

She asks Ken how she was injured. Ken tells her that people who exercise in that manner often get injured. Annoyed, she asks Ken why he did not use his knowledge to warn her.

Ken tells his mother: 'Before you exercise, it is your responsibility to learn everything about exercise. Since you did not ask me how to avoid being injured, you are responsible for failing to ask me the right questions. You did the exercise, so you are responsible for injuring yourself.'

Ken's mother replies angrily: 'I told you what I was doing because you are a sports trainer! I trusted you because I thought you knew the right exercises and would warn me! So, you did know the right exercises, and you decided not to warn me! You even know I cannot read and write, and yet you insist I must learn everything?! Yes, I am responsible for injuring myself because I exercised! Are you telling me that I am responsible for blindly trusting you to do the right thing? Are you telling me that you take no responsibility for this bad outcome?'

Ken tells her the 'truth' he has told himself all this while. 'Yes. You are responsible for what you do. You are responsible for what happens if you trust me. Even if I told you how to exercise properly, I cannot guarantee you would not injure yourself. Anything is possible. Hence, why should I be held responsible for something you chose to do, whether I told you what I thought? Imagine if I was a doctor and you paid me to cure you. It is your fault if you blindly trust me. I am not responsible for what happens to you after you see me. I am not responsible for what happens if you take the medicine I give you. There is no guarantee that the medicine would cure you or that the medicine would have no side effects, so holding me responsible for something I cannot guarantee, is absurd.'

Ken is demonstrating hypocrisy. He tells his mother she is responsible for what she does, and soon afterwards insists that he has no responsibility for what he does. Factually, he is right about being unable to provide guarantees, but he is using this fact as an illogical reason to evade *all* responsibility. Throughout his explanation, he sidesteps the real issue: responsibility comes from his choices too, not just the outcome alone.

Ken is pretending to talk about his responsibility, but the real subject of all his sentences is his mother. He is pretending that he has no responsibility to use his knowledge or fulfil his role. He is abandoning his responsibility for his choices, and pushing all responsibility onto her.

The real problem is not the words he has just said. The real problem is his intentional omission of reasonable advice, which contributed to the poor outcome. His words merely mirrored his behaviour.

Though this example may seem unreal to you, some doctors talk and behave towards their patients in a similar fashion, just like Ken is talking and behaving towards his mother.

I was taken aback the first time I was told about this style of counselling. Specifically, I was advised to use this style of counselling.

A colleague with a poor professional reputation and track record, advised me against giving specific advice to my patients.

I asked my colleague for the basis of their advice.

The answer was: 'If you keep it vague, there is leeway to argue about the interpretation of your advice in case the outcome is not so good.'

I was shocked. Once I considered my colleague as a whole, my surprise faded.

This colleague was giving me vague advice, by using vague words to describe a vague reason to give vague advice.

This doctor had probably done most or all of the following:

1. Never listened to themselves talking when they decided to be vague.

2. Never asked themselves if learning to be specific would help avoid the poor outcomes they feared.

3. Never realised that being knowledgeable and specific, builds confidence, trust, and a superior track record, which in turn helps with one's professional reputation.

4. Never paid attention to the implications of someone who thinks and speaks specifically. This meant being so inattentive to my speech and style, that it never occurred to them that poor or vague advice would be instantly recognised as such.

5. Never accepted full responsibility for the consequences of vague, unhelpful advice.

6. Decided that patients would not notice the unhelpfulness of vague explanations.

7. Decided that specific counselling was unimportant to the patient's outcome.

8. Decided that being vague to colleagues was an effective method of persuasion.

9. Decided that colleagues could not 'read' vague and noncommittal words to realise the truth of the speaker: someone who lacks knowledge, confidence, and specificity.

I replied: 'If I do not tell the patient exactly what to do and what to expect, how are they going to get the disease under control? How is the patient going to know when to come back if something goes wrong?'

The other doctor ignored the questions and walked away.

Deliberately choosing to be vague, locks the poor reasoner into a self-created vicious cycle. Instead of admitting that the root cause of the problem is their weaknesses, the poor reasoner instead focuses on the superficial actions (such as speaking vaguely) to try to conceal those weaknesses. They seem to assume (wrongly) that their actions will conceal their weaknesses from everyone else, and thus, there is no need to remedy their weaknesses. Thus, the weaknesses persist. The poor reasoner is stuck with the poor outcomes and is committed to speaking vaguely, perhaps forever.

Just like the example of Ken, the real problem is what was done instead of what was said. The real problem is not the vagueness of the counselling. The real problem is the underlying weakness that leads to poor diagnostic accuracy, poor decisions, and poor counselling. The weakness is already apparent from the problems created by the poor reasoner's ineptitude in diagnosis and decision-making, which patients and fellow doctors readily notice.

If your diagnosis and plans are already inappropriate, your words are unlikely to make much difference to the patient's outcome or to fool any attentive colleague. Instead, intentional omissions and vagueness in your counselling will reveal your self-serving and deceitful nature, which further increases the chance of a complaint or lawsuit.

Referrals

Making referrals

Referrals involve asking a colleague to assist you in the patient's care.

You will be disclosing information that is confidential to the patient. Thus, all referrals require informed consent.

All formal referrals require a formal letter, which includes, at a minimum:

1. A summary of the patient's clinical features and your diagnosis

2. Information from any tests or treatment provided and the response to treatment, if any

3. The task you are requesting of the letter's recipient

The task you are requesting, should either be to assist with:

- The diagnosis where this diagnosis is uncertain; or

- Treatment where the diagnosis is known, but help is needed.

If a delay in consulting your colleague is likely to lead to major harm or death, you must call your colleague immediately. Without attempting to directly contact your colleague, you will not know if they are available for an urgent consultation.

If requesting help with the diagnosis, always ask for the most likely diagnosis. You must furnish the patient's clinical features and if relevant, the risk factors.

The classic mistake is to ask your colleague to rule out a disease. The request to rule out can inflict tunnel vision on your colleague; this colleague proceeds to rule out that disease, often leaving the patient no better off than before.

You should receive a formal reply for the referral.

After making a referral, the common mistake is to assume 'someone else will take care of this properly' and forget about the original problem that prompted the referral.

Never assume that the patient will always consult the colleague you referred them to.

Never assume that the colleague who saw the patient will always get it right.

If the patient has consulted your colleague, continue to follow up on the patient for the original problem. Referrals are not excuses to be inattentive.

If your colleague gets it wrong, intermittent enquiry of the patient about the original problem will inevitably reveal this. A skilful and conscientious doctor can still rescue the situation.

Consider this example.

A 22-year-old man is referred to the haematologist for suspected lymphoma. He had lost 6 kilograms over 6 months. His appetite had remained normal. He looked cachectic. His full blood counts showed worsening thrombocytopenia and anaemia over the same period. He had a previous lymphoma, which had been deemed to be in remission.

At the consultation with the haematologist, he has an incidentally noticed fever of 38 degrees Celsius. Other vital signs are normal and there are no other clinical features.

The haematologist labels him as having 'sepsis' because 'the most common cause of fever is infection', and ignores the rest of the clinical information and the results of the previous full blood counts.

The haematologist insists that the patient must be hospitalised to undergo tests and antibiotic treatment for 'sepsis'. Tests 'to rule out lymphoma' are to be postponed 'until the sepsis is cured'.

The patient is admitted to the general ward, under the care of Internal Medicine. The doctors of the ward unthinkingly copy the label of sepsis, do not evaluate the patient themselves, do not read the referral letter that was originally written to the haematologist, and follow the haematologist's instructions.

The original doctor, Doctor S, calls the patient a week later to follow up. It is 5 p.m.; Doctor S has just ended his work day.

The patient's responses are horrifying to Doctor S. Despite being on a 2nd course of antibiotics, the patient complains that he is not getting better.

The patient is getting worse. He has begun losing his appetite too. He has developed a new flank pain, for which the ward doctors are giving him painkillers 'for symptomatic treatment', but the painkillers are not working. All microbiological cultures returned negative. The ward doctors told the patient: 'We do not know where the fever is coming from, but we will continue antibiotics.' This statement upset the patient's family.

Doctor S travels to that hospital immediately and introduces himself to the ward doctors. The doctors show him the documentation of their assessments and plans. He sees the patient for himself. It is baffling how the label of 'sepsis' (which is not a proper diagnosis anyway) can apply to this clinical picture.

Doctor S politely explains to the ward doctors the suspicion of lymphoma with malignant fever.

Doctor S then calls the haematologist. Doctor S reinforces the suspected diagnosis in the referral and explains that he thinks the fever and new symptoms are likely due to an increased tumour load, not an infection.

The haematologist concedes and orders the necessary investigations for lymphoma to be performed urgently. Had Doctor S not followed up and acted accordingly, the outcome would have been worse: prolonged suffering of the patient and a higher chance of death, due to a delay in appropriate care.

The most senior doctor of the ward team is a consultant about the same age as Doctor S. This ward consultant seemed courteous when talking with Doctor S. When Doctor S is walking away, this consultant remarks to her junior colleagues, 'That doctor is strange. Why bother to check on the patient? Why do more work? Why care so much for 1 patient? I would not do that.'

Being habitually inattentive, this poor reasoner does not realise how sharp the hearing of other humans can be.

Doctor S hears the comment and feels sad.

The answer to that consultant's questions would be obvious to any *human* who has even a shred of empathy or responsibility: to respect others as human beings; to properly do the job entrusted to you; to reduce unnecessary suffering; and to save lives if possible.

Doctor S realises the ward doctors are probably apathetic too; how else could such a comment be acceptable to the ward team?

To be fair to the ward doctors and to ensure that he heard correctly, Doctor S decides to check. Since Doctor S has not had dinner yet, he has a quick bite in the hospital canteen. He then walks back into the general ward.

He spots one of the junior doctors who had been standing with the ward consultant when he left, and approaches her. Her eyes widen when she notices him.

He asks: 'What did your boss say to you as I was leaving?'

As the junior doctor looks into his hard eyes, she realises they have underestimated Doctor S. She realises that he must have overheard her boss' words. She also realises that underestimating him further, such as trying to deceive him, would be dangerous.

She meekly repeats what her boss said, confirming Doctor S's suspicions. He thanks her and turns to leave.

She says, 'I hope you are not too insulted.'

He pauses and turns back to her. 'Why should I be? I am saddened by what I heard, but I am not insulted. I would have been insulted if your boss suggested I was like her. I am glad that I am not like her.'

'One day, when you are a patient and your doctors want the money and prestige that comes with the title of "doctor" whilst not caring enough about you to provide the excellent healthcare you paid for and trusted them to provide, perhaps you will understand. Each of us can choose to be part of the problem or part of the solution. I made the mistake of not checking in sooner on this patient. I will learn from it. I will not be part of the problem.'

Doctor S leaves. Doctor S considers getting the patient transferred to another team of doctors, perhaps to another hospital if necessary.

The next day, the patient is transferred to the care of another team of doctors, and Doctor S continues to follow up closely on the patient's condition and care.

Receiving a referral

When you receive a referral, carefully study the information provided. You should verify the clinical information and perform a proper clinical evaluation to decide on the diagnosis.

Never assume the referring colleague documented all the relevant information in the letter. Never assume your colleague's diagnosis is always correct.

If your colleague asks you to rule out a particular disease, do not do that. Instead, figure out the patient's most likely diagnosis, which decides optimal decisions and can indirectly fulfil your colleague's request simultaneously.

When you have completed your job for the patient, provide a formal reply to the referring doctor, updating him or her on the outcome. This is called 'completing the communication loop'.

This reply builds professional collegiality, gives your colleague the chance to learn from what you did, and encourages further referrals to you if your decision-making was optimal.

Capsule summary

- Informed consent is the foundation of shared decision-making, requiring customisation to each patient's situation and preferences.

- There are 3 styles of decision-making. The preferred style is shared responsibility.

- There are 3 categories of counselling. The preferred category is patient-centred, which requires considerable mindfulness and knowledge.

- Referrals require a clinical diagnosis and all relevant clinical information about the patient.

- If you receive a referral, approach the patient with an open mind. Complete the communication loop at the appropriate time.

DIAGNOSIS: DISEASE, SEVERITY AND TREATMENT

This chapter focuses on the 2nd and 3rd elements of the correct diagnosis: disease and severity. These elements decide optimal management.

To recap, the correct diagnosis should:

1. Explain all the patient's Clinical Features…(if 'all' is not possible, at least 'most'…while you learn more to try to explain 'all')

2. …with a Disease/Illness…

3. …and include your impression of the Severity of the illness.

Element	Importance for the immediate patient	The consequence for your learning, short-term and long-term
Explain all clinical features	You maximise your chance of being right about the Disease and its Severity.	If you cannot explain all clinical features, you are either wrong about the Disease, or you guessed the right disease but are ignorant of some of its clinical features. Or you are both wrong and ignorant. Adhering to this element prompts you to fix your weaknesses.

(Continued)

(Continued)

Element	Importance for the immediate patient	The consequence for your learning, short-term and long-term
Disease	The disease decides all potentially reasonable decisions. This element helps you to focus on these decisions, instead of wildly thinking of 'everything I can do'.	Follow up on this patient. If you were right, affirming the correct diagnosis and seeing the response to your management reinforces your mental processes. If you were wrong, committing to a Disease gives you the chance to identify the personal weaknesses that led to this mistake.
Severity	Among the potentially reasonable options (including tests and treatment), you select the best options: those that match the severity of your patient's illness. Estimating the correct severity, avoids excessive healthcare and inadequate healthcare.	You learn to clinically estimate the urgency and intensity of care that each patient needs. When you follow up with the patient, you then discover if your skill at assessing severity is accurate. If you were inaccurate, having previously committed to a severity level, you now get the chance to reflect and re-calibrate your assessment skill.

The specific disease

The specific disease dictates all potentially reasonable decisions. For example:

- The treatment for bacterial gastroenteritis is different from the treatment for acute appendicitis.

- The treatment for a stroke is different from the treatment of systemic lupus erythematosus.

Symptomatic treatment

Since symptoms arise from the pathophysiology of the disease, the pathophysiology of each unique disease dictates all effective treatments for that disease: symptomatic, curative or otherwise.

A common fallacy of 'symptomatic treatment' is that any medicine that may help with a symptom, can be freely used for all patients regardless of their disease. This fallacy ignores pathophysiology and tempts doctors to treat symptoms without making diagnoses.

To prescribe symptomatic treatment without the most likely diagnosis, is to guess wildly while hoping for the 'placebo effect' if your guess is wrong.

The placebo effect refers to the patient subjectively feeling better because they want to believe the treatment will work, not because the treatment does work.

Many patients do not succumb to the placebo effect. If the underlying disease persists, even those who succumbed to the placebo effect will eventually have the effect wear off.

Let us use fever as an example.

Three diseases include fever as a symptom: flu, heat stroke and neuroleptic malignant syndrome.

Symptomatic treatment of the fever depends on the underlying disease. The intent of treatment may differ for each disease.

If attempting to deal with the fever in a viral flu, the first choice would be Acetaminophen and sometimes Non-Steroidal Anti-Inflammatory Drugs (NSAIDs). The intent is to relieve discomfort from the flu.

If attempting to deal with the fever in a heat stroke, the first choice is immediate, intensive cooling. The intent is to prevent organ damage and death.

When dealing with fever in neuroleptic malignant syndrome (a rare adverse reaction due to antipsychotic drugs), the first choice is an antidote, such as Dantrolene. The intent is to prevent organ damage and death.

These diseases and their treatment in relation to fever, are summarised in the next table:

Disease (with fever)	Treatment (which also relieves the symptom of fever)	The intent of this treatment
Flu	Acetaminophen, NSAIDs	Reduce discomfort
Heat stroke	Intensive cooling	Prevent organ damage and death
Neuroleptic malignant syndrome	Dantrolene and other antidotes	Prevent organ damage and death

Another example would be the relief of itching.

The effective relief of itch depends on the underlying disease. The intent of treatment may differ for each disease.

If the itch is due to urticaria (itchy urticaria can be caused by allergic and non-allergic diseases), oral antihistamines are often the first choice. The intent is to reduce the discomfort.

If the itch is due to uremia from end-stage renal failure (ESRF), dialysis is the first choice. The intent is to reduce the discomfort, prevent deterioration, and prevent complications of ESRF.

If the itch is due to skin involvement in a graft-versus-host disease following a bone marrow transplantation, immunosuppression and immunomodulation is the first choice. The intent is to reduce the discomfort and cure the graft-versus-host disease.

Disease severity, disease activity and treatment intensity: the universal equation

Disease severity refers to the total severity level of the disease.

Disease activity refers to the presence and degree of symptoms, signs, and abnormal test results that represent active disease.

Treatment intensity refers to the sum total of all treatment measures that target the correct disease. These measures include medications, procedures, lifestyle measures, psychological counselling, and so on.

Proper use of the universal equation requires the doctor to make, or at least suspect, the correct diagnosis.

The universal equation

10 - ? = the difference

This is a basic mathematical equation, often taught in elementary and primary schools.

Translating this equation into healthcare, it becomes:

10	- ?	= the difference
(Disease severity)	minus (Treatment intensity)	equals Disease activity

This equation dictates an accurate estimation of disease severity and the correct interpretation of response to treatment, for all diseases on Earth.

Ideally, the patient's disease is cured or controlled. Equation-wise, disease activity should be zero. This requires treatment to at least match, if not exceed, the underlying severity of the disease. Otherwise, the patient is under-treated and disease activity will be more than zero.

When the patient is not on any treatment, such as when they first see a doctor for the onset of their new disease, the treatment intensity is zero. The disease activity is equal to the disease severity.

When a patient has been treated for the disease, disease activity is less than disease severity. You will see such patients; they have been treated by a previous doctor before they consult you.

However, the true severity of the disease is unchanged. Since the equation demonstrates that optimal management requires matching your management to the disease severity, how do you accurately estimate the disease severity in patients whose treatment has masked their true disease severity?

Getting it right: the true severity of the patient's disease

If you re-arrange the equation as per basic mathematics, you get (Disease severity) being equal to (Disease activity + Treatment intensity):

Disease severity	= Disease activity	Plus (Treatment intensity)

To get the true disease severity, add the treatment intensity to the disease activity (symptoms, signs, test results).

What we detect in the clinical evaluation (symptoms, signs) and on most tests, is disease activity.

Assuming what we see (clinically and on most tests) is always equal to the full disease severity, predisposes us to underestimate the true magnitude of the patient's illness. Underestimation leads to inadequate management: testing, treatment, monitoring, disposition, and so on.

When disease severity is not equal to disease activity, severity decides most of the intensity of the management plan, not activity. Thus, to rely on disease activity alone without recognising the difference between severity and activity, is to invite disaster.

Let us illustrate this with an example: asthma.

Patient A is a 20-year-old man who presents to the Accident and Emergency Department in the early morning, with breathlessness and wheezing that began the night before. This is accompanied by cough and rhinorrhea, which also began the night before. There are no other symptoms. He is hypoxic, with oxygen saturation at 92% on room air. He is speaking in short phrases and has chest retractions. He has fair air entry on both sides of the chest, with prominent rhonchi.

All of the above is disease activity.

As per many international guidelines and textbooks at the end of 2022, he would be classified as having a 'moderate-severity asthma exacerbation' and treated accordingly. After treatment, Patient A feels and looks much better.

Patient B then walks in an hour later. Patient B looks like a clone of Patient A: same demographics, same clinical presentation.

Using the same guidelines and textbooks, Patient B is also classified as having 'moderate-severity asthma exacerbation' and treated accordingly. Patient B worsens and develops respiratory failure. He is put on non-invasive ventilation and transferred to the Intensive Care Unit.

If both the doctor and Patient B are lucky, Patient B does not worsen so catastrophically but continues to suffer. The doctor wonders why the treatment for 'moderate-severity asthma exacerbation' as per the textbooks and guidelines, fails to work as expected.

Patients A and B looked virtually identical. What went wrong with Patient B?

The difference was the omission of treatment intensity.

Let us try the same 2 examples, this time factoring in treatment intensity.

Patient A comes in as before, with the same findings on history and examination. The doctor knows the universal equation and its implications: prior treatment could have reduced the disease activity, resulting in this patient *looking* like a moderate asthma exacerbation.

Thus, the doctor wants to know if the patient had recent treatment for asthma.

This doctor asks one more question: 'How much Salbutamol/Albuterol/other bronchodilator did you receive in the last 2 hours?'

Patient A says he has received no treatment for the asthma exacerbation. As per the universal equation, treatment intensity is zero. Therefore, the disease activity is equal to the disease severity. Patient A has a moderate-severity asthma exacerbation.

Patient B now comes in with the seemingly same presentation as Patient A. The doctor asks the same question about recent treatment.

Patient B says he self-administered 4 puffs of Salbutamol twice in the past hour. As he only felt slightly better despite the Salbutamol, he came to the Emergency Department.

(A common variation of this scenario is Patient B having seen their general practitioner, received Salbutamol without much improvement, and is then referred to the Emergency Department.)

Patient B's recent treatment intensity is noted. The doctor mentally adds his moderate-asthma-*activity* to his treatment intensity, and then realises that Patient B has a *severe*-severity asthma exacerbation.

This doctor orders more intensive treatment and closer monitoring for Patient B compared to Patient A, orders Patient B to be admitted, and considers alerting the Intensive Care Unit.

Patient B is likely to be cured rapidly. Deterioration and further suffering are unlikely when the doctors recognise the true severity of his exacerbation and know how to manage it well.

When disease severity is not equal to activity, does disease activity contribute to decisions?

When disease severity is not equal to disease activity, severity drives most of the decision-making; activity affects decision-making to a minor extent.

In the earlier example, Patient B had a severe asthma exacerbation with moderate disease activity, prompting the doctor to make plans that match the true severity: intensive treatment, close monitoring, admission and consider alerting the Intensive Care Unit.

Let us bring in Patients C and D to further illustrate the interplay between severity and activity.

Patient C comes to the Emergency Department. This patient had a moderate asthma exacerbation but had self-treated himself so intensively that he now has mild disease activity. The doctor should still factor in both the underlying disease severity (moderate asthma exacerbation) and disease activity (mild activity currently, because of intensive recent treatment) in the overall management plan.

Thus, Patient C is similar to Patient A in disease severity, but the current disease activity is milder. Since overall management must match severity, Patient C might be hospitalised and watched carefully. The doctor who intends to send Patient C home without hospitalisation, must 'break' Patient C out of the asthma exacerbation and be certain that Patient C will not worsen afterwards.

Since the disease activity in Patient C is less than in Patient A, the closeness of monitoring can be reduced earlier and Patient C may be ready for discharge sooner.

Patient D comes to the Emergency Department with a mild-activity asthma exacerbation. There was no recent treatment. Therefore, Patient D has a mild-severity asthma exacerbation.

Compare Patient D to Patient C. Both patients had mild disease activity upon presentation to the Emergency Department. However, Patient C had a *moderate*-severity asthma exacerbation whereas Patient D had a mild-severity asthma exacerbation. Would Patient D be hospitalised or require the same intensity of overall management as Patient C? No. They had the same activity, but severity dictates most of the management.

--

The same equation and considerations apply to all other diseases.

A patient with anaphylaxis (severe allergic reaction) receives an intramuscular injection of adrenaline. Thirty minutes later, the only sign of disease activity is a patch of hives on the forearm. This is mild allergic disease activity. This patient had a severe allergic reaction, but the disease activity after the treatment was mild. Should the patient now be classified as a 'mild allergic reaction', because there are residual hives in keeping with mild *activity*? No.

The next patient walks in with hives on the forearm, caused by an allergic reaction. There was no prior treatment. Their mild disease activity is equal to the severity. The first patient with more severe acute disease (anaphylaxis) whose treatment reduces their disease activity to mild, continues to be managed more carefully than the second patient whose acute disease activity is also mild.

When a patient presents to the Emergency Department and is diagnosed with viral gastroenteritis with severe dehydration, intravenous rehydration is administered. Upon review 6 hours later, the patient's signs of dehydration have decreased to 'mild activity' due to treatment. Should the patient now be classified as having 'mild-severity dehydration', and the intravenous rehydration reduced or stopped entirely to match this activity? No.

Disease activity includes results of most tests: another reason (pun intended) why reliance on numbers and tests alone, cannot replace the reasoning-based universal equation

Since disease activity includes test results, the same implications of the equation apply to the interpretation of the results of tests. Most of the tests used in healthcare, including blood tests, urine tests and imaging, demonstrate disease activity instead of disease severity.

However, these tests are commonly taught, and thought, to show disease severity. How is the doctor going to be consistently right if they do not realise that most tests show disease activity instead of severity?

Some tests truly demonstrate disease severity instead of activity. However, these tests are rare.

For example, doctors may track the elevated urea and creatinine in a patient with severe dehydration. They think the results show disease severity. After initial fluid administration, the subsequent improvement in these lab results leads some doctors to think: 'Oh, the treatment was good enough. The patient now has mild dehydration according to the current numbers. Let us reduce the intensity of the intravenous rehydration, to treat mildly severe dehydration.'

The numbers have improved because of the treatment's effect, which reduces the apparent disease activity. The underlying severity of the illness is unchanged. If the doctors now reduce the treatment intensity as if the current activity is equal to the severity of the disease, they will under-treat the patient.

Most patients' dehydration is clinically evident. They do not require tests for tracking dehydration. It is not a coincidence that poor reasoners skimp on the clinical evaluation, tend to order tests to 'track dehydration', and then proceed to misinterpret the results in this fashion.

As another example, doctors may track the patient's fever, hypoxia and C-reactive protein (CRP) in a patient who has septic shock due to severe pneumonia. The patient was admitted to the Intensive Care Unit. The improvement in vital signs and the CRP the next day leads some doctors to think: 'The treatment is ample! The disease is milder now. Let us reduce the treatment intensity by "rationalising the antibiotics". We will send the patient to the general ward. Everything will be fine.'

The patient is sent out whilst on insufficient treatment. The doctors did not understand the difference between severity and activity. If the doctors in the general ward also do not understand this difference or assume the preceding doctors are always correct, nothing will be done to rescue the situation.

The patient then deteriorates over the next 2 days and returns to the Intensive Care Unit.

The consequences of failure to recognise the universal equation

The essence of disease activity (what you see) being not always equal to the true disease severity (what you get), is:

- What you see, is not always what you get.
- What you see, is sometimes less than what you must get.

Commonplace teaching, documents, and scoring systems

Much of conventional teaching as of the end of 2022 does not recognise this universal equation. Many documents and scoring systems conflate disease activity with disease severity.

Scoring systems use clinical markers alone, or test results alone, or clinical markers in combination with test results, with the apparent aim of estimating disease severity.

If a scoring system aims to be truly accurate for disease severity regardless of treatment, the system must use the rare clinical features and/ or test results, which are unchanged by treatment.

However, the usual indicators in the scoring systems represent disease activity. When a patient has received treatment for that disease before performing the scoring, underestimation of disease severity is frequent.

If many doctors follow such documents unthinkingly, is it a surprise that patients' illnesses are often underestimated?

Is it a surprise that audits of disastrous outcomes often leave doctors wondering what went wrong, 'because according to the document, the management was appropriate for the symptoms, signs and test results that the document insists are equal to the disease severity'?

This is 1 reason I discourage unthinking, unquestioning obedience to documents written by someone else. The responsibility for the patient falls upon you, not the documents.

Humans can think straight, but it is easier not to.

Humans can ask themselves if authors are always correct, but it is easier not to.

Many guidelines and documents suggest 'step-up' treatments when the response to treatment is unsatisfactory. More treatment is needed.

How much more?

If the patient does not respond to Step 2 of treatment, should the next intensification be Step 3, Step 4, or Step 5?

Should the doctor go up 1 step at a time and let the patient suffer until 'the document gets it right'?

Does the patient need treatment halfway between Steps 2 and 3, like a Step 2.5, which avoids the higher costs and risks of Step 3?

This is where the equation makes all the difference for every patient. The doctor proficient in this equation can immediately escalate the treatment up to the necessary intensity.

The alternative is to unthinkingly follow the documents or wildly guess, and then hope for a good outcome.

Impact of the failure to recognise the universal equation, in different settings around the world

Recall Patient B, who had a severe asthma exacerbation but showed moderate activity when the doctor saw him. A poor outcome occurred because of the doctor conflating disease severity with disease activity.

Now consider the consequences of that mistake, to every patient on Earth with a potentially dangerous-if-underestimated disease. These patients could have been self-treated or treated by another doctor before they met the next doctor. When a patient is treated in the Emergency Department and is then hospitalised, the next doctor may not recognise that the reduced disease activity in the patient is due to the recent treatment, and may not recognise that this reduced activity is less than the true severity of the patient's disease.

If even one-fifth of such patients worldwide are managed whilst conflating disease severity with activity, the implications are staggering.

A common example is the patient treated for a presumed bacterial infection. The patient does not respond satisfactorily. The doctor must first question the diagnosis: was it correct? Treating for the wrong diagnosis usually leads to treatment failure. Should the diagnosis be correct on rechecking, the next question is: was the treatment intensity adequate for the disease severity?

If the doctor decides that the treatment intensity is inadequate, they must *add* the existing treatment intensity to the disease activity to estimate the overall disease severity. This doctor must then match the intensity of the entire management plan to this disease severity, instead of escalating only the treatment intensity. Disease severity affects all management, not just treatment.

Another classic example is the patient who was initially managed in the Emergency Department, is hospitalised, and then worsens. The next doctor did not realise the importance of factoring in prior treatment, such as the treatment administered by their predecessor in the Emergency Department.

At best, the patient continues to suffer and is unhappy. At worst, the patient collapses or dies. Infectious diseases, cardiovascular disorders, respiratory disorders, skin diseases, acute diseases and chronic diseases, and so on. Whatever you name, this conflation shows up catastrophically.

When Mortality and Morbidity (or Quality Assurance, or any other name for sessions intended to identify and learn from healthcare mistakes) rounds take place, ignorance of this equation explains some of the poor outcomes and the confusion of the attending doctors.

When clinical reasoning (including this equation) is ignored, these Mortality and Morbidity rounds can completely miss the root cause of the poor outcome.

Instead, various unthinking (and thus, ineffective) solutions are often offered, including:

- Do more tests
- Review the patient more often
- Call other specialists for complex patients.

None of these 'solutions' prevent the next preventable collapse or death, because the doctors have failed to recognise and fix the root cause of their mistakes: lack of reasoning, and lack of recognition of this universal equation.

Pushing the blame for a poor outcome after reducing treatment intensity, due to ignorance of the universal equation

Sometimes, the doctors who take over the care of an inadequately treated patient are blamed for the deterioration 'because the patient deteriorated whilst under your care'.

However, the main fault lay with the previous doctor who reduced the treatment to inadequate intensity. The previous doctor can become hostile when questioned about their decision to reduce treatment intensity, their reply reflecting variations of 'how dare you imply I made a mistake?' This is unacceptable on many levels.

Mistakes do occur. Denial of mistakes is bad. Pushing blame to colleagues for one's mistakes, is worse.

The doctor who pushes blame is not admitting their mistake, and thus will not learn from their mistake: ignorance of an elementary-level maths equation for healthcare.

Would you trust such a doctor to take care of you?

What is the difference between intuitively knowing treatment can mask disease severity, versus fully understanding the equation?

It is important to be aware that the treatment can mask disease activity. It is even more important to fully understand the equation to compensate for this masking effect.

Some students mention that when they are shown a patient with an 'infection partly treated with oral antibiotics', the doctors often escalate the treatment to a standard intravenous dose of a common antibiotic.

I ask the following questions:

- 'Are you sure it is an infection?'
- 'How do you know if the infection is bacterial or viral? If bacterial, what are the likely pathogens? Which antibiotics would work on these?'
- 'If the treatment intensity must be increased, how much must the increase be to match the disease severity?'
- 'If the disease is more severe than what the patient is showing you, is treatment intensity the only decision that is affected?'

These questions are often met with the students checking their assumptions. Sometimes, it is not an infection at all.

If it is an infection, it is often unclear if it is bacterial or viral.

If the treatment is escalated, the notion of different levels of intensification is often novel. The puzzled response I often get is: 'We can do something other than give intravenous Ceftriaxone?' Use of the equation to estimate 'how much more' is demonstrated later in this chapter.

The last question about the true disease severity affecting all management, not just treatment, always takes the students aback.

In every patient, the proper clinical evaluation reveals the disease activity.

Always enquire about the patient receiving any recent treatment for that disease. If there is recent treatment, obey the equation and add the mental estimate of disease activity to the treatment intensity. The total is the true disease severity.

Some doctors intuitively realise the existence of the equation for some diseases and can apply it to these diseases, but cannot apply it to other diseases.

Sufficient treatment

Sufficient treatment for most patients aims to bring the disease activity to zero.

$$10 - ? = 0$$

Using the same universal equation, the components become:

10	- ?	= zero
(Disease severity)	minus (Treatment intensity)	equals Disease activity

Therefore, for disease activity to be zero, the treatment intensity must be at least 10 points.

When the sum total of treatment intensity matches or exceeds the severity of the disease, the disease activity becomes zero.

The degree by which the treatment intensity exceeds the disease severity, is seen in the speed of resolution of clinical features and test-based indicators of disease activity. This speed is the 'velocity of improvement'.

The degree to which the treatment intensity exceeds the disease severity, correlates with the velocity of improvement up to a certain limit. Beyond this upper limit of treatment intensity, more treatment confers no additional benefit.

Cases #24 and #25 illustrate this concept of velocity of improvement:

CASE #24: Del

Del is a 40-year-old lady with migraine. She is experiencing an acute flare of migraine for the past 2 days. Her pain score is 8 out of 10.

She is prescribed analgesia.

(Continued)

(Continued)

If she is prescribed 1 tablet of Paracetamol 4 times a day, and the treatment is sufficient, her pain score drops gradually to zero over the next 5 days.

If she is prescribed 1 tablet of Paracetamol 4 times a day and 1 tablet of Ibuprofen twice a day, her pain score drops gradually to zero over the next 3 days.

If she is prescribed 1 tablet of Paracetamol 4 times a day, 1 tablet of Ibuprofen twice a day, and the trigger of insufficient sleep was identified and countered through adequate sleep, her pain score drops to zero after 1 day.

CASE #25: Jerry

Jerry is a 75-year-old man who presented to the hospital with fever, cough and breathlessness. He is admitted for *Streptococcus pneumoniae* pneumonia.

Oral Amoxycillin is prescribed for him.

If he is given a dose of 500 mg thrice a day, he recovers in 5 days, as evident by the symptoms and signs. The cough may take a longer time to resolve fully, because of post-infection tissue recovery.

If he is given a dose of 1,000 mg thrice a day, he recovers in 3 days. The cough may take a longer time to resolve fully.

If a C-reactive protein (CRP) was obtained at admission, the speed at which it drops toward 'undetectable' will correlate with the speed of clinical recovery. Thus, the CRP adds no value to a proper clinical evaluation.

Reducing treatment intensity for acute diseases: when and how

Since the velocity of improvement correlates with excessive treatment intensity, this velocity helps you safely decide whether treatment intensity can be reduced. Treatment intensity just needs to be enough, not excessive. Though excessive treatment can improve the patient's rate of recovery, the disadvantages of excessive treatment can be considerable and are discussed later in this chapter.

Example: Rationalising the use of antibiotics

Recalling the earlier, disastrous example of 'rationalising the antibiotics': the patient returned to the Intensive Care Unit because of the ignorance of the universal equation.

'Rationalising the antibiotics' usually refers to altering the dose, route or choice of antibiotic being used for the patient. This rationalisation depends on new information. This new information includes improvement in the patient's status and the return of positive cultures.

Commonplace healthcare uses the 3 points below for rationalising antibiotics:

1. The patient seems to be getting better.

2. Positive culture results, which can suggest which antibiotics seem to work *in vitro*.

3. Epidemiological knowledge, in the absence of any positive cultures. The doctor guesses the pathogen causing the patient's disease. The usual antibiotic that works on that pathogen is then used.

If you aim to be right all the time, these 3 points are insufficient. Recognising the patient's severity of disease and velocity of improvement are necessary, and at least as important as laboratory results and epidemiological guessing.

Alterations in the dose, route or choice of the antibiotic, address at least one of these 2 areas:

1. Narrow the spectrum of coverage against potential pathogens

2. Decrease the intensity of the antibiotic against the suspected pathogen

The spectrum of coverage is the theoretical list of pathogens against which the antibiotic is effective.

Intensity is the antibiotic's effectiveness on the suspected pathogen and severity of infection in that patient.

The doctor who decides to rationalise antibiotics must think through both areas.

Patients who rapidly improve are the patients in whom you might be able to safely 'rationalise the antibiotics'. Thus, rationalisation of antibiotics is usually a viable consideration (unless dealing with a severe infection, in which case you must be doubly careful) if there is a marked improvement in any of the following within 24 hours of commencing antibiotics:

- Intensity of fever (if present)

- Intensity of other symptoms and signs, which will often accompany improvement in fever intensity if fever is present. If fever is present and seems unchanged whilst other symptoms and signs seemingly improve, the doctor must recheck the diagnosis

- Patient's function.

If improvement is detected only between 24 and 48 hours after commencement, rationalisation of antibiotics requires more caution.

If there is no significant improvement after 48 hours of commencing antibiotics, the doctor must ask themselves, even if the cultures imply the antibiotics should have worked:

- Was their diagnosis correct?

- If they identified the correct disease, pathogen and site, are they underestimating the disease severity?

- Did the patient receive the antibiotics?

Other factors affecting decisions to reduce treatment intensity

Disease severity is the most important deciding factor when planning to reduce treatment intensity. The velocity of improvement is an indirect reflection of the adequacy of the treatment relative to the disease severity.

For example, if you are treating a patient whose cancer is likely to be fatal if untreated, the severity of the cancer is 'severe'. Even if the patient rapidly improves with initial treatment, the savvy oncologist does not reduce the treatment intensity purely because of rapid improvement.

This oncologist remembers the underlying disease severity. As cancer treatment can result in significant and dangerous side effects, the oncologist must balance the underlying disease severity, the velocity of improvement, and the risk of the side effects of treatment.

Chronic diseases and control

The same equation applies to chronic diseases. Control is evident from the resolution of the disease activity.

One example is shown in Case #26.

CASE #26: Ayra

Ayra is a 30-year-old lady with persistent, uncontrolled asthma. She smokes 10 cigarettes daily. In the past 6 months, she has had 2 hospitalisations for asthma exacerbations, 2 lesser exacerbations requiring outpatient treatment by her regular doctor, and nocturnal cough twice a week for every week.

If no controller treatment is provided, this pattern of asthma activity continues.

If she is prescribed an inhaled corticosteroid — Fluticasone propionate, 100 micrograms (mcg) twice daily — her nocturnal symptoms resolve. Instead of the 4 exacerbations previously, she has 2 exacerbations in

(Continued)

(Continued)

6 months, one of which requires hospitalisation and the other requires treatment by her regular doctor.

If she is prescribed Seretide (a combination of Salmeterol and Fluticasone propionate) 25/50 mcg concentration at 2 puffs twice a day, she improves even more than if she had been only given Fluticasone propionate alone. Her nocturnal cough may resolve more rapidly. Her only clinical feature of disease activity is 1 hospitalisation for a moderate-severity asthma exacerbation, once per 6 months.

If she is prescribed Seretide at the same dose and also stops smoking cigarettes, she has no symptoms of disease activity over the next 6 months. The regular smoking of cigarettes was a trigger and thus, was temporarily increasing the severity of her disease.

If spirometry was performed at all reviews, the improvement in her forced expiratory volume tends to correlate with the decrease in disease symptoms. There can be a point where the spirometry seems normal, but mild disease activity is still present as evident from the presence of ongoing symptoms.

Some chronic diseases have multiple aspects. These diseases require different treatments for different aspects. Control of 1 aspect is evident from the resolution of the disease activity of that aspect. An example is end-stage renal failure, where dialysis alone can deal with some aspects of the disease, but will not control the aspects of hypertension or mineral bone disease.

Case #27 demonstrates 1 example of a disease with multiple aspects.

CASE #27: Samuel

Samuel is a 70-year-old man with end-stage renal failure. His disease is accompanied by hypertension and anaemia. He is itching, nauseous and lethargic.

(*Continued*)

If no controller treatment is provided, he will remain in terrible shape.

If he undergoes haemodialysis once a week, he will continue to feel unwell, though less than before. His uremia and acid-base abnormalities will improve with each session of dialysis, but will be marked just before each session of dialysis.

If he undergoes haemodialysis thrice a week, he will feel much better. His uremia and acid-base abnormalities will improve and may normalise by the end of each session of dialysis. If the uremia and acid-base status are rechecked just before each session of dialysis, these abnormalities will be far less marked than if he was undergoing haemodialysis only once a week.

Since dialysis does not treat the aspects of his hypertension and anaemia, his hypertension and anaemia do not improve. Separate treatment is needed for the hypertension and anaemia.

The universal equation can also be demonstrated graphically.

The next 2 bar graphs depict the relationship between disease severity, disease activity and treatment intensity.

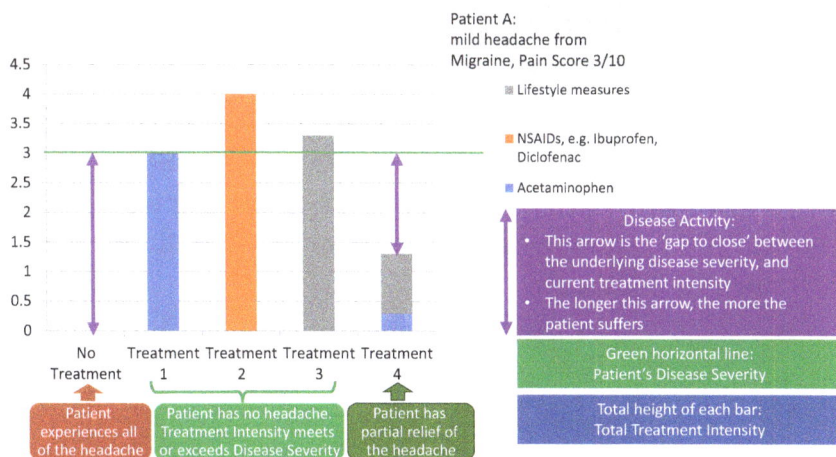

Patient A:
mild headache from
Migraine, Pain Score 3/10

▨ Lifestyle measures

▨ NSAIDs, e.g. Ibuprofen, Diclofenac

▨ Acetaminophen

Disease Activity:
• This arrow is the 'gap to close' between the underlying disease severity, and current treatment intensity
• The longer this arrow, the more the patient suffers

Green horizontal line:
Patient's Disease Severity

Total height of each bar:
Total Treatment Intensity

No Treatment — Patient experiences all of the headache

Treatment 1, Treatment 2, Treatment 3 — Patient has no headache. Treatment Intensity meets or exceeds Disease Severity

Treatment 4 — Patient has partial relief of the headache

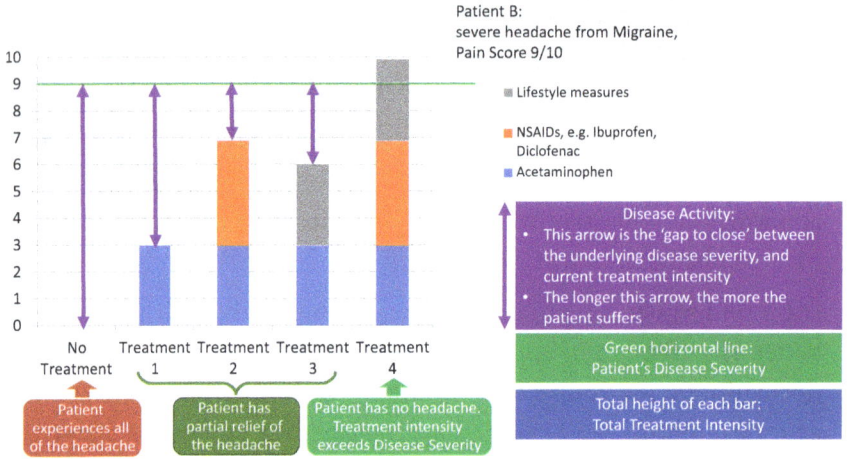

Patient B:
severe headache from Migraine,
Pain Score 9/10

■ Lifestyle measures

■ NSAIDs, e.g. Ibuprofen, Diclofenac

■ Acetaminophen

Disease Activity:
• This arrow is the 'gap to close' between the underlying disease severity, and current treatment intensity
• The longer this arrow, the more the patient suffers

Green horizontal line: Patient's Disease Severity

Total height of each bar: Total Treatment Intensity

No Treatment / Treatment 1 / Treatment 2 / Treatment 3 / Treatment 4

Patient experiences all of the headache

Patient has partial relief of the headache

Patient has no headache. Treatment intensity exceeds Disease Severity

Each graph depicts a patient with a disease (described in the grey text box).

The y-axis is the severity scale. The horizontal green line depicts the patient's disease severity.

The x-axis represents different scenarios for the same patient. Each vertical bar corresponds to 1 scenario.

Each treatment type is assigned 1 colour. The height of the bar of 1 colour, represents the amount of that type of treatment.

Multicoloured bars represent 'stacking' of different types of treatment. The total height of the multicoloured bar is equal to the total treatment intensity in that scenario.

The gap between the horizontal green line (disease severity) and the top part of the vertical bar (treatment intensity) corresponds to the disease activity. This gap is shown by the double-sided purple arrows. The longer the purple arrow, the bigger the gap and thus, the greater the disease activity.

Descriptions of the disease activity are at the bottom of each graph.

The first graph shows Patient A. Patient A has mild migraine.

The second graph shows Patient B. Patient B has severe migraine.

If both receive no treatment, they suffer the full severity of their symptoms. Patient A will have far less pain than Patient B.

As effective treatment is instituted, the symptoms decrease.

When the total treatment intensity matches or exceeds the disease severity, the top of the vertical bar meets or surpasses the horizontal green line. The patient has no disease activity and thus, no symptoms.

More treatment is needed to control severe disease in comparison to mild disease. This is the basis for stacking (or piling on) different treatments for severe migraine, whereas mild migraine may be controllable with enough of just 1 treatment type. Patient A needs less treatment than Patient B to abolish all symptoms of their migraine.

These graphs apply to both acute and chronic diseases. Regardless of whether you were considering the acute migraine attack or the long-term control of the underlying migraine over months, the graphs are the same.

Though these graphs used migraine as examples, the concepts in these graphs apply to all diseases.

The next figure depicts an example focused on long-term control. The patient has moderately severe persistent asthma.

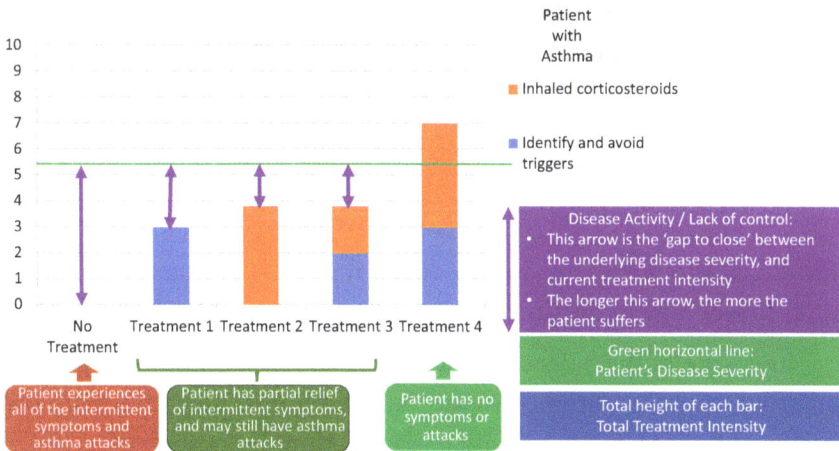

When there is no treatment, the patient experiences the full severity of their asthma.

When there is treatment, the degree of the patient's suffering reflects the 'gap' between their asthma severity and the sum total of treatment intensity.

When the total treatment intensity meets or exceeds the severity of the patient's asthma, the patient has no disease activity, and thus no symptoms of asthma.

Chronic disease: adequate treatment, and why it matters

Most chronic diseases cause troublesome symptoms. Patients want doctors to control the disease and wipe out the symptoms. Thus, the prudent doctor always aims for zero disease activity, unless major barriers for that patient require a 'balance point'.

A balance point arises when there are costs, risks, or side effects of treatment, or other major barriers, which may make zero activity unsustainable or dangerous for the patient.

Any compromise on a balance point that allows disease activity to be present, should only come after:

1. The realisation of the barriers that prevent cure or full control of the disease, and

2. These barriers have been discussed with the patient, and

3. The new (non-zero activity) goal of treatment has been discussed with the patient.

The doctor should not unilaterally decide if it is okay for patients to suffer 10%, 20% or 50% of the time.

The issue of the balance point usually arises when patients are still suffering from the chronic disease, but find it difficult to intensify the treatment further due to expense or danger from the treatment.

One example is the patient with epilepsy, who is already on 3 antiepileptic drugs that make the patient intermittently drowsy. Despite being on these drugs, the patient still has 2 brief seizures every month. Treatment less intense than this results in the patient having status epilepticus every month. Increasing treatment may reduce the seizure frequency, but is deemed too dangerous and leaves the patient non-functional. The neurologist and the patient discuss the 'balance point', and mutually agree to the current treatment regime.

Some chronic diseases may be asymptomatic whilst active. The absence of symptoms does not mean that the chronic disease can be left uncontrolled. Since complications are separate, often disastrous diseases, which tend to occur when the original disease is uncontrolled for a sufficiently long period, the asymptomatic-but-active chronic disease must be controlled. Hypertension is the most common example. Uncontrolled hypertension predisposes to myocardial infarction and stroke.

In some chronic illnesses, which are considered 'benign', very mild disease activity does not appear to significantly increase the chance of complications. One example is mostly controlled allergic rhinitis, where the occasional sneezing does not seem to increase the chance of developing complications such as acute sinusitis or obstructive sleep apnea. In these situations, mild disease activity can be allowed if the patient does not wish to burden themselves with additional treatment.

Partial response to treatment: how to interpret this response to estimate disease severity

If you have given the treatment enough time to show its full effect on the disease but disease activity is still present, the treatment is insufficient.

The proportion of improvement from the patient's baseline symptoms and signs can provide an estimate of the underlying disease severity. By extension, this partial response also allows an estimate of the additional treatment intensity needed to cure or control the disease.

The interpretation of the partial response can be demonstrated using the universal equation. Consider the next 3 examples.

First example: 10 (severity) — 1 (treatment) = 9 (remaining disease activity)

The patient improves by a tiny bit, which implies the disease severity is much greater than the doctor had initially estimated. The doctor must dramatically intensify the treatment and review all other management decisions, including testing, disposition, monitoring and counselling.

Second example: 10 (severity) — 5 (treatment) = 5 (remaining disease activity)

About half of the patient's baseline symptoms and signs are gone, or reduced to half of their initial magnitude/frequency. If the symptom was pain, the pain could be half as severe or half as frequent as before. This 50% improvement implies that the treatment intensity must be doubled to control the disease. As with the first example, the greater-than-initially estimated disease severity should also prompt the doctor to reconsider all other management decisions.

Third example: 10 (severity) — 8 (treatment) = 2 (remaining disease activity)

Most of the patient's baseline symptoms and signs are gone. If the symptom was pain, the pain intensity and/or frequency is dramatically reduced. This dramatic-yet-not-total response implies that the treatment intensity must be increased slightly more, to control the disease. As the true disease severity is only slightly greater than the doctor's initial estimate, all other initial management decisions usually do not need major adjustments.

Without this equation, wildly guessing about the intensity of escalation can be harmful in 2 ways:

1. The doctor can fail to adequately increase the treatment intensity, leaving the patient to suffer. The patient may develop a complication.

2. The doctor increases the intensity of treatment too much, leaving the patient to suffer unnecessary side effects.

No apparent response to treatment

10 (severity) — 0.3 (treatment) = 9.7 (remaining disease activity)

Suppose a patient in status migrainosus, has a pain score of 10/10. This patient takes 1 tablet of Acetaminophen. The medicine reduced the pain by 3%.

Can the patient tell the difference between 100% of pain (their original pain) and (100–3=) 97% of pain? No.

Thus, if the patient has an apparently zero response to treatment, you may have underestimated the disease severity *tremendously*.

This situation is like moving a street bus.

Moving the street bus needs enough force. If you push the street bus by yourself, it may move 1 micron. Can you see this movement? No. You lack the strength to visibly move the bus. You might need eight other people to help you push the bus to get a visible movement.

You should be worried if the patient's disease does not seem to 'move' at all. Reasons for apparently zero response to treatment include treating for the wrong diagnosis and the treatment being grossly insufficient.

Thus, recheck the diagnosis. If you are sure the patient has this disease, consider the universal equation. Sorely underestimating the disease severity requires you to alter the intensity of your entire management plan.

Precise and customised doses of treatment

The universal equation allows precise, customised doses of treatment that match the disease severity in each patient, instead of only using the standard quantities suggested in guidelines and textbooks. Earlier, I mentioned some guidelines suggesting discrete Steps of treatment, such as from Step 1 up to Step 5. In addition to helping the doctor recognise when some patients need more treatment, this equation also enables accurate estimation of the necessary treatment intensity. Examples include:

- 'Step 2.4': 40% of the difference in treatment intensity between Steps 2 and 3 of the guideline, above Step 2
- 'Step 3.8': 80% of the difference in treatment intensity between Steps 3 and 4 of the guideline, above Step 3
- 'Step 0.3': 30% of the treatment intensity suggested by Step 1 of the guideline

These precise treatment estimates allow disease control with doses in between the 'standard' Steps. In-between-Step treatment doses that cure or control the disease can confer additional benefits such as lower cost, less risk and fewer side effects of the treatment compared to the next-higher standard Step.

For example, the patient who only needs 'Step 2.4' equivalent of treatment, may spend less money and have fewer side effects than if they had been bumped straight up from Step 2 to Step 3 of treatment.

Chronic disease: when to wean treatment

Doctors and patients are often keen to wean down or wean off, treatment for chronic disease.

As per the universal equation, zero disease activity is only possible when treatment intensity matches or exceeds the disease severity.

Therefore, weaning treatment for most patients is viable only when the disease activity is zero. When disease activity is zero, the treatment intensity may be greater than the disease severity. Thus, the patient might remain well on less treatment.

When weaning treatment, check for previous treatment intensity, which was less than the current, satisfactory treatment intensity. If previous lower doses of treatment led to unsatisfactory outcomes, it is often imprudent to try the failed doses of treatment again. The patient may discover this themselves if they have tried weaning down to the next-lower-treatment dose and then became symptomatic. Alternatively, the doctors may have achieved 'zero disease activity' because they have just *increased* the treatment intensity. Do not reduce the treatment intensity back to a known, inadequate level.

For example, if the patient's hypercholesterolemia is controlled on 20 mg daily of Atorvastatin, but attempts to control this disease on 10 mg daily of Atorvastatin were unsuccessful 3 months ago, it is often imprudent to try weaning down to the 10 mg dose again.

The velocity of improvement contributes to the decision on weaning.

The disease severity and frequency of disease activity alter the interval of follow-up when weaning.

Let us use asthma as an example. Consider patients E, F and G.

Patient E has episodic asthma, which results in 2 hospital admissions for asthma in an average 6-month period. The aim of asthma control is zero episodes in 6 months. Patient E is currently not on controller therapy.

Controller therapy is instituted. Patient E is followed up once at the 4-month mark to check if there were zero admissions by the 4-month mark.

If there were no admissions for asthma at the 4-month visit, the patient is seen again at the 7- to 8-month mark after starting control therapy to ensure there were zero admissions in slightly more than 6 months, which amply ensures the aim of treatment was met. If there was no disease activity by the 7- to 8-months-later mark, weaning treatment can be considered.

If the patient had at least 1 hospital admission at either visit, a review of the overall care and escalation of treatment intensity should be discussed.

If you weaned treatment much earlier — say, at the 4-month mark despite the goal being no hospitalisations in 6 months instead of 4 months — you must be supremely confident that your initial controller intensity has greatly exceeded the underlying asthma severity.

Patient F has exercise-induced asthma, with 8 episodes of cough and mild breathlessness every month when exercising. The aim of asthma control is zero activity every month. Controller therapy is instituted, and the patient is reviewed 1 to 2 months later:

- If either the patient or the doctor is dissatisfied because of ongoing disease activity, a review of the overall care and escalation of treatment intensity should be discussed.

- If the patient has zero disease activity for at least 1 month, thereby proving there are no episodes out of the original 8 every month, weaning control therapy can be considered.

Patient G has 1 asthma exacerbation every year requiring admission into the Intensive Care Unit. Thus, their underlying asthma is severe. Intensive control therapy is needed to reduce the number of asthma exacerbations to zero every year:

- The controller therapy must be continued for at least 15 to 18 months even if there is no exacerbation after 12 months. This is because of the Law of Central Tendency (described later in this chapter); the once-a-year is an average. The next exacerbation could be 10 months later, or 14 months later.

- If disease activity is zero for at least 15 to 18 months, weaning can be considered.

- Given his severity of asthma, weaning must be slow and careful. As a comparison, weaning this patient's control therapy is far slower than weaning the control therapy of Patient E or F.

If treatment was weaned too early to conclude whether a particular treatment intensity was optimal, any flare in disease activity makes it hard to discern the optimal treatment intensity. You had not given yourself and the patient enough time to be certain if a particular treatment intensity would have sufficed to meet the goal. Let us illustrate this by going back to Patient E.

Patient E has episodic asthma, which results in 2 hospital admissions for asthma in an average 6-month period. You know this patient has an average of 1 hospital admission for asthma every 3 months. There is a time-based variation for all diseases; patients do not have their flares at perfectly timed intervals.

Your aim for asthma control is zero episodes in 6 months. Suppose you use treatment regime X at the beginning, then halve the treatment intensity 3 months later. The patient then has another hospitalisation due to an asthma exacerbation, a week after you halved the intensity of treatment regime X.

This exacerbation raises questions:

- Did the patient have their exacerbation just a little over 3 months into treatment regime X because the treatment was already insufficient, or was the exacerbation due to halving the intensity of treatment regime X?

- Was treatment regime X sufficient to ensure no exacerbations in 6 months? You do not know the answer, because you reduced the treatment too early.

Over-treatment

Given that treatment intensity must match disease severity, and given the faster resolution of disease with higher treatment intensity, it is tempting to use the maximum 'safe' dose of treatment for every patient.

However, over-treatment can cause problems.

The dose-dependent relationship of treatment effect applies to risks and side effects too.

Higher drug doses predispose to higher costs, and more frequent and severe side effects of those drugs.

For example, if you were to double your usual dose of beta-lactam antibiotics for your patients whilst keeping to the maximum limit described in the literature, more patients will develop nausea, abdominal pain or diarrhoea. Those who would have these symptoms on the standard dose would have more severe symptoms on the double dose.

Furthermore, there is an upper limit to the effectiveness of each treatment type (drugs, lifestyle measures, and so on). Above this limit, any increase in the treatment intensity of that type confers no benefit whilst increasing the risks and side effects. For example, if someone with migraine needs adequate sleep, increasing their current 6 hours of sleep per night to 9 hours, works wonders. Increasing the 9-hour sleep duration to 14 hours is unlikely to confer any extra benefit whilst depriving them of 5 more hours each day to work and relax.

These problems extend to the treatment of chronic diseases too. Unnecessary, additional control therapy imposes an unnecessary chronic burden upon the patient.

Over-treatment has consequences on a larger scale. For example, antibiotic resistance is a huge problem in areas where broad-spectrum antibiotics have been prescribed indiscriminately. This indiscriminate prescription increases the prevalence of bacteria which are resistant to multiple antibiotics, such as methicillin-resistant *Staphylococcus aureus*. The inability to treat infections caused by such bacteria increases morbidity and deaths. Researchers spend huge amounts of time and money to develop more potent drugs to treat these bacteria. When doctors indiscriminately prescribe new, more potent antibiotics, bacteria adapt and become resistant to the new drugs too. This fuels the vicious cycle of increased resource expenditure, further drug resistance, and avoidable deaths. Stopping this vicious cycle requires government officials, pharmaceutical companies, and leaders of healthcare to work together to make the hard decisions that require the relevant, strict prescription of these drugs whilst ensuring the development and testing of these drugs remain affordable for everyone, and profitable for the company.

Indiscriminate prescription of antibiotics does not spare the doctor, either. With easy access to broad-spectrum antibiotics, the doctor can delude themselves into believing that they do not need to reason, do not have to know the spectrum of pathogens for each infection, do not have to perform tests to determine the identity and sensitivity patterns of pathogens, and are safe. These delusions lead to ignorance, complacency, and sometimes, outright disaster. By telling themselves there is no apparent need to learn or reason, the doctor misses all other dangerous diseases, and becomes less competent at recognising or treating bacterial infections.

Triggers

Triggers are factors that temporarily increase the severity of the disease. The term 'trigger' is usually applied to chronic diseases.

The first equation shows the disease without the trigger.

$$10 - ? = 0$$

The next equation shows the trigger contributing to the disease severity.

$$12 - ? = 0$$

Broken down into its components, the equation is

12 (Disease severity plus trigger)	- ? minus (Treatment intensity)	= zero equals Disease activity

Since disease activity is equal to the difference between the disease severity and the treatment intensity, the disease activity will increase when a trigger is present. This increase in activity often manifests as greater suffering in the patient. Hence, patients often notice the presence of the trigger.

When a trigger is present, the temporarily increased severity of the disease means that more treatment is necessary to control the disease. Removing the trigger is preferable to using more treatment to control the disease. However, removing the trigger does not remove the disease; some treatment is still needed to control the disease. Case #26 demonstrated the effect of removing the trigger, whilst recognising that removal of the trigger alone would be insufficient for disease control.

Without reasoning, it is easy to mistakenly assume that the increased disease activity is due to 'the treatment has stopped working on the disease'. Patients who make this assumption, often stop the treatment on their own. However, poorly reasoning doctors also make this assumption and stop the treatment. Stopping the treatment that was suppressing the disease, results in an even greater worsening of the patient's condition.

When a trigger is present, the disease severity may increase so much that treatment intensity cannot be safely increased enough to control the disease. The classic example is the breastfed infant who has eczema and food allergies. The infant's food allergies are so severe that exposure to the tiny amounts of allergen through breastmilk, causes the infant's eczema to be uncontrolled. No topical steroid seems able to control the allergic inflammation. The distressed parents often wander from doctor to doctor, trying in vain to control the eczema using different topical steroids these doctors prescribe, until the parents meet a doctor who deduces the presence of the trigger.

Therefore, triggers should be identified, and then avoided. When triggers cannot be avoided, they must be mitigated. Let us use eczema to illustrate this concept.

Eczema is a chronic disease where patients suffer from itching due to an impaired skin barrier. The primary sign correlating to the degree of itching for most patients, is the dryness of the skin from localised water loss. Adequate moisturisation alone can stop most patients from scratching.

A patient may require 5 applications of moisturiser daily to the eczematous areas to remove all itch. If this patient undertakes a 5-kilometre run, they will lose more water through the skin. The exercise is the trigger. The patient scratches their skin after the run, even if they have already applied the moisturiser 5 times earlier that day.

The solution is to educate the patient on mitigating the trigger. I usually tell patients who have eczema to compensate for dryness-inducing triggers by applying their moisturisers twice more whenever they anticipate or encounter these triggers; once before (or at) the appearance of the trigger, and once afterwards. These extra applications are on top of their daily treatment regime for their eczema. Advising these patients to avoid the trigger ('Please stop exercising') is unhealthy.

Chronic disease: the Law of Central Tendency

Disease activity waxes and wanes around a true average, from hour to hour, from day to day, and sometimes from week to week.

This is the Law of Central Tendency:

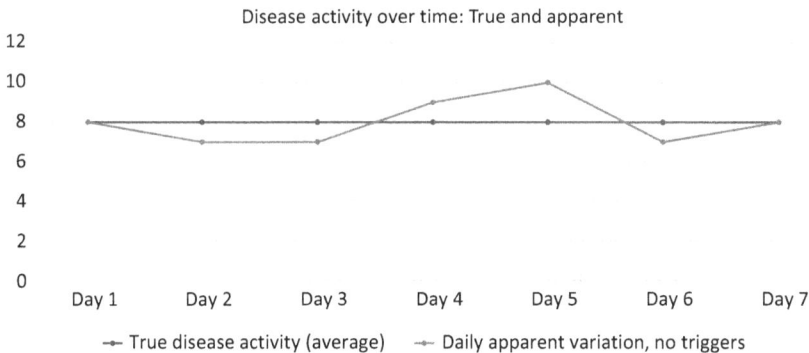

Disease activity over time: True and apparent

The y-axis represents the amount of disease activity.

The x-axis represents time.

The blue line represents the average of the disease activity. In chronic diseases, disease severity often remains unchanged or changes slowly. Therefore, if the treatment intensity remains constant, the average disease activity remains constant. The blue line representing this activity, is horizontal.

Since the disease activity is the difference between disease severity and treatment intensity, an unchanging treatment intensity decides the position of the horizontal blue line relative to the y-axis: a lot of disease activity on average, a little, or none.

The orange line represents the daily, spontaneous oscillation of the symptoms, signs and test-based markers of disease activity around the true average of activity.

If the patient in the graph had eczema, this patient would scratch their skin an average of 8 times per day. However, the spontaneous variation means that they may scratch 7 times a day on days 2–3, 9 times on day 4, 10 times on day 5, 7 times on day 6, and so on.

Using asthma as an example, the frequency of intermittent symptoms and exacerbations can spontaneously oscillate around the average of the current disease activity. Earlier in this chapter, Patient G was described as having 'brittle asthma' whose average of 1 hospitalisation per year does not occur exactly every 12 months. The actual interval between hospitalisations for asthma could be a range of 10 to 14 months, every year.

The Law of Central Tendency has implications for healthcare:

- Hourly or daily variation in the disease activity of a patient, is not always due to triggers. The variation can be spontaneous.

- A doctor who learns of apparent, even transient, worsening of the chronic disease must recheck the treatment intensity and search for triggers. However, if both efforts do not turn up any answers, the explanation is likely to be the Law of Central Tendency.

- Assessment of the average disease activity must be over a sufficiently long period, to get an accurate picture of the disease activity. Assessing intermittent symptoms of chronic diseases should be over 1 week at a minimum, whilst assessing for exacerbations of chronic diseases should be over 1 month at a minimum.

Outgrowing

Some chronic diseases, especially those in children, can be apparently 'outgrown'.

Outgrowing is the spontaneous improvement or resolution of the disease over time, usually taking months to years. Classic examples are food allergies, chronic urticaria, asthma and eczema.

Outgrowing manifests as the gradual decrease in disease severity over time. Thus, if the patient is not on any controller therapy, they will notice their symptoms decreasing gradually.

If the patient is on controller therapy, outgrowing manifests as them requiring less controller therapy over time, to 'match' the decreasing disease severity and suppress all symptoms. This is the basis for weaning or stopping controller therapy periodically, such as in perfectly controlled chronic idiopathic urticaria.

The next figure depicts this decrease in severity over time.

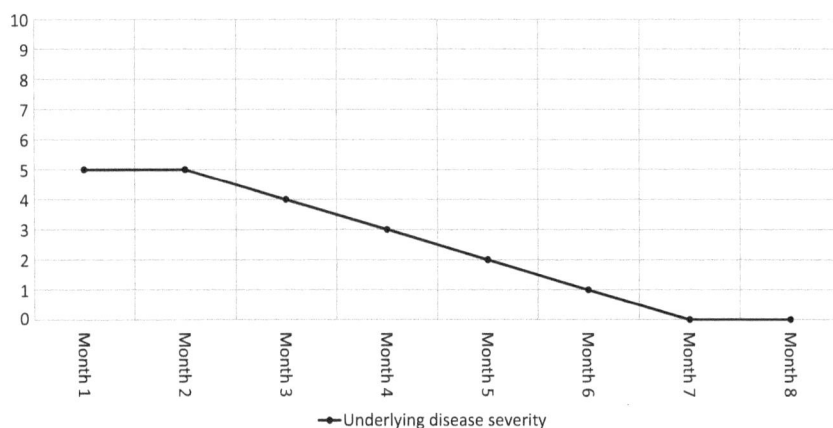

—●—Underlying disease severity

In some patients, outgrowing does not lead to a complete resolution of the disease. For example, in many children with moderate eczema, the severity of eczema spontaneously decreases, but the milder eczema persists for life. These children require greater quantities of moisturising in early childhood, then require less moisturising in later years to control eczema. If they attempt to stop all treatment for eczema in adulthood, the symptoms and signs corresponding to their new eczema severity in adulthood, will re-appear.

Capsule summary

- All effective treatment (including symptomatic treatment) targets the specific disease.
- The universal equation decides effective treatment, and accurate interpretation of the response to treatment.
- As disease severity is part of the diagnosis, excellent decisions are dependent on accurately estimating this severity.
- Always equating disease activity (symptoms, signs and most test results) with disease severity, predisposes to under-treatment and avoidable tragedies.

Frequently asked questions

Q: Do you need to track test-based disease activity to decide on treatment?

A: No. Most diseases have symptoms and signs that mirror the changes in test results: C-reactive protein, procalcitonin, X-ray changes, and so on. When these diseases always demonstrate symptoms and signs, the resolution of the disease will equate to the resolution of all symptoms and signs. In these diseases, the test results often correlate with the symptoms and signs. Thus, performing these tests in these diseases will add no value when the doctor bothers to perform a proper clinical evaluation.

Unfortunately, poor reasoners tend to neglect a proper clinical evaluation, order these tests unnecessarily, then misinterpret the results, and then make erroneous decisions.

If the disease can be present but clinically occult, tests are useful for adjusting treatment.

Q: If the concept of velocity of improvement of the patient's clinical status is applied to the treatment duration, would this application allow a doctor to identify patients who need more or prolonged treatment?

A: Yes. Many books and guidelines suggest standard treatment durations for various diseases, such as 14 to 21 days of antibiotics for bacterial meningitis. These durations will work for most patients.

I believe the doctor should get it right for all patients, not most patients. Thus, I track the velocity of improvement in the patient's clinical features and function, using this velocity to titrate the treatment intensity and duration.

Some patients do not need the full standard treatment duration for a cure. Conversely, a minority of patients need a much longer duration of treatment than the standard recommendation. In this minority, inflammatory markers such as ESR and CRP are often masked by antibiotic treatment and thus, cannot be relied upon to identify such patients. Their slow clinical velocity of improvement identifies them as patients who will relapse after completion of a standard treatment course.

Without this skill, a recurrence, re-hospitalisation and restarting of an antibiotic regime (now far more prolonged than the previous regime) often occurs in patients who need more than the standard treatment.

Some clinical indicators are more important than others for certain diseases when interpreting 'velocity of improvement'. The specific indicators for each disease require time-based illness scripts and advanced clinical reasoning to use properly, which I will not cover in this book.

Q: What are the implications of the universal equation for research studies on treatment (called 'therapeutic studies')?

A: Many therapeutic studies are randomised controlled trials. These trials often have 2 groups. One group, called the intervention arm or intervention group, receives the treatment of interest. The other group, called the control arm or control group, takes the control/comparator, which is often a placebo. The trial aims to demonstrate the treatment is beneficial, by showing superior outcomes in the intervention group in comparison to the control group.

The design of therapeutic studies must account for the universal equation to produce accurate conclusions. When researchers are unaware of the universal equation, there are 2 common ways these studies can be fatally flawed:

1. Masking of disease activity

2. Insufficient difference in treatment intensity between the groups, relative to the disease severity in most study participants

Masking of disease activity is due to treatment. Without this realisation, therapeutic studies can be conducted unnecessarily, and draw the wrong conclusions too.

The DREAM study, published in the Lancet in 2006, was a randomised controlled study that included over 5,000 participants. Half of the participants received daily rosiglitazone (a drug used to control diabetes mellitus); the other half received a placebo (no active drug). They were followed up for a median of 3 years. The main outcome being compared between the 2 groups was the development of diabetes mellitus as defined by the *measurement of the activity of diabetes mellitus*. The participants who received rosiglitazone were still taking the drug when the outcomes were measured. At the end of the study, the participants who were still on rosiglitazone, were less likely to have active diabetes mellitus than the participants in the placebo group.

The authors behind DREAM concluded that rosiglitazone prevents the development of diabetes mellitus.

The universal equation points to the truth: when you treat someone for the disease you are trying to detect, you are masking the disease and thus, are less likely to detect that disease.

Rosiglitazone does not prevent the development of diabetes mellitus; it prevents the *detection* of diabetes mellitus whilst the patient is on the drug.

To be fair to the authors of the DREAM study, the Discussion section of their article showed awareness that their conclusion could be mistaken.

Thus, they enrolled the 3,366 DREAM participants who did not seem to have diabetes mellitus by the end of that trial, into another trial where the rosiglitazone was stopped, and they were followed up for a median of 3 years to check for unmasked diabetes mellitus. After rosiglitazone was stopped and its effects had worn off, the incidence of diabetes mellitus was the same across both groups. Rosiglitazone did delay the onset of diabetes mellitus in some participants, but did not prevent these participants developing diabetes mellitus anyway.

Thus, the final and accurate conclusion is that rosiglitazone masks detection of diabetes mellitus, and taking this drug can delay its onset for up to as long as the patient is on the drug. A friend of mine pointed out that, if a patient does not yet have diabetes mellitus, asking them to receive treatment for diabetes mellitus in the hopes of delaying the onset of the disease, is nonsensical.

If a doctor tried to advise a patient to take rosiglitazone to try to delay the onset of diabetes mellitus, the conversation could go like this:

Doctor: 'You do not have diabetes mellitus. You should take rosiglitazone. This drug is taken every day. This drug is usually used to treat diabetes mellitus.'

Patient: 'Why should I take that drug? You just said it treats diabetes mellitus, and I do not have diabetes mellitus.'

Doctor: 'Because it may delay you getting diabetes mellitus.'

Patient: 'Uh, it *may* delay me getting diabetes mellitus?'

Doctor: 'Yes.'

Patient: 'Okay, suppose I take this drug for this disease I don't have anyway, for the sake of hoping I don't get the disease. What happens after I stop the drug?'

Doctor: 'If you have diabetes mellitus, it will show up. The drug masks the signs of the disease.'

Patient: 'And if the disease shows up because it was being masked?'

Doctor: 'I will treat you for diabetes mellitus. I might ask you to continue taking the rosiglitazone.'

Patient: 'And how long is the delay in getting diabetes mellitus if I take the drug every day for 2 years?'

Doctor: 'Up to 2 years. Probably less.'

Patient: 'Does the drug prevent me from getting diabetes mellitus?'

Doctor: 'No.'

Patient: 'Okay, so let me summarise what you have said. You want me to take a drug for a disease I do not have, for an unspecified duration in hopes that the drug may delay the onset of the disease by up to that duration I am taking the drug? Doctor, are you mad?'

--

Other studies have made similarly mistaken conclusions. In 2014, 2 studies were published in the *Journal of Allergy and Clinical Immunology*. Both studies subjected young babies to frequent moisturising, comparing the rates of detectable eczema in those who were moisturised versus those who were not moisturised. The moisturisers were not stopped in the intervention arm when the babies were assessed.

At the end of both studies, the authors mistakenly suggested that early frequent moisturising prevents the development of eczema.

The universal equation provides the foregone conclusion even before conducting these studies: when you treat someone for the disease, you mask the disease activity, making it harder to detect that disease.

Thus, moisturising people does not prevent the development of eczema. Instead, moisturising people prevents the *detection* of eczema whilst the patient is on treatment, and until the effect of treatment fully wears off.

To prove moisturising could prevent eczema, the moisturising must be stopped, and the participants followed up (with almost no dropouts) for at least several more months whilst off treatment.

Subsequent studies demonstrated the equation: when the babies who were moisturised had their treatment stopped, their previously masked eczema appeared. The rates of eczema in the moisturised versus non-moisturised group were similar. Studies that continued a low intensity of moisturising in the treatment group while assessing for eczema, showed that the low intensity of moisturising could not mask the detection of more-than-mild eczema.

<u>Insufficient difference in treatment intensity between the groups, relative to the disease severity in most study participants</u> can also lead to inaccurate conclusions.

This concept is demonstrated by the analogy of moving a street bus.

To move a bus a visible distance, enough force must be applied. A tiny amount of force will not result in any visible movement.

The amount of force in a therapeutic study, is the difference in treatment intensity between the intervention group and the control group. The equivalent of the weight of the bus, is the severity of the disease in most of the participants.

The treatment intensity in the intervention group may be significantly greater than in the control group. However, the analogy of the street bus points to something even more important: Since the disease severity in most of the study participants decides the intensity of treatment needed to make a visible difference in the outcome, is the difference in treatment intensity between the groups enough to make a visible difference in the outcome?

Demonstrating a visible benefit requires matching the difference in treatment intensity, to the disease severity of most of the study participants.

If the difference in treatment intensity between the intervention versus the control arms fails to match (or even come close to matching) the disease severity in most of the participants, a visible difference in outcome between both arms is unlikely.

Imagine that I am comparing the strength in my little finger, to an Olympic weightlifter's strength in their little finger. I am in the control arm of the study. The Olympic weightlifter is in the intervention arm of the study. The outcome of interest is the visible movement of a street bus. Though the strength of the Olympic weightlifter's little finger is several times greater than the strength of my little finger, would you see any visible movement if we each tried to push the bus with our little finger?

You would not see either of us move the bus.

You would not see any difference between us when we tried to move the bus.

The difference between the strength of my little finger and the Olympic weightlifter's little finger is considerable, but that difference is insignificant in comparison to the weight of the bus.

If you did not consider this factor, you might wrongly conclude that the strength of my little finger and that of the Olympic weightlifter's little finger, is equal.

Many studies, such as studies on dust mite avoidance in dust mite allergy-related diseases, demonstrate this fatal flaw. When these studies demonstrate no apparent benefit, most authors and readers do not realise the reason is the insufficient difference in treatment intensity between the study groups, relative to the disease severity in most of the study participants. Hence, the usual conclusion is: the treatment is totally ineffective in most patients regardless of the disease severity.

When other studies on the same treatment demonstrate visible benefits, this mixed picture confuses many readers. One common explanation, which is often offered for this mixed picture, is 'random error'. Random error refers to differences in results that are mostly due to chance. The fatal flaw I am describing is not a random error; it is a systematic error.

When studies demonstrate mixed results, scrutinise for clues to the disease severity in the study cohorts. Sometimes, this scrutiny reveals this exact flaw in the studies that seemed to show no benefit.

Power calculations cannot compensate for this fatal flaw. Power calculations involve estimating the minimum number of participants to show a statistically significant difference, based on the assumption that the treatment will show a benefit of at least a certain magnitude. However, the number of participants is irrelevant if there is insufficient difference in treatment intensity between the study groups, relative to the disease severity in most of the study participants.

The irrelevance of the number of study participants once this fatal flaw goes unnoticed, is explainable by the earlier analogy of comparing the strength in my little finger to that of the Olympic weightlifter's little finger, by trying to move a bus. Is there going to be any visible difference in the outcome regardless of whether we 'participate' in this contest 1 time, 10 times, or 10,000 times?

Thus, therapeutic studies need to recognise and report the true disease severity in at least most of the study participants. On top of this, they must also match the difference in treatment intensity between the different groups in the study, to that disease severity. Another intervention group employing significantly greater treatment intensity than the 'standard treatment intensity' group, may be necessary.

Once you consider the universal equation, even the existing studies that reported benefits may have underestimated the true effect because the difference in treatment intensity between the groups of study participants was inadequate to match the disease severity in a significant minority of the participants.

When I use the universal equation to try treatments for diseases where different studies report mixed results (some report benefit, others report no benefit), my patients consistently (90% or more) report a marked benefit when the treatment intensity is matched to their disease severity. This benefit cannot be explained by the placebo effect.

When studies showed a benefit for a treatment, matching that treatment's intensity to my patients' disease severity resulted in even greater benefit than the studies reported. I describe this result for asthma, in the next chapter.

Clinical reasoning must form the foundation of clinical research, especially research about diagnosis or treatment. Without this foundation, the effort and money spent designing, approving, conducting and reporting such research are often wasted. The universal equation reveals a mere fraction of the insights that researchers need. Applying the entire foundation of clinical reasoning to existing research, would require significant changes to the current methodology of clinical research worldwide.

Q: What are the implications of the universal equation for research studies on diagnostic tests?

A: Diagnostic studies usually compare the accuracy of a cheaper, faster or more convenient test to the accuracy of a 'gold standard' test. Both tests are applied to the participants in the study cohort, all of whom should have a significant chance of having the disease. Since most tests, including gold standard tests, are not 100% accurate, the best 'gold standard' is the revelation of the true disease through follow-up. Thus, robust diagnostic studies often include a follow-up period, which is long enough to detect undiagnosed disease, in the participants whose 'gold standard' test result was negative.

Like therapeutic studies, studies on diagnostic tests should account for the universal equation. However, many do not.

Why does the equation matter for diagnostic studies?

Most tests, including diagnostic tests, report disease activity instead of severity.

Since untreated milder disease has less activity than untreated-and-more-severe disease, milder disease is more difficult to detect on diagnostic tests.

Diagnostic studies usually recruit patients with moderate or severe disease. Patients with mild disease tend to form the minority of the cohort.

When the study is conducted on these participants who often have more-than-mild disease, the disease activity that is seen, used and reported to make the conclusions in the study, is often more prominent than the activity seen in mild disease.

When researchers propose criteria or cutoffs for the diagnosis of that disease, based on the average disease activity shown in that diagnostic study, the proposed criteria and cutoffs tend to be accurate for most of the study participants, but not so for the participants with mild disease.

Even if researchers did report the spectrum of severity of the disease in the study cohort and accounted for this spectrum in their study, poorly reasoning readers may not realise that the patient's disease severity matters when interpreting the results of these tests.

I have seen this confusion in many diseases, where the disease was mild but clinically obvious. Many experienced doctors and specialists are confused by the 'standard test' result, which seems to be negative based on the standard cutoffs. They do not realise that many cutoffs reported in diagnostic studies are representative of patients with moderate or severe disease. These cutoffs, if applied to patients with mild disease, would lead to many of these patients' results being interpreted as negative.

These doctors can refuse to believe the patient has that disease because they do not understand that the test and the cutoff are less accurate in mild disease. They then refuse to treat the patient. The patient continues suffering until they find a doctor who can reason properly. The subsequent response of the patient to the treatment for their disease 'rules in' that disease.

For example, exhaled nitric oxide and spirometry are diagnostic tests for asthma. Patients whose asthma tend to be mild, such as the historically named 'cough-variant asthma', tend to be more difficult to diagnose using these tests in comparison to the average patient with asthma. Spirometry often returns with normal results in patients with cough-variant asthma. Although exhaled nitric oxide has been reported to be useful in the diagnosis of patients with cough-variant asthma, it is less accurate in patients with cough-variant asthma compared to the average patients with 'asthma'.

Q: What is your opinion on scoring systems for patient care? How do you score disease severity?

A: Some scoring systems were created to standardise reporting of research findings. Others purport to be useful for patient care, but are impractical for patient-centred care. Many conflate disease severity with disease activity.

These limitations preclude their use if you are truly serious about excellent patient-centred care.

I generally split my 'severity' grades for all diseases into 3 categories: mild, moderate, and severe.

The deciding criteria for each category are:

- Description of the symptoms, such as frequency, duration and general intensity (e.g. pain scores)
- Degree of impairment of the patient's daily function
- Likelihood of complications if inadequately treated
- Threat to life if inadequately treated.

These categories focus on the patient in your locale. Being patient-centred, they facilitate decision-making and discussion with your patient and with colleagues, in a simple manner that everyone can understand.

Disease of mild severity has minimal symptoms which are often tolerable, cause little to no functional impairment, and does not threaten the patient's life. There is a nearly zero chance of complications if inadequately treated. Thus, some cancers and chronic diseases would never receive this descriptor.

Disease of moderate severity has significant symptoms that usually impair function. There is a significant chance of complications if the disease is inadequately treated. If the disease can threaten the patient's life, there is a small chance of premature death if the disease is inadequately treated.

Disease of severe severity usually has crippling symptoms. There is a high chance of complications if the disease is inadequately treated. If the disease can threaten the patient's life, there is at least a moderate chance of premature death if the disease is inadequately treated.

Does this 3-category classification overlap with some of the common grading systems for specific diseases in use worldwide? Yes. If you wish to use the common grading systems, many of which describe disease activity instead of severity, you can compensate somewhat by adding the treatment intensity to the disease activity to ascertain the true disease severity, and then manage the patient accordingly.

Q: Does clinical reasoning apply to decisions to withhold ongoing treatment for chronic diseases?

A: Yes. When patients present to the doctor with a new illness, some patients are already on treatment for one or more chronic diseases.

Some of the chronic treatments may pose problems for the safe management of the patient's new illness. Optimal decisions to withhold chronic treatment require the following:

1. The correct diagnosis must be made as soon as possible.

2. The doctor must weigh the pros and cons of withholding chronic treatment, as chronic treatment is often crucial to keeping the patient healthy.

3. Withholding chronic treatment is undertaken with the informed consent of the patient (or patient's representative, if the patient is unconscious or uncommunicative).

The 3 requirements ensure the patient's safety, and minimise the risk of perceived malpractice. Failure to meet all 3 requirements results in preventable harm to patients, and unhappy patients.

Poor reasoning predisposes to disastrous decisions regarding the withholding of chronic treatment.

Poor reasoners often fail to make the correct diagnosis. Furthermore, they tend to fixate upon their fears, such as fear that a symptom or test result abnormality may make the medication dangerous to use. Failure to recognise the correct diagnosis causing the symptom/abnormality, leads to failure to resolve the symptom/abnormality. Thus, the poor reasoner continues to be afraid and withholds the chronic medication for days, weeks or even months.

Poor reasoners often fail to weigh the pros and cons of withholding chronic treatment. Attempting to start a discussion with them on the pros and cons is often interrupted by repeated declarations of their personal fear: the symptom or test result abnormality they have fixated upon.

Poor reasoners tend to be inattentive. Even when they are told the correct diagnosis and advised to restart the chronic medication, they tend to ignore this advice.

The astute observer who watches the poor reasoner being advised on the correct diagnosis and appropriate management, will notice that the poor reasoner can appear to be superficially agreeing, but is not really listening. If the poor reasoner says anything in reply, at least half of the response is often fixated on their fear of the symptom or test result abnormality. When the doctor who told them the correct diagnosis goes the extra mile to explain how that disease causes the symptom or test result abnormality, the poor reasoner often reveals ignorance of the principle ('the diagnosis dictates the optimal decisions') by insisting that the medicines must be withheld because of the symptom or test result abnormality. Worst of all, the poor reasoner often does not treat the correct diagnosis that has been given to them, demonstrating they truly were not paying attention to their colleague or did not believe their colleague anyway. Thus, the symptom or test result abnormality remains, and the chronic medication continues to be withheld.

To the astute observer, the entire display is ironic: the poor reasoner is paralysed by their poor reasoning, and needs help. However, when given the help they need, they have such poor reasoning, and are so consumed by fear, that they readily ignore this help. After receiving the help they need, the poor reasoner often continues to be afraid and withholds the medication.

Examples include the patient with:

- Diabetes mellitus for more than 5 years. This patient has been on an unchanging dose of Metformin for years without any side effects. The patient now presents with abdominal discomfort of a few days' duration. The doctor stops the Metformin for the duration of the abdominal discomfort, because 'Metformin theoretically can cause abdominal discomfort'.

- Ischemic heart disease. This patient has been on an unchanging dose of Aspirin for a year without any side effects. The patient now presents with dizziness. The Aspirin is stopped because 'of the risk of bleeding if the patient has a fall'.

- Hypercholesterolemia. This patient has been on an unchanging dose of Atorvastatin for years without any side effects. Monitoring of the liver panel in the patient has always returned with normal results. The patient now presents with fever and neck pain. A battery of tests reveals mild transaminitis on the liver panel. The Atorvastatin is held off for weeks because 'transaminitis may be caused by Atorvastatin'.

In all 3 (real) examples, the correct diagnosis was not used as the basis for the decision. Thus, the chronic treatment was withheld without valid justification.

Such mistakes are often compounded by ignorance of the universal equation for treatment. For example, the doctor knows the patient is on diuretics because of their chronic heart disease. Since the patient is not in obvious heart failure, the doctor stops the diuretics without a valid reason. Their rationale can go like this: 'Anything is possible. What if the patient becomes dehydrated during the hospital stay? Stopping the diuretics will prevent any chance of dehydration. There is no respiratory distress or hypoxia now. Therefore, the heart condition is not severe. Maybe the patient was wrongly diagnosed with that heart disease because I do not see any sign of it now.'

When patients with chronic heart disease require diuretics to control their disease, unthinkingly stopping the diuretics often makes them breathless, and they can become hypoxic. Poor reasoners often seem oblivious to the predictable consequences of their actions. Instead of making the correct (obvious) conclusions, a common reaction is to 'treat only the number' and place the patient on oxygen, and then walk away. If so, such patients end up in the Intensive Care Unit soon afterwards.

You may think: 'How could any doctor be so illogical and callous? Are you inventing these examples?' Unfortunately, I am not inventing these examples. Several reliable junior doctors have independently and repeatedly told me the same bizarre, illogical explanations furnished to them by peers and seniors for withholding chronic medications. They simultaneously described the pattern of poorly reasoning behaviour in these peers and seniors. Worrisomely, other junior doctors have tried defending such behaviour and illogical explanations by saying: 'Just obey your seniors. Do not question them.' When these patients inevitably deteriorate in front of the robustly reasoning junior doctor, and their peers and seniors continue to seem clueless and uncaring about the problems they are creating through their reckless withholding of chronic treatment, this junior doctor has to do more work to save these patients.

Valid, informed consent to withhold chronic treatment becomes a problem when any of the first 2 requirements are not met. If the doctor does not know the correct diagnosis or fails to think of the adverse outcomes of withholding chronic treatment, how can they counsel the patient accurately?

Thus, doctors who fail to fulfil either of the first 2 requirements often fail to adequately counsel patients (the 3rd requirement) as well, illustrating the disastrous chain of dominoes.

When disaster strikes the patient, the failure to disclose such withholding-chronic-treatment decisions before the poor outcome, increases the patient's unhappiness with the doctor. This is particularly dangerous when the poor outcome can be perceived to be linked to the unilaterally decided and undisclosed decision, such as withholding aspirin, which was prescribed for ischemic heart disease in a patient, who then suffers a heart attack.

Many doctors are reluctant to fulfil the 3rd requirement of informed consent. I have heard senior doctors proclaiming aloud that 'I do not hear other doctors explaining their decisions to patients. Why should I?' This is often accompanied by 'I am too busy to explain things to patients.' These statements cannot be justified. The final decision belongs to the patient, and consequences of such decisions also fall upon the patient. Thus, informed consent to withhold chronic treatment, is a must.

In an emergency, the decision to withhold chronic treatment can be made unilaterally by the doctor. The discussion for informed consent is still important, but can be postponed until the patient is stabilised.

Even if the patient fully trusts the doctor to make all the healthcare decisions, this trust does not remove any of the 3 requirements.

If the current doctor is unfamiliar with the chronic disease, the primary doctor managing the chronic disease must be contacted for a discussion. Thereafter, the treatment should be restarted as soon as is safely possible.

APPLIED CLINICAL REASONING FOR IMPROVED HEALTHCARE

This chapter will illustrate the combination of the components of universal clinical reasoning, for 2 common diseases.

Acute asthma exacerbation in children

Acute asthma exacerbation: clinical differentials and difficulties with the diagnosis

The usual differentials for a child with wheezing are:

- Acute asthma exacerbation
- Viral bronchiolitis/bronchitis
- Rare causes

Rare causes of wheezing include 'cardiac wheeze' due to heart failure from various causes, aspiration into the lungs due to various causes, and inhaled foreign bodies. The details of the clinical features of these rare differentials, are different from the details of the clinical features of asthma and viral bronchiolitis/bronchitis.

Thus, in most patients with the 'classic' presentation of cough and wheezing heard on both sides when auscultating the lungs, asthma and viral bronchiolitis/bronchitis are the most relevant differentials. Other clinical features often accompany this classic presentation for these 2 diseases.

Asthma is a chronic disease that often manifests as episodes of cough, breathlessness, wheeze or chest tightness.

Asthma which is unrecognised or undertreated, can leave the patient coughing, wheezing and breathless for days to weeks.

Failure to recognise asthma, with the corresponding failure to diagnose and treat these children, is compounded by 3 issues:

1. Absence of detailed illness scripts

2. Loosely using the term 'viral-induced wheeze'

3. Tunnel vision

The abundance of information on risk factors — atopic history, family history of asthma, history of premature birth, and so on — in many guidelines, tempts doctors to abandon clinical features and clinical observation when trying to diagnose asthma. Without such observation, they lack detailed illness scripts and thus, cannot distinguish asthma from viral bronchiolitis/bronchitis.

Many young children with asthma do not have supportive risk factors such as an atopic history or positive family history. Thus, reliance on risk factors inevitably leads to missing such children whose asthma is obvious from their clinical features.

Popular umbrella terms worsen the problem. Umbrella terms are descriptors, not diagnoses. One such term is 'viral-induced wheeze'. Years ago, this phrase was often synonymous with viral bronchiolitis/bronchitis. 'Multi-trigger wheeze' was used almost synonymously with 'asthma'.

In recent years, more websites and journal articles are using the term 'viral wheeze' to refer to all children who wheeze and may have a viral infection, and then suggest trying treatments for both asthma as well as viral lung infections. These misleading suggestions can be interpreted to mean that doctors do not need to make the correct diagnosis.

Bronchiolitis/bronchitis and asthma are different diseases. However, many doctors argue 'common things happen commonly is the same thing as common things happen always'. For example, the doctor argues that infection is the most common cause of wheezing they know, so they must always diagnose infection. The doctor then labels all wheezing toddlers as having bronchiolitis/bronchitis. The doctor then watches these children suffer and wheeze for days to weeks, all the while insisting that this is the natural course of the infection, and thus their diagnosis must be correct.

However, undiagnosed and under-treated asthma *also* leaves the patient (adult or child) suffering and wheezing for days to weeks in the same fashion. Thus, the doctor who refuses to consider the differential of asthma and does not treat the child when the child truly had an asthma exacerbation, has seen only what they wanted to see *and* created the situation where they can continue seeing only what they want to see.

These doctors will probably never learn if they were wrong. Sadly, poorly reasoning doctors often seem unwilling to learn if they are wrong. The consistent refusal to change their behaviour or beliefs even when they were proven wrong, suggests that they find it immensely difficult to accept that they were mistaken.

Diagnostic tests could help. However, young children cannot cooperate with spirometry or exhaled nitric oxide. Furthermore, spirometry is not accurate in some children. Poor reasoners who misunderstand and misinterpret these tests often tell parents of children with asthma: 'The child does not have asthma because the test result is normal'.

A common suggestion rooted in poor reasoning, is to use epidemiology: diagnosing asthma only when the child is more than 5 years old. That means every asthmatic child below 5 years of age, keeps suffering from mismanagement until they meet a doctor who knows the folly of relying on arbitrary cutoffs. Furthermore, the rare causes of wheezing can also persist beyond 5 years of age. Thus, believing that asthma is the only possible diagnosis in the older child who is wheezing, is a fallacy based on tunnel vision.

Another common suggestion rooted in poor reasoning, is to diagnose asthma after the patient has had a large enough number of wheezing episodes. However, the number of wheezes does not differentiate between asthma and the other differentials. Consider the following:

- Some children are predisposed to recurrent, viral lung infections ('recurrent viral wheezers'). These children do not have asthma.
- Rare causes of wheezing, if untreated, often lead to recurrent wheezing.

To assume the child who wheezes repeatedly must have asthma and nothing else, is a fallacy based on tunnel vision. From a patient's perspective, the notion of waiting for enough wheezes before trying to do the right thing, is horrifying: let the patient suffer multiple times before the doctor deigns to start thinking. At the point this doctor should start thinking after the patient has suffered multiple times, the doctor refuses to think and instead automatically assumes the patient has asthma. The doctor seems only to care about doing what they want, instead of getting the correct diagnosis.

Asthma exacerbation: the clinical diagnosis

Two clinical features usually differentiate between an acute asthma exacerbation and a viral lung infection:

1. Absence of fever
2. The time lag between the onset of 'upper respiratory tract symptoms' and the development of wheezing/breathlessness

The first clue that suggests an asthma exacerbation in many wheezing children, is the absence of fever.

In children aged 2 years and above, a universal clinical feature of viral bronchiolitis/bronchitis is fever. In children who are at least 1 year old but below 2 years old, fever is a near-universal feature of viral bronchiolitis.

From my observations, at least 98% of children above 1 year of age with a viral lung infection, have fever. The fever can be low-grade.

Thus, if a toddler has a cough and has wheezing sounds in both lungs, but no recent fever, you should be wary about diagnosing 'viral bronchiolitis/bronchitis'. If there are no clinical features to suggest the rare differentials of wheezing, by elimination, the only likely diagnosis is an asthma exacerbation.

The second clue that strongly suggests an asthma exacerbation, is the time lag between the onset of 'upper respiratory tract symptoms' and the development of wheezing/breathlessness.

In this two-phase clinical pattern of illness — symptoms of involvement of the upper respiratory tract, followed by the development of lung involvement — the time lag in an asthma exacerbation is usually less than 24 hours. In viral bronchitis/bronchiolitis, the time lag is universally more than 24 hours. Thus, in this context, a time lag of fewer than 24 hours is a secondary specific feature of asthma in children.

Either of these clues is sufficient to clinically diagnose asthma and commence the correct treatment.

There are 2 caveats to relying on these clues:

- The history must be accurate. Ensure you are speaking to the child's main caregiver.
- I am describing how I recognise and handle asthma in Singapore. In theory, one could argue that asthma in Singapore might look different from asthma in the rest of the world, which is dubious but impractical to disprove: I must have seen asthma in every healthcare facility worldwide to do so. If you make this argument, you may want to try the 'trial of treatment' (described later) before taking my words as truth.

Some children with acute asthma exacerbations do not present with either of the 2 clues. In these uncertain situations, a trial of sufficient treatment intensity with inhaled salbutamol/albuterol may help to clarify the diagnosis.

Acute asthma exacerbation: the optimal treatment route

The phrase 'break the asthma cycle' refers to giving enough treatment to ensure the patient is broken out of the vicious cycle of untreated (or inadequately treated) asthma: perpetual wheezing and breathlessness that goes up and down for days. Sufficiently intensive treatment 'breaks' the acute asthma exacerbation.

Thus, 'break the asthma cycle' is the asthma-specific translation of the universal equation: treatment intensity must match or exceed disease severity.

The key points are:

- Inhaled bronchodilator, administered via a spacer and facemask, must be used. In comparison, nebulisation has a significantly higher chance of failure.

- A mild-severity asthma exacerbation will resolve with the weight-appropriate dose (100 mcg for every 3 kg body weight, up to a maximum of 1,000 mcg) of Salbutamol/Albuterol, administered up to 6 times, at 30-minute or shorter intervals.

- A moderate-severity asthma exacerbation will resolve with the weight-appropriate dose of Salbutamol/Albuterol, administered 7–12 times. The first 6 times are administered at 15-minute intervals. The next 1–6 times are administered at 30-minute intervals or less. A minority of children require a repeat of this treatment regime to cure the acute asthma exacerbation.

- Upon achieving 'resolution', stop all bronchodilator treatment and observe the child for 4 hours. Usually, the child remains well and can be discharged at the end of the observation period, with no need for another healthcare visit for the current exacerbation.

Nebulisation of salbutamol/albuterol is a popular practice. However, I discourage the use of nebulisers for asthma. There are 3 reasons why the nebulised route is inferior to the inhaler-and-spacer route.

The first reason is existing evidence on efficacy. Studies demonstrate that the inhaled route is superior to the nebulised route, for treating asthma in children. These studies (Iramain et al., 2019; Payares-Salamanca et al., 2020) are listed in the References section of this book.

The second reason is the mechanistic evidence from studies on nebulised and inhaled medications. At least 70%, and often more than 90%, of the nebulised medication escapes the mask through the vent holes instead of reaching the patient. In contrast, more of the medication administered via the inhaler route, even without accessory aids such as spacers, reaches the lungs of the patients.

The third reason is my observation of children hospitalised for moderate asthma attacks. As a first-year Paediatrics trainee in 2006, having been taught that the inhaled and nebulised routes were equally effective for administering drugs for asthma, I decided to verify this teaching. I also reasoned that though I had been taught that the 2 routes were equally effective across a cohort, their efficacy might differ between unique patients.

Children were being admitted daily for the treatment of asthma exacerbations.

When I managed a child newly admitted for asthma, some were prescribed inhaled Salbutamol via a spacer and facemask. Others were treated with nebulised Salbutamol. The doses used were age- and weight-appropriate, similar to doses used in children's hospitals in other parts of the world.

Each child would receive 3 to 6 doses of Salbutamol at dosing intervals which ranged from 15 minutes apart to 1 hour apart. My observations of prevailing practice before 2006 had already suggested that intervals longer than 1 hour apart, were rather ineffective. Even doses 1 hour apart, could be of questionable value.

As the velocity of improvement would vary based on the universal equation, I had to assess the children serially during the course of treatment. This meant frequent reviews over the first few hours after commencing treatment.

As it would be difficult to draw accurate conclusions about a given treatment intensity if I did not give that treatment enough time to work, I had to keep the intervals between Salbutamol dosing unchanged until I had enough information from my frequent reviews, to draw those conclusions.

With initial treatment using 1 route, after a few hours, the status of these children often improved: they were less breathless. Some 'broke out' of the asthma exacerbation within this time.

More of the children who received nebulised Salbutamol continued to be breathless and exhibit respiratory distress, compared to those on inhaler Salbutamol. Switching the still-breathless-on-nebuliser children over to the inhaler route often led to rapid recovery.

Conversely, if there were any children who were not recovering rapidly whilst on inhaler Salbutamol, switching them over to nebulised Salbutamol often led to them worsening.

If you are familiar with the recent literature, which compares the efficacy of the inhaler versus nebuliser route, you may wonder why the results I describe from long ago, sound even more one-sided in favour of the inhaler-and-spacer route than the recent studies suggest. It is tempting to dismiss my observations, or insist the observations must be biased because I did not perform a randomised controlled trial. Though a randomised controlled trial would have been ideal, an absence of randomisation does not automatically render an observed effect of treatment, biased or moot.

I had no pre-conceived notion of the efficacy of the nebuliser versus inhaler route. I was not deliberately choosing to use the nebulised route instead of the inhaler route for patients with more severe asthma exacerbations, or vice versa.

If my observations whilst I was comparing the 2 routes were to alter my behaviour in a biased fashion, I would probably have swung towards using the nebulised route in patients with less severe asthma exacerbations and the inhaler route in patients with more severe asthma exacerbations, to try to convince myself the two routes were equivalent in outcome. However, if I had been subconsciously doing this, based on the outcomes, the inhaler route clearly remained superior to the nebuliser route.

It could be argued that, despite what I had been taught previously and would have been tempted to believe, I could still have subconsciously used the nebulised route more often in patients with more severe asthma exacerbations, and the inhaler route more often in patients with less severe asthma exacerbations, thereby leading to the outcome falsely suggesting the inhaler route was superior to the nebuliser route. This argument cannot overturn the observations that switching still-breathless patients from the nebuliser to inhaler route often led to rapid recovery, whereas switching still-breathless patients from the inhaler to nebuliser route often led to them worsening.

The marked difference in outcome was so consistent that I found it difficult to justify continuing to use the nebuliser route to treat an asthma exacerbation in children.

The same universal equation, which applies to any 'comparison of treatment' for all diseases on Earth, may further explain this discrepancy between my observations and the literature.

Recall the analogy of using enough force to move the bus. If the force is sufficient to move the bus, greater force leads to greater movement.

Since appropriate treatment intensity provides a greater response than half-adequate treatment, the more study participants there are whose disease severity is at least matched by the treatment, the greater the apparent benefit in the study cohort.

I used this universal equation back then, when choosing the initial dosing regimes for both inhaler and nebulised Salbutamol.

Most of the children would have received adequate or near-adequate treatment via at least 1 route. Thus, the comparison between both routes would demonstrate the superior route, with the difference in benefit being more apparent because more children were receiving treatment at the necessary intensity relative to the severity of their exacerbation, to show that difference.

At this point, you may be thinking: If this evidence points to the inhaler route being superior to the nebuliser route for delivering treatment for asthma in children, does the same concept apply to adults?

A Cochrane review in 2013 on the therapeutic studies in asthmatic adults, suggested no difference between the inhaler-and-spacer versus nebuliser routes. However, I suspect that many of the therapeutic studies in adults with asthma did not account for the universal equation. It may be worth repeating the therapeutic studies in adults, this time incorporating the equation, to see the truth in adults.

I say 'may be worth repeating', because it is almost certain that the inhaler route would prove superior to the nebuliser route in adults too. I have not seen 1 patient or study prove the universal equation wrong, across patients of different ages and diseases, and across therapeutic studies for multiple diseases around the world. In fact, combining pathophysiology and the universal equation often predicts the results of many therapeutic studies before they are even conducted; it is hard to believe that asthma in adults can magically be an exception to the equation.

Even if you disbelieve the universal equation and my observations, it is impossible to logically dispute the implications of the mechanistic studies mentioned earlier in this chapter, which show that more of the medication from the inhaler route reaches the patient's lungs in comparison to the nebuliser route. It is also impossible to logically dispute that the same drugs are effective in most children and adults with asthma, even if the doses are different and a minority of adults with asthma may have a different phenotype from most patients with asthma.

If you ask me whether I think the therapeutic studies for the inhaler-versus-nebuliser route in asthmatic adults are worth repeating, I would say, "No". The result is a foregone conclusion. Wasting time and money to satisfy sceptics (or poor reasoners, or doctors who ignore pathophysiology) or to add to one's resume for self-promotion, should not be the aim of research. There are genuine questions that remain unanswered, that this time and money can be better spent on.

Since 2008, I have used inhaler Salbutamol near-universally. The one time I tried nebulisation in a patient, between 2010 and 2020, led to a poor outcome.

Acute asthma exacerbation: the optimal treatment regime

My regime employs inhaled Salbutamol administered at short intervals, ensuring an intense burst of bronchodilators within a short time. This regime accounts for another observation: when the bronchodilators were administered with time intervals that were too far apart, such as 1 hour or more, the child tended to stay in the asthma cycle of breathlessness, wheezing and hypoxia. If the intervals were lengthened when the child still had clinical features of an active acute asthma exacerbation, the child often worsened. The clues from this observation demonstrate the universal equation: disease activity increases when the treatment intensity decreases.

Recognising the optimal route and universal equation, points to the next questions:

- How many doses of Salbutamol are needed to match the severity of the exacerbation, thereby achieving 'resolution/breaking out' of the exacerbation?

- How can you safely ensure your assessment of breaking them out of the exacerbation, was accurate?

- What are the clinical features that define the 'resolution/breaking out' of the exacerbation?

For mild asthma exacerbations, a regime of up to 6 doses was sufficient to break the child out of the exacerbation. The usual range was 3 to 6 doses.

For moderate asthma exacerbations, 6 doses administered 15 minutes apart, were insufficient. After some tweaking and observation, a total of 12 doses (6 doses 15 minutes apart, then 6 doses 30 minutes apart) was optimal for most patients. Some patients needed less than 12 doses. A minority (10% or less) needed up to a total of 24 doses; the extra 6 to 12 doses on top of the initial 12 doses, were given using the same dosing intervals as the initial 12 doses.

For example, a child who needed a total of 18 doses, would receive 6 doses 15 minutes apart, then 6 doses 30 minutes apart. Upon being deemed to still have the active exacerbation, this child is given another 6 doses 15 minutes apart.

This treatment regime breaks most children out of their acute asthma exacerbation within 10 hours.

Severe asthma exacerbations usually cannot be resolved using this regime. Upon recognising a severe asthma exacerbation, greater intensity of treatment, such as intravenous Magnesium Sulphate in addition to the 12-or-more-doses described earlier, should be commenced immediately.

Acute asthma exacerbation: when the child is broken out of the exacerbation

The clinical features (criteria) that define the 'resolution/breaking out' of the acute exacerbation are:

- The main caregiver says the child's breathing is fully back to normal
- If asked for breathlessness, the child (if they can understand the question) replies 'No'
- There is no tachypnea, retractions or use of accessory muscles of breathing
- On auscultation, the air entry is equal bilaterally
- The oxygen levels are 95% or more on room air.

Though wheeze and rhonchi are signs of disease activity, their presence seemed to have no impact on the outcome. Therefore, I left these out of the criteria, and do not use wheeze or rhonchi when assessing for breaking out of the exacerbation.

A child who fulfilled the criteria for 'resolution/breaking out' of the exacerbation was well enough to be discharged. To be doubly sure, I usually stop all bronchodilator treatment and recheck the child 4 hours later, thereby ensuring the child remained in the 'resolution/breaking out' state without masking any of the disease activity.

If the child fulfilled all criteria by the no-bronchodilators-for-4-hours mark, they could be discharged.

The parents of these discharged children, are advised to administer a low dose of Salbutamol inhaler (usually 100 mcg or 200 mcg) once every 4–6 hours for the next 2–3 days. Once you consider the universal equation and the intensity of treatment needed to break the asthma exacerbation, this very low dose of Salbutamol after discharge is probably unnecessary in most patients. However, as local practice often involves advising *some* Salbutamol treatment for 3 days after discharge, and I have not yet conducted a trial to see if these children need any treatment after my intense treatment regime, I stick to this aspect of local practice. For now.

Most of these children with moderate exacerbations also complete a 3-day course of oral steroids. Most of these children would become symptom-free within the next few days (unless they had a flu that precipitated the asthma attack, in which case the flu symptoms may still be present).

Side effects of treatment

Over the years, I watched the children treated with this intense regime, for side effects of Salbutamol treatment, including signs of overdose/toxicity.

By matching the treatment intensity to each patient's severity of their asthma exacerbation, including treating severe exacerbations appropriately (instead of giving them scores of doses of Salbutamol in vain), I have not yet seen 1 child with Salbutamol toxicity.

Hypokalaemia is a side effect of Salbutamol treatment. Having used this 12-to-24 dose regime for hundreds of children and having checked the serum potassium levels of many of these children at the end of the regime,

I count less than 10 children (all needing more than 12 doses) whose serum potassium levels dropped significantly because of this therapy. The drop was less than 1 mEq/L, which was often left alone because the new potassium level was normal, or was near-normal and would spontaneously return to normal within 24 hours. A few of these children received 1 oral dose of potassium supplementation.

Only 1 child had transient tremors.

Thus, I no longer check the serum potassium for children with a moderate asthma exacerbation, unless they needed more than 12 doses and their appetite was poor enough (which can predispose them to hypokalaemia) to worry me.

The literature comparing the side effects between these 2 routes supports the use of the inhaler route over the nebuliser route. Bronchodilators administered through the inhaler route have fewer side effects, such as tremors and tachycardia, compared to the nebuliser route.

Burger et al. (2021) reported skeletal muscle weakness being more common in the group who received bronchodilators via the nebulised route compared to the bronchodilator route. They postulated the muscle weakness was caused by hypokalaemia. However, the serum potassium of the study participants was not measured.

Conclusions about asthma treatment: inhaler versus nebuliser route

In summary, the inhaler route is superior in efficacy to the nebuliser route. This is evident both from my personal experience and the literature. The literature also suggests the inhaler route is superior to the nebuliser route in terms of side effects.

Many students often ask: 'Why do so many doctors try nebulisation in children with asthma? Surely, they must have a good reason!'

The real, unspoken question is: 'Are you saying the common practice of many doctors is not optimal?'

They do not want to believe the answer to their often-unspoken question, which would shatter their belief that doctors always do what is right. However, by the time they ask this question, they already know the answer.

Humankind often indulges in common behaviours that are dubious or harmful. These behaviours can be fuelled by beliefs and ignorance. Beliefs can cause unnecessary harm if they are so rigidly followed that reality is ignored. Doctors are no exception.

Commonplace treatment and outcomes for asthma exacerbations

Healthcare practice is varied. Even with the literature pointing to the inhaler route being superior to the nebulised route, nebulisation continues to be common in the treatment of acute asthma exacerbations.

Regardless of whether the route of bronchodilator administration is nebulised or inhaled, the dose intervals vary widely too. A common practice is to administer 3 weight-appropriate doses of the bronchodilator with an arbitrary time interval between each dose, review the patient clinically after the 3rd dose, and then decide the time interval between the next 3 bronchodilator doses. This pattern is continued until the patient recovers, or deteriorates enough to be sent to the Intensive Care Unit. The initial intervals can range from 15 to 30 minutes apart, which are then increased stepwise to 1 hour apart, then 2 hours apart, then 3 hours apart, and so on.

When doctors are unaware of the universal equation, a common mistake is to assume 'improvement' is the same as 'good enough'. After the initial treatment for an asthma exacerbation, there is often some improvement in the child's condition. This improvement is assumed to be 'good enough'. However, the initial treatment intensity is insufficient to break the child out of the exacerbation. At this point, the doctors often make one of 2 choices:

1. Maintain the same dosing interval even though the child still has increased work of breathing. As per the universal equation, the

same insufficient treatment intensity leaves the disease activity unchanged: the child remains in the same state for several hours or days.

2. Lengthen the dosing interval (e.g. 1 dose every 30 minutes is 'stretched' to 1 dose every hour instead), thereby reducing the intensity of bronchodilator treatment over the next 2 to 6 hours. When questioned, the doctors declare the patient's improvement shows that the treatment is ample. The child usually worsens afterwards, demonstrating the universal equation: when insufficient treatment intensity is reduced further, the disease activity increases.

These doctors often bounce between either of these 2 choices over the next few days, never realising that neither choice is optimal.

Many patients who are treated in this way, recover in 2 to 5 days. Some are discharged from hospital prematurely without being cured; their asthma activity rebounds after they stop the bronchodilator treatment at home, and they end up re-attending the hospital's Accident and Emergency Department.

What junior doctors ask upon seeing my treatment regime, and what I teach about it

Medical students and junior doctors often rotate to different hospitals and consultants. When they encounter me, either as part of my ward team or during teaching, my regime seems novel to them. Some declare this outright, with variations of 'No one else does this!' They go on to explain that my treatment regime is much more intense in a shorter period, than the other treatment regimes they have seen.

Initially, many of these students and doctors found it hard to accept this treatment regime. This reluctance is understandable: humans often want to fit in with others. Doctors often want to do the common thing that other doctors do. Seeing something novel, is uncomfortable for many people.

Despite the varying levels of acceptance, none of them can dispute reality: the child recovers within the span of several hours. When they see this happen consistently, they are forced to accept that the results are not a fluke.

They are uncomfortably aware that the other doctors they have observed and learnt from, are not getting the same results: their patients remain unwell for days.

As observation alone is not enough for consistent learning and full understanding, I explicitly teach the concepts in this chapter to these students and junior colleagues.

Only a few are bold enough to tackle the unspoken gorilla in the room. They ask: 'How did the basis of giving 3 doses every 30 minutes, then stretching to every 1 hour, then every 2 hours, then every 3 hours, come about? Why are so many doctors doing that?'

I explain that if the doctor has never realised the existence of the universal equation, any 'stepwise' regime (optimal or not) can seem logical in any disease. It does not matter whether the disease is asthma, or any other disease where stepwise regimes have been suggested in guidelines and protocols.

I advise the medical students and junior doctors who are part of my ward team, to come by every 1 to 2 hours to review the patients treated with my regime. This allows them to observe the changes in the child's condition when the treatment is optimal, so that they learn the time-based clues that point to optimal treatment of an acute asthma exacerbation, and the lack of reliability of the less-reliable clues (such as the presence of wheeze or rhonchi) for predicting recovery.

This advice is also based on mindfulness: The medical students and junior doctors will see that I do not always review my patients every 1–2 hours, due to reasons such as me being in my busy clinic for the next 4 hours. They can wrongly assume that frequent reviews are unnecessary, especially if they keep seeing these patients 'break' out of the asthma exacerbation whilst their teacher (me) never seems worried enough to keep reviewing the child. This assumption leads to complacency.

If learners want to get the same results consistently and safely, they must acquire the reasoning and attentiveness that allow them to deliver the right treatment to the right patients.

Poorly reasoning doctors who misuse my lessons

I caution you against taking the 'easy way out' and indiscriminately administering 12–24 doses of Salbutamol to every child who wheezes.

I have taught junior doctors about the clinical recognition of asthma and shown them the results of this treatment in children with asthma exacerbations, including children who were misdiagnosed or labelled as having a 'viral wheeze'.

After my teaching, some proceed to skimp on the clinical evaluation and instead administer this treatment indiscriminately to all wheezing children they see. Others have heard of my results and started doing the same unthinking 'trial of intense treatment' whilst skipping the evaluation or proper diagnosis for the patient.

I cannot condone this behaviour.

Research studies that tried indiscriminate treatment with different routes in wheezing children without a proper diagnosis, often showed no difference in efficacy between the routes. This result is unsurprising, because effective treatment targets the diagnosis and its severity, instead of treating a symptom or sign. However, many doctors and researchers seem oblivious to the fact that the correct diagnosis is the anchor for excellent decisions. Effective treatment targets the diagnosis; ineffective treatment treats a symptom, sign or test result abnormality whilst ignoring the diagnosis.

Treating children with bronchiolitis or bronchitis using salbutamol through an inhaler and spacer is often futile. This was stated openly until doctors began using the label 'viral wheeze' to conflate asthma exacerbations with viral lung infections. By conflating the 2 diseases, the label of 'viral wheeze' then allowed the claim that treating anyone with 'viral wheeze' with salbutamol could be beneficial. This conflation has led to many children with bronchiolitis and bronchitis being treated for asthma, with a predictable lack of significant improvement.

Bronchiolitis and bronchitis tend to resolve on their own after several days. Thus, poor reasoners who label children with viral lung infections as having 'viral wheeze', can provide treatment for an asthma exacerbation, see the child recover a few days later due to spontaneous resolution of the lung infection (the asthma treatment having shown no effect for days), and then erroneously declare that 'viral wheeze does respond to asthma treatment'.

When questioned, poor reasoners often reply that they are 'treating a wheeze'. When asked *why* they are treating a wheeze, they claim other doctors and seniors are doing the same and thus, they can do it too. If their claims are true, the argument that 'I can do what I see other people doing, regardless of what happens afterwards' is usable if you are only interested in copying others, instead of providing excellent healthcare. This argument is also used by some criminals to justify their crimes.

Upon exploration of what these poor reasoners saw of 'other doctors doing the same', the description is always the disastrous chain of dominoes: scant clinical evaluation, no proper diagnosis, routine batteries of tests, and indiscriminate treatment.

To lack reasoning, is bad. To decide to unthinkingly copy others instead of fixing one's poor reasoning, is worse. When the 'others' being copied also lack reasoning (and are unthinkingly copying others too), the entire situation demonstrates the saying: The blind leading the blind.

Wasting resources is foolish. Moreover, unthinkingly 'treating a wheeze' is dangerous. Doctors who treat a symptom or sign will usually skimp on the clinical evaluation, and thus will miss dangerous diseases. These poor reasoners routinely miss the rare causes of wheezing. Some of these poor reasoners indiscriminately order batteries of tests to try to 'rule out' the rare causes of wheezing, mistakenly believing that normal test results rule out all rare causes of wheezing.

Poorly reasoning doctors who know the proper treatment for an asthma exacerbation, but refuse to treat it optimally

Sometimes, doctors know the child has an asthma exacerbation and know the first-line treatment is Salbutamol administered through an inhaler and spacer, but insist on using nebulisers instead. Their explanations often include:

- 'The patient is hypoxic. The saturation is less than 93%. The nebuliser allows me to give oxygen at the same time, which will make the oximeter number look good.'

- 'The parents want to use the nebuliser.' When asked if they explained the importance of the inhaler and spacer route to the parents, the doctor says 'No' or remains silent.

In a patient with an acute asthma exacerbation, whose hypoxia is caused by the asthma exacerbation, the doctor should provide treatment with enough intensity to 'break' the asthma exacerbation, thereby getting rid of the hypoxia.

If the poor reasoner truly cared about getting rid of the abnormal oximeter number rapidly and permanently, should they not properly treat its cause?

Furthermore, the use of the inhaler and spacer does not preclude the administration of supplemental oxygen in between giving doses.

Insisting on using a route for treatment that the doctor knows is inferior to the alternative, for fixing the 'number' the doctor claims to care about, while pretending that only the nebuliser route allows adequate provision of oxygen supplementation, reveals the truth: the doctor is using specious arguments to justify doing what they want.

Giving the child's parents what they want whilst knowing it is inferior to the alternative, and without doing the right thing such as explaining and offering the superior alternative, is the decision-making style of abandonment of responsibility.

Imagine that the doctor diagnoses a patient as having acute appendicitis. This patient asks for antibiotics as the definitive treatment. The doctor knows that antibiotics are not the gold standard for the treatment of appendicitis. The doctor prescribes these antibiotics anyway, deliberately fails to inform the patient of the higher chance of a poor outcome when using antibiotics alone, and deliberately fails to inform the patient of the gold standard treatment for acute appendicitis.

Who has the expertise in the disease? Who has the responsibility to use that expertise?

A variation of the apparent fixation on numbers involves reducing the treatment in a child who was already mildly tachycardic from the asthma exacerbation, because 'the child is tachycardic'. The doctor says 'the child is more tachycardic when we give Salbutamol. I don't like the higher heart rate. Let us reduce the Salbutamol frequency.'

If the tachycardia is due to the asthma exacerbation, 'breaking' the asthma exacerbation resolves the tachycardia, and simultaneously reduces the need for further Salbutamol treatment the doctor professes concern over.

Thus, if the poor reasoner truly cared about the abnormal number, should they not take effective action to resolve the abnormality quickly and effectively? Giving inadequate treatment ensures the child continues to suffer and remains tachycardic for days to weeks.

When asked how they can justify withholding the treatment that would cure the asthma exacerbation rapidly and simultaneously resolve the tachycardia they claim to care about, the poor reasoner often goes silent. The silence reveals much: the poor reasoner does not really care about the number. They are using the number to try to conceal their true aim: to do what they want.

Experience with young children with asthma: over the years

Being able to break all mild and virtually all moderate asthma exacerbations in less than half a day is useful. These children can be treated and discharged from the Accident and Emergency Department and clinics. Unnecessary hospitalisations are avoided.

I have intervened many times in these toddlers with asthma who were labelled as 'viral wheeze'. When I see them in the morning rounds in the children's ward, intervention at that point means their asthma exacerbation is rapidly 'broken'. They are often discharged by the same evening. Follow-up reveals they often become symptom-free within the next few days at home (unless they had a flu that precipitated the asthma attack, in which case the flu symptoms may still be present).

The effect is dramatic for parents whose toddler had been bedbound for days, wheezing away from an undiagnosed moderate asthma exacerbation. Many of these toddlers are labelled as 'viral wheeze' or misdiagnosed with bronchiolitis/bronchitis. The parents witness the effects of the 12- to 24-dose burst of Salbutamol via the inhaler-and-spacer route. By evening, the child is up and running.

As parents should not go home with the mistaken impression that they should routinely perform such intense treatment themselves — safety lies in a proper clinical evaluation, which most parents cannot perform — I caution them not to try the same intense regime at home in the event of another wheezing episode. Instead, they should consult the doctor first.

Promptly recognising children with asthma also facilitates the discussion on controller therapy in those children who need controllers.

Consider the usual rates and length of stay of hospitalisation for asthma.

If children with asthma exacerbations were routinely diagnosed and treated this way, the rates of hospitalisation would plunge.

If children with moderate asthma exacerbations were routinely hospitalised (which is probably unnecessary) regardless of their initial response to treatment, this regime would drastically shorten the length of stay.

The real difference in asthma: a recent example

I saw a 2-year-old girl, Abby, in early 2023 in my clinic for the first time, for her previously undiagnosed atopic diseases. A few weeks later, her parents reached out via email to request my input. The tone in the email was frantic. I saw the email in the morning when I arrived at work, and called her parents at 7.30 a.m.

Her mother unhappily told me:

- Abby had been admitted with fever, cough, breathlessness and noisy breathing to another hospital. This was the first time she had ever developed breathlessness and noisy breathing.

- For the past 2 nights in that hospital, she had been given various treatments, including inhaled Salbutamol once every 2 hours.

- She was improving minimally. She was still hypoxic (saturations 90% or so on room air) and breathless.

- As of that morning, her parents had been told the diagnosis was still acute bronchitis.

I asked a few questions, and then explained that Abby's diagnosis was probably a moderate asthma exacerbation triggered by an upper respiratory tract infection, with a 99% certainty. Though I would have preferred to also examine her myself, the clinical features were convincing and specific for asthma, and did not fit acute bronchitis. I explained that I could speak to Abby's doctor and advise them on the optimal treatment. If they were not comfortable providing this treatment, I mentioned the option of transferring Abby over to my hospital, where I would then break her out of the exacerbation the same day.

Mindful of the perceptions and ego of her doctor, and also of her parents' unhappiness, I asked to speak to her doctor. After we chatted for a bit, I explained that Abby's parents were unhappy, repeating the information her mother had provided earlier. I explained the most likely diagnosis of a moderate asthma exacerbation instead of 'acute bronchitis', and specified the exact optimal treatment regime to break Abby out of her moderate asthma exacerbation.

As I also knew that some doctors prefer to adhere to their existing plans or protocols instead of considering a new perspective, I mentioned that if they were uncomfortable following my advice, Abby could be transferred to the hospital I was in. I explained that they could either follow my advice and break her out of the asthma exacerbation by that same afternoon, or transfer Abby over for me to break her out of the exacerbation.

Almost an hour later, Abby's mother called me back and told me: 'The doctor does not agree with you. They want to keep following their protocol and do the same thing they were doing. They advise that Abby stays tonight in this hospital again, to see what happens.'

I replied, 'Then you know what to do. She should come to the Children's Emergency at my hospital. I'll see you soon.'

I then pre-empted the senior doctor of the Children's Emergency, of Abby's arrival and my treatment regime. When Abby arrived near noon, she was independently reviewed by that doctor, and the clinical diagnosis of asthma was affirmed.

The doctor at the Children's Emergency called me, sounding puzzled: 'Abby's mother is expecting admission.'

I apologised to him, and explained that I had told Abby's mother that the point of the transfer was to promptly break Abby out of her asthma exacerbation. I had not mentioned admission; thus, her mother could have thought that since Abby had been admitted to the other hospital, I had intended to admit Abby too. I explained that admission would probably not be necessary, and I would clarify this personally with Abby's parents after my morning clinic.

Abby was commenced on the regime of weight-appropriate Salbutamol via inhaler and spacer, every 15 minutes, for 6 consecutive doses.

Near 1 p.m., I visited Abby in the Children's Emergency. Abby had just received her 3rd of the first 6 doses of Salbutamol. Her parents said she was still breathless. On examination, she was quiet. She was still hypoxic at 90–92% on room air. She was tachypneic with intercostal recessions, with bilateral rhonchi and patchy decreased air entry over her right chest.

I considered her clinical diagnosis, current findings on examination and the treatment received thus far. I then told Abby's mother that Abby would be broken out of the exacerbation by 3 p.m. (the 9th dose of my 12-dose regime, described earlier in this chapter). I explained that she would see it for herself, as Abby's breathing would return to her normal pattern.

Abby's mother was worried enough to request admission to the hospital ward. I explained that I routinely broke other children out of their asthma exacerbations within hours, and thus an admission would probably be unnecessary. After I had explained this to both of Abby's parents, they decided to wait and see if my prediction was accurate.

At 2.20 p.m., en route to the canteen to grab a quick (and late) lunch, I stopped by the Children's Emergency again. By then, Abby was back to normal, smiling and playfully bouncing on the small bed. She had just received her 7th dose of my 12-dose regime. Her parents were happy. Abby was discharged from the Children's Emergency later that afternoon.

This example demonstrates all the earlier points in this book, and this chapter:

1. It is important to perform a proper clinical evaluation, and understand the significance of the information gathered.

2. The correct diagnosis dictates the optimal treatment.

3. The optimal chain of dominoes comes with robust reasoning; the disastrous chain of dominoes shows itself through poor reasoning.

4. If you do not treat for the correct disease, you can create the situation that facilitates your seeing only what you want to see.

5. Doctors may not want to learn, even when reality shows the outcome is poor, they are aware the patient is unhappy, and specific advice was given to them to 'rescue' the situation.

6. It is foolish to do the same thing over and over again, and expect a different result.

7. Casual, genuine confidence in accurate decision-making, counselling and prediction, comes from robust reasoning backed up by years of consistent, patient-centred success.

Do patients with acute asthma exacerbations really need steroids? If so, how much?

I am unsure if patients with asthma exacerbations truly need steroids. Calling upon the pathophysiology of asthma and the universal equation, I suspect patients who receive a severity-matched bronchodilator regime to 'break' them out of their asthma exacerbation, would either require no steroids at all or a 1-day course at most.

To answer the question about the need for steroids, a randomised controlled trial with at least 3 groups is optimal. A bronchodilator treatment regime, matched to the subjects' individual exacerbation severity, is administered to all groups. One group receives no steroids, 1 group receives 1 day of steroids and 1 group receives more than 1 day of steroids. The subjects must then be followed up for at least 2 weeks to monitor for a relapse of the asthma exacerbation.

It can be argued that doctors who cannot match their treatment regime's intensity to their patients' asthma severity, would not obtain the same results as this trial would reveal. Thus, why bother with the trial?

This argument falls flat once we remember that doctors are supposed to match their treatment intensity to the severity of their patients' disease. Arguing that a trial is not applicable because doctors should be assumed to be incompetent, conveniently reinforces the next indefensible argument: if there are no trials that require doctors to be competent for clinical application, then trials do not need to be designed around effective healthcare because doctors should be deemed incompetent.

If a doctor has not learnt the clinical skill of recognising disease severity and then making optimal decisions around that severity, the problem does not lie with the trial. Instead, the problem lies with the doctor.

Giving more treatment in other areas to try to compensate for an inability to recognise the disease severity, does not address the doctor's weakness. In asthma exacerbations, some doctors propose trying a 5-day course of oral steroids instead of 3 days, 'in case the patient needs more treatment'. I disagree with this proposal. Giving more treatment in other areas should be done only when necessary, and only after optimising the most important treatment for the disease.

Commonplace practice in many diseases, including asthma, demonstrates this 'give more treatment in other areas, just in case' behaviour. A bit of everything is prescribed to the patient. However, the most important treatment is not optimised. The coexistence of suboptimal treatment optimisation and polypharmacy is not a coincidence. Doctors who understand treatment optimisation do not need to resort to polypharmacy unless it is necessary. Doctors who do not understand treatment optimisation, often resort to polypharmacy in the vain hope that doing a bit more of everything, can substitute for treatment optimisation. Some patients do require multiple drug treatments for optimal care, but polypharmacy should not become an excuse to ignore learning the skills to optimise treatment.

When the most important treatment for their disease is not optimised, the patient's outcome is often poor. Everything else in the treatment regime, thrown in without understanding the disease, cannot compensate for the failure to optimise the most important treatment.

This commonplace 'throw the kitchen sink' polypharmacy-type treatment regime with its attendant poor outcomes, is explained in the next disease in this chapter: Eczema.

Optimising asthma treatments: how this affects our world

Reducing greenhouse gas emissions is important for sustainability and slowing the pace of climate change.

Pressurised metered dose inhalers are 1 mode of delivery for asthma medications. These inhalers contribute to greenhouse gas emissions more than other inhalers, such as dry powder and soft mist inhalers, because they contain propellants made of hydrofluorocarbon. Greenhouse gas emissions are detrimental to the environment and speed up climate change.

Widespread substitution of the less-environmentally-friendly inhalers for the more environmentally friendly inhalers would reduce greenhouse gas emissions.

Inhaler type aside, the most important factor in healthcare that reduces greenhouse gas emissions all around, is the reduction of wastage. The production of many healthcare resources and treatments, contributes to greenhouse gas emissions. Wastage of resources requires new production of these resources, which increases greenhouse gas emissions. Having patient-centred doctors who can optimise care and simultaneously reduce wastage because they do not order unnecessary tests and treatments, would go a long way towards the goal of sustainability and preserving the environment, for ourselves and future generations.

Eczema

Eczema: clinical differentials

Eczema is a common chronic disease that causes itching.

The potential differentials for eczema include:

- Seborrheic dermatitis of infancy
- Scabies
- Fungal infections of the skin
- Various benign skin diseases
- Systemic diseases with skin manifestations: juvenile dermatomyositis, celiac disease, psoriasis, and so on.

Eczema: the universal equation applied to the reasons to itch

There are 3 reasons for a child with eczema to be itchy. These reasons for itchiness, are aspects of eczema. Instead of expounding on the many pathophysiological theories, I will cut to the chase:

1. Dry/rough

2. Inflamed

3. Bacterial infection

Each child has one or more aspects (reasons to be itchy). Most patients will have dryness and roughness as the main aspect and the root cause. If inadequately treated, the child develops additional skin inflammation due to them scratching their skin. If this scratching continues, the child can develop bacterial infection on the skin.

The entire 'itching' relationship looks like this:

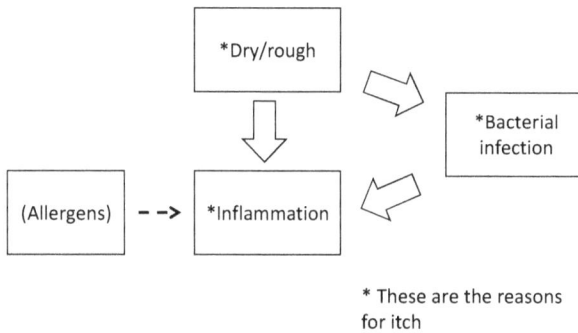

```
        ┌──────────────┐
        │ *Dry/rough   │
        └──────────────┘           ⇨
              ⇩                        ┌──────────────┐
                                       │ *Bacterial   │
                                       │  infection   │
┌────────────┐   ┌──────────────┐      └──────────────┘
│ (Allergens)│--->│ *Inflammation│   ⇦
└────────────┘   └──────────────┘

                        * These are the reasons
                          for itch
```

Obtaining an estimate of the average number of days a week that the patient scratches their skin, is a useful marker of overall disease activity.

Ascertain the disease activity of the aspect of dryness/roughness. Disease activity is evident from the symptoms (frequency and functional disturbances caused by itching) and signs (the feel of the skin on touch). This activity is added to the intensity of the existing moisturising regime, to obtain the severity of this aspect. This severity must be matched by the total intensity of moisturising.

Ascertain the disease activity of the aspect of inflammation. Disease activity is evident from the symptoms (frequency and functional disturbances caused by itching) and the signs (degree of skin pigmentation, weeping, flaking, and sometimes papulation). This activity is added to the intensity of the potency and frequency of the topical steroids being used, to obtain the severity of this aspect.

Since inflammation is often driven by the activity of the aspects of dryness/roughness and bacterial infection, treating the dryness/roughness and bacterial infection aspects adequately will dramatically reduce or abolish the need for any topical steroid or immunomodulatory therapy.

If the inflammatory activity remains significant despite ensuring both (dryness/roughness and bacterial infection) aspects are either adequately treated or absent, allergens must be suspected as drivers of the inflammation.

The 3rd aspect, bacterial infection, is not the classic rapidly progressive fever, golden crusting or pustules described as 'impetigo' in many references. Instead, the usual scenario is the patient who has been scratching their skin for years, and then develops a new-onset itchy rash lasting weeks to months (rarely, infants can develop this too). More moisturising and topical steroids of increasing potency confer little or no improvement. The doctor who sees the patient presenting with this scenario, has 3 options:

1. Ignore the history, and assume the patient needs more of the usual skincare. Increased moisturising, potent steroids, immunomodulators or phototherapy inevitably fail. The patient looks for another doctor.

2. Jump to the wrong conclusions, such as assuming the patient has developed eczema herpeticum and treating for this disease. Some doctors 'treat for everything', including using antibiotics. When the doctor fails to recognise the aspect of bacterial infection, the prescribed antibiotics are inadequate and only serve to mask the disease activity until the antibiotic course is completed. Afterwards, the symptoms recur in full force. The patient looks for another doctor.

3. Use robust clinical reasoning, and recognise the rash for what it is (see below).

On inspection, the new rash comprises punctate scabs and excoriations with surrounding erythema, often over the years-long eczematous areas and previously uninvolved areas of skin. This rash spreads slowly. If untreated for long enough, the pustules and golden crusting of classic impetigo eventually appear. Application of an appropriate topical antibiotic and the use of an antiseptic wash once a day, works wonders within a week.

The activity of bacterial infection is estimated from both the symptoms (frequency and functional disturbances caused by itching) and the extent of the skin involvement. This activity is added to the existing use of antiseptics and topical antibiotics, to ascertain the severity of this aspect of bacterial infection. This severity then dictates the total treatment intensity targeting the bacterial infection.

Bacterial infection is a complication of uncontrolled eczema. Therefore, such infection is a clue that the underlying eczema is usually uncontrolled. The poor control is usually due to insufficient moisturising. Without tackling this root cause driving the complication, the itching will continue and the bacterial infection tends to recur once the antibiotics and antiseptics are stopped.

For long-term control and eventual eradication of the bacterial infection, both the antiseptic intensity and the moisturising must be adequate. Recurrence of itching or spots points to one or both being inadequate. The antiseptic wash may be needed for a few months to prevent relapse.

Thus, treatment of eczema should be titrated to the severity of each aspect in each patient. Optimal eczema care shares the same principles as care of other chronic diseases with multiple aspects, where effective care requires titrating treatment to each aspect of the disease in each unique patient.

By recognising the relationship between each reason to scratch, and the contributions of the aspects of dryness/roughness and bacterial infection to the aspect of inflammation, 2 goals can be accomplished:

1. Control the eczema by reducing the itching and scratching to approximately zero, through patient-centred assessment and management.

2. Accomplish such control whilst dramatically reducing or abolishing entirely, the use of topical steroids or more expensive/ risky treatments.

Eczema: commonplace care as of the end of 2022

Commonplace care for eczema and 'eczema action plans' are limited by various factors. One is the abundance of literature with many confusing hypothetical descriptions of eczema types and pathophysiological theories.

Poor clinical reasoning is common. One manifestation of poor reasoning is the 'throw the kitchen sink' strategy, also known as 'try a bit of everything': a bit more moisturising, more potent topical steroids, antibiotics, antihistamines, and so on.

With this 'try a bit of everything' strategy, most patients will improve somewhat since the regime would cover a bit of every potential aspect.

However, the poor reasoner often has no idea of the presence and severity of each aspect. Thus, this doctor cannot tailor the treatment to match the aspects of eczema in each unique patient. The 'try a bit of everything' strategy is attempted, not because polypharmacy is necessary, but because the doctor cannot fully understand and thus, cannot adequately assess the patient's eczema.

Common variations of the 'try a bit of everything' strategy include:

1. 25% moisturiser, 25% steroids/immunomodulators, 25% antiseptic wash/antibiotics, 25% oral antihistamine

2. 33% moisturiser, 33% steroids/immunomodulators, 33% oral antihistamine

3. 50% moisturiser, 50% steroids/immunomodulators

4. 25% moisturiser, 75% steroids/immunomodulators

Unfortunately, if even 1 reason to scratch (such as dryness/roughness) is not adequately treated, the patient continues to scratch. Since most patients do not have equal proportions of severity of each aspect of their eczema, and since most patients who would benefit from topical steroids need more moisturising than steroids for effective control, most of these patients continue to scratch.

Are they feeling better compared to no treatment? Yes.

Is their feeling better, the same as good enough? Probably not.

The doctor's eczema action plans often mirror the ineffective, static 'throw the kitchen sink' strategy of the doctor. The presence and magnitude of reasons to scratch can vary with each day and each flare. Thus, a static treatment strategy and action plan cannot account for this variation.

I identify the reason(s) the child scratches, and then teach the child's parents (and the child, if possible) to assess the reason(s) for scratching. This is followed by teaching them how to increase the corresponding treatment for each aspect.

Since the universal equation that drives this assessment is the same as an elementary maths equation, this teaching is easy for most patients to understand and use.

Eczema and unnoticed food allergies in children

Of the children who have eczema, a minority also have unnoticed food allergies. Ongoing exposure to the food allergen renders their eczema uncontrollable. Even when specialists attempt to use potent topical steroids or immunomodulators outside of the standard recommendations for use, the eczema remains refractory to treatment.

These patients fulfil 3 clinical criteria:

1. Infant-onset of eczema, and

2. An overall severity of moderate-or-higher, and

3. The severity of skin inflammation matching or exceeding the severity of the dry/rough skin when the eczema first began. For this criterion, just ask the child's parents which was more prominent: the dryness/roughness of the skin, or the colour changes?

A child who fulfils all 3 criteria is almost certain to have one or more food allergies. A careful dietary history (in breastfed infants with this type of eczema, the mother's dietary history is important) and correlation with the temporal pattern of eczema activity, often reveal the allergens before any testing is performed.

Being able to clinically diagnose the food allergies in these patients even when there is no history of IgE-mediated reactions, facilitates prompt testing and effective treatment for these patients, and simultaneously avoids unnecessary testing in everyone else with eczema.

The optimal treatment regime for eczema-with-food-allergies is slightly different from the common eczema seen in most other patients. The natural history of a child with eczema and food allergies, which drives the chance of outgrowing eczema and each food allergy, is complex. I will not discuss the treatment regime or prediction of outgrowing in these patients, in this book.

Eczema: common fallacies

The common fallacies regarding eczema and its treatment include:

1. Topical steroids cannot be applied for more than 1 week continuously, because they are harmful.

2. Topical treatments for eczema must be applied in a fixed sequence for all patients.

3. Topical treatments for eczema must be applied one at a time, with several minutes between each type of treatment.

4. The illness known as topical steroid withdrawal, does not exist.

1. Topical steroids cannot be applied for more than 1 week continuously, because they are harmful.

If the doctor has made the correct diagnosis and is treating an inflammatory flare of eczema, the appropriate topical steroid will often remove the inflammation within a few days.

If the patient feels they need to use the topical steroid continuously beyond 1 week, it is usually safe to continue the topical steroids for a total of 2 weeks. However, the optimal reaction to the patient needing to use the topical steroid continuously beyond 1 week, is not to continue the topical steroids alone.

If a patient feels compelled to apply the topical steroid daily for over a week, they are still suffering.

If they are still suffering after a week of this treatment, the disease is not eczema or the doctor has missed the reason(s) causing the flare.

In this situation, the correct move is to promptly get a second medical opinion and hope the doctor can get it right, be it the same doctor or a different doctor the second time.

Without this knowledge, the suffering patient may stop the topical steroid at the 1-week mark, because they were told to use the steroid for 1 week without any explanation as to why the recommended duration was 1 week. They can then assume the medicine is dangerous, which is untrue and does not solve the patient's problem. Thus, the immediate harm in believing this fallacy comes from the failure to advise patients appropriately.

Failure to advise the patients appropriately can create more harm: The patient may wildly guess that the steroid must be dangerous, which can perpetuate steroid phobia and phobia about medications in general. Widespread phobias, compounded by doctors failing to explain their plans in full, fuel non-compliance and distrust of the healthcare profession.

2. *Topical treatments for eczema must be applied in a fixed sequence for all patients.*

When this fallacy is believed, the doctor insists that the moisturiser must always be applied before the topical steroid, or vice versa.

Neither is true.

In many patients, the sequence of application makes no difference to efficacy or safety. I have stopped asking my patients to try the different sequences and tell me the better sequence, because the answer was almost always 'there is no difference'.

In a minority of patients, all topical treatments for the skin must be applied simultaneously for maximum efficacy. Thus, insisting on sequential instead of simultaneous application can reduce the benefit of the topical treatments for these patients.

3. *Topical treatments for eczema must be applied one at a time, with several minutes between each type of treatment.*

This fallacy is based on the belief that topical treatments can interfere with each other. This is untrue for most patients.

As mentioned earlier, a minority of patients require all topical treatments to be applied simultaneously for maximum efficacy. This simultaneous application seems to have a synergistic effect for these patients, much greater than the expected sum of its individual parts. This is like 1 (treatment A) + 1 (treatment B) = 4 (final effect of both treatments).

Some experts in eczema, and recent studies, echo my experience. However, this minority of patients usually encounter doctors who tell them this fallacy. Only a few in this minority eventually stumble upon a doctor who recognises their eczema subtype, and knows the importance of simultaneous application of topical treatments.

4. *The illness known as topical steroid withdrawal, does not exist.*

It is usually impossible to prove a sweeping negative. Furthermore, humans who want to believe something does not exist, often ignore all proof of its existence. Doctors are no exception.

Topical steroid withdrawal is a condition where the frequent (daily or almost daily) and prolonged use (often, for at least several weeks) of steroids on the skin, creates discomfort instead of helping the patient.

In topical steroid withdrawal, the usual chronological sequence is: The patient notices the topical steroid, applied continuously or near-continuously for several weeks or longer, has a diminishing effect on their skin on consecutive applications.

Eventually, there is no improvement with the use of the steroid.

When the application of the steroid continues, the topical steroid begins worsening the skin condition instead of helping. The patients often describe burning pain over the sites of steroid application.

On physical examination, topical steroid withdrawal usually leaves signs of florid, homogeneous inflammation over each area the patient had applied the topical steroids.

At this point, the patient usually stops the topical steroid and consults a doctor. At the consultation, the signs on physical examination may be fading, especially if the patient has stopped the topical steroid for at least 2 weeks before the consultation.

Though topical steroid withdrawal does exist and patients will describe it in graphic detail, many doctors dismiss the patient's concerns. Some doctors pretend to agree with the patient, which does not fool the perceptive patient. These doctors often tell the patient to continue the steroids, or prescribe even stronger topical steroids instead! Some doctors prescribe topical immunomodulators as a substitute for the topical steroids, and then struggle to control the eczema.

The patients who consult me usually have seen 3, 5 or more doctors; some have seen 'skin specialists' in different countries. These patients are often unhappy with these doctors for 2 reasons: the doctors did not believe them and could not control their eczema.

Though the universal equation suggests that the stopping of topical steroids in ongoing inflammation will result in a recurrence of disease activity, topical steroid withdrawal is a separate problem that is unrelated to the universal equation's explanation of topical steroids and inflammation.

The robust reasoner who hears a history from the patient that somewhat resembles the chronological description for topical steroid withdrawal, does not instantly assume the patient has topical steroid withdrawal. The other differential to consider is a new skin disease. A proper clinical evaluation distinguishes between a new disease and topical steroid withdrawal.

Applying the entirety of clinical reasoning to other diseases

Are the concepts described for these 2 diseases, applicable to other diseases? Yes.

Are fallacies common across diseases? Yes.

The discussion on acute asthma exacerbations demonstrates the need to be clinically observant, have detailed illness scripts, make the correct diagnosis promptly, and then institute proper treatment. The universal equation also demonstrates the adverse consequences of underestimation of treatment effect relative to disease severity, for patients and for therapeutic studies.

The concepts illustrated for eczema mirror effective care for all chronic, complex diseases with many aspects, such as advanced chronic kidney disease. Such diseases require the doctor to identify each aspect of the disease and the severity of that aspect, and then match the treatment accordingly. For example, not every patient with end-stage renal failure needs the same intensity of treatment in their dialysis regime, medications to prevent renal bone disease, and medications to control anaemia.

Would outcomes superior to commonplace healthcare outcomes (as of end-2022) be achieved, merely by applying all the basic concepts in this book? Yes.

Would clinical research be less confusing and more accurate, by applying the relevant concepts in this book to each study type? Yes.

Would these benefits be realised without requiring more technology or vast financial expenditure? Definitely.

Capsule summary

- The universal clinical reasoning method can dramatically improve healthcare and clinical research worldwide.
- Safely recognising and treating asthma requires the entire reasoning process, instead of misuse of individual components whilst ignoring the rest of the process.

- Effective eczema care requires treatment to target each aspect in each unique patient.

Frequently asked questions

Q: Why didn't you publish your insights into treatment, much earlier?

(This is the common refrain from students and colleagues, especially after they consistently see the results of my not-published-in-journals treatment regimes for multiple diseases. I only mentioned 2 diseases in this chapter. One could argue that I only discussed one-and-a-half diseases because I did not describe my treatment regimes for control of the different clinical phenotypes of asthma.)

A: To publish 1 study at a time, is to deliver these insights in a piecemeal and potentially incomplete fashion. Publication requires a formal application for a study, and then money and manpower to conduct the study. This consumes a lot of time and energy for just 1 study. Expending the time and energy to publish each discovery for each disease would require me to sacrifice something else in return.

If I had tried to publish these during my traineeship, the sacrifice would be the honing of my reasoning, which enabled these discoveries in the first place, or my official training.

Furthermore, the refinement of clinical reasoning to come up with these treatment regimes, required a deeper understanding of the clinical evaluation and the concept of reasoning, than what was known prior to the publication of this book. If you look at the years between 2006 and 2023, there have been many publications about external descriptors of clinical reasoning, but little progress in the understanding of clinical reasoning. Without providing that deeper understanding, many readers would immediately reject treatment regimes that seem novel, regardless of their efficacy.

Even if every reader was prepared to try a treatment regime to see for themselves, describing these regimes without providing the clinical approach and clinical reasoning for these diseases would limit the applicability of these regimes. If the doctor struggles to deduce the correct disease or estimate its severity, their patients would be frequently mistreated anyway.

Thus, understanding and then describing the process to maximise the chance of getting the correct diagnosis, was necessary. Simultaneously, understanding the applications of the universal equation was necessary; readers must understand how the same clinical evaluation needed to maximise the chance of getting the correct diagnosis is also necessary to optimally use any treatment, including my treatment regimes.

Even now, I am still honing my clinical reasoning and making other discoveries. My time is better spent on more valuable purposes than filling out my resume with publications, for the sake of self-promotion.

If my students or colleagues want to conduct studies using my insights on various diseases, I am happy to share these insights with them, so they can conduct the formal study itself to verify the insight and then publish the results.

Earlier, I alluded to more valuable purposes than filling out my resume. One 'more valuable purpose' was the assembly of the insights and lessons, followed by the massive effort expended to describe this method fully, simply and clearly for the world.

To those who kept asking me to publish my insights: this book would be equivalent to *at least* 30 journal articles describing novel, crucial and immediately applicable concepts in medical education.

Once you recall the book's audience includes doctors across all specialities and settings, all healthcare workers other than doctors, government health officials, and researchers, and then add up the effect of the book across all these readers, '30 journal articles' is a gross underestimate of the impact.

Until the concepts in this reasoning method are incorporated universally, the flaws in many clinical studies will persist. A researcher cannot reliably counter a flaw if they are unaware of its existence. Doctors who unthinkingly copy and apply the results of flawed research studies, will automatically copy the mistakes.

Even if reasoning-centred clinical studies were conducted, the second major barrier remains: the readers. Without systematic training in clinical reasoning, readers often misuse the results of these studies, just as some have misused my treatment regimes by skimping on the clinical evaluation.

Q: Can we join you in your clinic or ward rounds to see what you do, for ourselves? Can you demonstrate this method in patients and diseases outside your professional specialities?

A: You are welcome to join me to observe, assuming my current employer (if any) is also agreeable. I can be reached at my electronic mail address in the 'Additional resources' chapter.

When something seems too good to be true, it is often untrue. This wisdom is important for protecting oneself against frauds and misleading opinions. I live by this wisdom too. Thus, some who request the chance to observe, are sceptical and perhaps rightly so. If I were in their shoes and were not convinced despite reading this book, I would want to see for myself if the seemingly too-good-to-be-true claims are indeed true.

The many benefits of robust reasoning were described in the FAQ section of the earlier chapter 'Common mistakes in the clinical approach'. If such reasoning was applied to the care of all patients in a ward, benefits include short ward rounds, everyone understanding what is going on in their patients, effective management, shorter hospital stays, fewer (or no) tests ordered, few (or no) test results to wait for, and less work all around. The doctors get more time for themselves and can go home sooner.

Asking me to travel to your workplace to demonstrate this method, will require discussion.

I demonstrate this reasoning method during the Universal Clinical Reasoning teaching sessions, on patients outside my professional specialities. You are welcome to observe these sessions. More information on these sessions is provided in the chapter 'How this came about'.

COMMON MISTAKES IN TREATMENT

Common mistakes in treatment can be divided into:

1. Having no (or misplaced) goals of treatment, and

2. Incorrect interpretation of the response to treatment.

These can be further subdivided into:

1. No (or misplaced) goals:

    - Treating without any diagnosis

    - Treating after making a diagnosis, but without recognising the goal of the treatment.

2. Incorrect interpretation of the response to treatment:

    - Reacting wrongly to 'failure to respond to treatment'

    - Wrongly equating 'the patient is better' to 'this is good enough'.

Categories of Mistakes

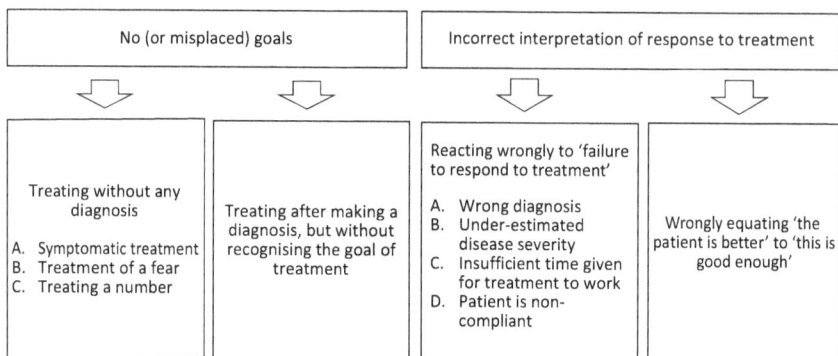

No (or misplaced) goals		Incorrect interpretation of response to treatment	
Treating without any diagnosis A. Symptomatic treatment B. Treatment of a fear C. Treating a number	Treating after making a diagnosis, but without recognising the goal of treatment	Reacting wrongly to 'failure to respond to treatment' A. Wrong diagnosis B. Under-estimated disease severity C. Insufficient time given for treatment to work D. Patient is non-compliant	Wrongly equating 'the patient is better' to 'this is good enough'

1. No (or misplaced) goals

Treating without any diagnosis

There are 3 common manifestations:

    A. Symptomatic treatment

    B. Empirical treatment of a fear

    C. Treating a number

Often, a proper clinical evaluation is not performed. This omission of a proper clinical evaluation is both cause and effect of these manifestations: the doctor who decides not to treat diagnoses would see no reason to perform a proper clinical evaluation to obtain a diagnosis. Since there is no diagnosis, the doctor randomly picks something else (a symptom, fear, or number) to treat.

Missing the diagnosis increases the risk of disaster.

A. *Symptomatic treatment*

This mistake occurs when the doctor looks at the patient's symptoms and signs in isolation, and then treats each symptom or sign in isolation.

The choice of the treatment often comes from wild guessing, or copying what they saw other doctors do for their patients without understanding why those doctors gave that treatment.

Examples include:

- Fever is treated with antipyretics
- Itch is treated with antihistamines
- Cough is treated with cough syrup
- Pain is treated with analgesia
- Rash is treated with topical steroids
- Ulcers are treated with antiseptic cream
- Wheezing is treated with Salbutamol

Disaster can strike because there is no diagnosis. For example, the patient consults a doctor for the symptoms of fever and cough. The doctor decides to treat each symptom in isolation. The clinical evaluation is omitted or performed carelessly. Having missed the signs of pneumonia, the doctor prescribes Acetaminophen 'for fever' and cough syrup 'for cough', and then tells the patient to go home. The patient deteriorates, and is then hospitalised for pneumonia.

Another example is the doctor who sees a patient with a fever and headache. The history is scant and the physical examination is lacking. The doctor prescribes Acetaminophen and Ibuprofen. The patient is hospitalised the next day with septic shock due to bacterial meningitis.

B. *Treatment of a fear*

Some doctors assume patients can have a disease they fear, and then let their personal fear consume them. This doctor then treats the patient as if the patient has that disease. Thus, they are treating their fear instead of the patient. A doctor who is often consumed by fear will often be treating their fears at the expense of most of their patients.

The classic example is the doctor who prescribes antibiotics to every patient with fever, high fever, fever for more than (insert a number of 3 to 7) days, sore throat, or any symptom presumed to be related to bacterial infection.

When consumed by these fears, the doctor also tends to order tests that can be linked to that fear. For example, the doctor who fears bacterial infections tends to order a full blood count or CRP readily, thinking 'a high total white cell count or C-reactive protein must mean there is a bacterial infection'. Even when the test results are normal, the doctor often treats the patient for the feared diagnosis anyway. This behaviour reveals the true intention of ordering the tests: the tests were not intended to aid in the diagnosis, but to find some superficial (illogical) justification for ordering treatment and persuading the patient to agree to the treatment.

Treating a fear is the same as wildly guessing about treatment, with the same problems of complacency and masking. The consequences of complacency and masking were described in the chapter 'Diagnostic puzzles: how to handle them'.

C. *Treating a number*

The doctor treats a number, be it a vital sign or test result. The usual aim of treatment is to 'make the number normal'. Examples include:

- Tachycardia: the patient is given intravenous fluids
- Hypoxia: the patient is given supplemental oxygen
- Uremia: the patient is given intravenous fluids
- Hyponatremia: the patient is given intravenous sodium chloride.

These treatments can seem to imply the doctor has a diagnosis in mind. For example, in a patient who has tachycardia or uremia, the administration of intravenous fluids can imply the suspicion of intravascular hypovolemia caused by a disease.

However, when the medical notes lack documentation of any clinical evaluation or diagnosis, or even record findings that directly contradict the implied condition, these clues demonstrate that the doctor has no diagnosis. Instead, the doctor is probably (unthinkingly) copying what they have seen other doctors do. Whether those doctors who were copied were also unthinking, is unknown.

To find out whether the doctor is managing a diagnosis or a number, ask the doctor for their diagnosis. If they do provide a diagnosis, ask them the difference between treating the number versus treating the diagnosis. A robust reasoner consistently furnishes the correct diagnosis and can always explain the difference between treating that diagnosis and treating the patient's numbers. A poor reasoner inevitably struggles with the first question or second question.

Treating numbers without knowing the correct diagnosis, can greatly increase the danger of major harm or death, if the treatment:

1. Directly worsens the severity of the disease, or
2. Is directly contraindicated in that disease

If a patient has tachycardia due to acute viral myocarditis, aggressive intravenous fluid boluses to 'normalise the heart rate' often do not normalise the heart rate. Worse, these fluid boluses overload the already compromised heart to the point that the patient develops acute pulmonary oedema. The patient may collapse or need ventilatory support (or both). The consultant in the Intensive Care Unit and the cardiologist are unlikely to be happy with this outcome, because they must treat the patient's myocarditis *and* they have to deal with the pulmonary oedema that was disastrously precipitated by their colleague. The doctors who deal with this mess get even more upset when they detect the obvious clinical features of acute myocarditis in the patient, which their poorly reasoning colleague did not bother to look for. The doctor who made this mess may face an official enquiry or a lawsuit from the unhappy family of the patient (or both).

Another dangerous example is the poor reasoner who sees a patient with unexpected hyponatremia. Instead of using clinical reasoning, this doctor follows an arbitrary checklist that is mostly based on wishful thinking and wild guesses.

The usual first step is to check that the lab result was assigned to the correct patient.

When the lab result is proven to have been correctly assigned, the next step is to recheck the patient's serum sodium in hopes that the hyponatremia is a laboratory error.

When the repeat sodium level is similar to the first, thereby crushing that hope, the next step often is to order a workup for the syndrome of inappropriate antidiuretic hormone (SIADH). The doctor has no idea why the patient has hyponatremia, and has a vague notion that SIADH occurs when the patient has puzzling hyponatremia.

The doctor is ignorant of the fact that hyponatremia is often not puzzling when interpreted in the clinical context. When this doctor decides to ignore the clinical context, a SIADH workup is often unhelpful even if they could understand the results.

Poor reasoners often cannot understand the results of the SIADH workup. The results either:

1. Do not suggest SIADH, thereby implying the cause of the hyponatremia would be clinically obvious if the doctor bothered to evaluate the patient clinically and reason (if this doctor had already done a proper clinical evaluation and reasoned properly, the SIADH workup would probably not have been performed in the first place), or

2. Do suggest SIADH, leaving the poor reasoner to order another battery of tests targeting the long textbook list of causes of SIADH, whilst still ignoring the patient's clinical context.

Regardless of whether a SIADH workup was performed, the doctor wildly guesses about the appropriateness of treating the hyponatremia.

If the patient has sufficiently severe acute hyponatremia regardless of the underlying disease, the hours spent performing and waiting on tests whilst failing to recognise symptomatic acute hyponatremia, may culminate in a seizure, perhaps even status epilepticus.

Unthinking treatment of hyponatremia is not safe, either. To aggressively 'treat the number' in a patient with chronic hyponatremia can lead to central pontine myelinolysis, which can cause permanent brain damage and death. This mistake has killed patients and the careers of the doctors who made this mistake.

Figure out the diagnosis first, and fast. Do not unthinkingly treat a number!

Treating after making a diagnosis, but without recognising the goal of treatment

This mistake usually occurs when a diagnosis has been made, but the treatment is administered without truly understanding if and how the treatment helps the patient. Advice on such treatment often focuses on measuring and treating a number.

This is often seen in Paediatrics, where parents are concerned about the child's fever. The doctor diagnoses the child with the flu and prescribes antipyretics: Acetaminophen and Ibuprofen. The parents are told: 'These medicines treat fever. The Acetaminophen must be given every 6 hours and strictly, and is used for temperatures below 38.5 degrees Celsius. If the temperature is 38.5 degrees Celsius or higher, use Ibuprofen instead. If you use both medicines, you should alternate the Acetaminophen and Ibuprofen with 3 to 4 hours between using either medicine.'

From the perspective of superficial theory and numbers, the above advice can seem logical. However, from the perspective of robust reasoning, all of the advice is inappropriate.

The child's parents keep spooning the medications into the child based on the thermometer reading, waking the child up at night every 6 hours if they only use 1 antipyretic, or every 3 hours if they use both antipyretics. This can be tiring, even annoying to the child and their parents.

This behaviour makes no sense if the child was sleeping comfortably that night. Why wake the comfortably sleeping child up (which is uncomfortable) to give antipyretics, which were supposed to help make them comfortable?

The goal of treatment for the common flu is to relieve discomfort. The doctor should ascertain if there is discomfort, and advise the child's parents accordingly on the proper use of the antipyretics. Effective patient-centred use of antipyretics, regardless of the number of antipyretics, is not dictated by the thermometer. The optimal timing of the antipyretics is not decided by relying on a vague notion of pharmacokinetics while forgetting the goal of the treatment.

A common fallacy that drives the treatment of the thermometer number, involves febrile seizures. Many people, including doctors, assume that the name 'febrile seizures' means that the fever causes the seizure. This is not true. Instead, the fever is seen with the seizures. Association is not the same as cause and effect.

Consider this analogy. The weatherman is seen walking around with an umbrella just before the rain begins.

The weatherman did not make it rain. His carrying an umbrella and the rain are seen in association, not a cause-and-effect relationship.

Likewise, the results of studies that administered antipyretics to try to prevent febrile seizures, corroborated with the pathophysiology: the antipyretics would bring down the number on the thermometer, but would not prevent the seizures anyway. This is because the antipyretics do not stop the immunological response that precipitated both the fever and the seizures. By applying pathophysiological reasoning, this result would be predictable even without these studies. A robust reasoner would ask: why were these studies even performed?

I do not use temperature cutoffs when I advise parents on the use of antipyretics. I educate them on the intensity of each antipyretic for the treatment of the child's discomfort. The timing of the antipyretics is based on the child's discomfort, whilst respecting safe limits dictated by pharmacokinetics.

2. Incorrect interpretation of response to treatment

Reacting wrongly to 'failure to respond to treatment':

The worst possible reaction by the doctor, is to ignore the surprising failure to respond to treatment. Since this surprise is usually part of the disastrous chain of dominoes, inattention and a sloppy clinical evaluation often precede this surprise. The same inattentiveness towards the patient predisposes to the doctor failing to detect, or outright ignoring the surprise. Instead, the doctor often insists 'give the treatment more time' despite ample time having passed to prove that the doctor was wrong.

There are 4 reasons for this surprise. Reason A is a stand-alone. Reasons B to D can coexist, albeit rarely. Move through the 4 reasons in this sequence:

A. Wrong disease

B. Under-estimated disease severity

C. Insufficient time is given for the treatment to work

D. Patient is non-compliant

A. *Wrong disease*

This is the most important, and first reason you must consider. Failure to think of the 'wrong disease' can be lethal.

The failure to respond to treatment satisfactorily is a warning that your treatment could be wrong, which then implies your diagnosis could be wrong. Since the mainstay of the correct diagnosis is the clinical approach and reasoning, you may have missed something in your initial approach. Recheck your history and examination, and then re-analyse the information.

For example, you see a patient presenting with cough, wheeze, and breathlessness. You diagnose him with chronic obstructive pulmonary disease. You treat the patient, and then wonder at the lack of improvement over the next few hours.

By retaking the history and re-examining the patient, you realise the patient instead has a 'cardiac wheeze': myocarditis with heart failure. You commence appropriate management, potentially saving the patient's life.

B. *Underestimated the disease severity*

If you are sure the disease was correctly identified, the next reason to consider is the underestimation of the disease severity.

There are 2 variations. The patient seemingly has:

1. Zero response, or
2. Partial but inadequate response

You need to recheck the true disease severity and total treatment intensity the patient has received.

Recall the analogy of moving a street bus. If you pushed the street bus alone, it may move such a tiny distance that you cannot see the response.

You should be worried if the patient's disease did not seem to 'move' at all. This could mean your treatment was grossly insufficient. The reflex action would be to dramatically increase your treatment intensity. However, since your entire management plan is predicated on the estimated level of severity, the realisation that you could have sorely underestimated the disease severity should prompt you to re-think your entire management plan.

Before you assume under-estimation is the only reason, quickly check for the other 2 reasons: insufficient time given for response, and the patient not receiving the treatment. Sometimes, these other reasons also coexist and if so, they would alter your decisions.

Failure to recognise the true (greater) disease severity can be lethal.

If the patient has a partial but inadequate response, the degree of improvement in disease activity, gives insight into the true severity of the disease. The universal equation can be employed for this purpose, as discussed in the earlier chapter 'Diagnosis: disease, severity and treatment'.

C. *Insufficient time is given for the treatment to work*

You must know how long the treatment takes to work.

Ignorance is no excuse; the time to effect of most treatments is well-described.

However, the actual speed of response also varies with the degree to which the treatment intensity matched or exceeded the disease severity. A very slow response is a warning about the disease severity being potentially greater than you thought.

If you have not given the treatment enough time to work, you will not see the expected effect. Patients who are not counselled about this time to effect, or who are too impatient, may stop the treatment prematurely. When the doctor fails to realise that insufficient time has elapsed to see the treatment effect, this doctor often changes the treatment prematurely.

D. *The patient is non-compliant*

The treatment will not work if the patient is not receiving the treatment. When patients refuse to comply with the treatment plan, this is called non-compliance.

Non-compliant patients may tell the doctor that a given treatment did not work. Many patients will not openly admit to their non-compliance. Careful enquiry is needed to ferret out the truth.

Sometimes, the error lies in the provision of medication, especially if the patient was hospitalised. Sometimes, the doctor forgot to prescribe the medicine.

Sometimes, the doctor assumes that their verbal or hastily-keyed-in electronic order for the medication to be administered by someone else, like the nurse, was obeyed. However, the order may not have been executed due to various reasons, such as the busy subordinate forgetting the verbal order because they were swamped with other duties, or the electronic order not being 'confirmed' by the ordering doctor.

If the doctor has strong reason to suspect the patient was indeed non-compliant, various measures to address this non-compliance can be undertaken. These measures include requiring hospitalisation or clinic visits for direct observation of the patient taking their treatment.

Wrongly equating 'the patient is better' to 'this is good enough'

This mistake occurs when the doctor assumes an improvement in the patient's condition means that the treatment is adequate.

When 'the patient is better' is not the same as 'this is good enough', disease activity is still present. The patient still has pain, stiffness, breathlessness, or impaired vision. The laboratory tests, such as HbA1c for diabetes mellitus and iron panel indices in iron deficiency anaemia, are still abnormal.

Patients want disease activity (symptoms) to become zero. As soon as possible.

If the disease remains active, the doctor should not unilaterally decide that the patient's improvement is 'good enough'. If the doctor intends to allow the disease to remain active, the barriers to disease control must be assessed and discussed with the patient, so as to decide on a balance point between treatment costs and side effects, versus the problems caused by disease activity.

When patients are half-treated for diseases, avoidable problems arise:

- The half-treated acute disease takes a long time to cure, resulting in prolonged convalescence (sometimes in the hospital).

- Relapses requiring more treatment create more work for everyone and readily anger patients: 'Why did you fail to treat my illness properly?'

- The half-treated chronic disease leaves patients suffering and increases the risk of complications. Asymptomatic patients with uncontrolled chronic disease, even if they are not suffering daily, still face the risk of complications. One example is a patient with uncontrolled hypertension who develops a stroke.

It should be obvious that the usual goal patients want is 100% cure and control, or at least want their doctor to put in a decent effort to achieve this goal.

However, my experience whilst teaching doctors, some trained outside of Singapore, and some whose parents are doctors themselves, suggests otherwise.

Here is one such discussion:

Me: 'What is the outcome you should aim for when treating a chronic disease?'

Doctor D: 'A balance of safety and cost.'

Me: 'That's part of the process, not the outcome. I repeat: what is the outcome you should aim for when treating a chronic disease?'

Doctor D says tentatively: 'Er…make them feel better?'

Me: 'I see you are unsure. Let us try this. If the patient has symptoms from their chronic disease — such as pain, dizziness, breathlessness or immobility, how much relief are you aiming for? Give me a percentage.'

There is often a long pause lasting at least 20 seconds. Doctor D has never thought about the outcome before. Eventually, Doctor D says: '50% is good enough.'

Me: 'If you were the patient, would you be happy with suffering 50% of the problems?'

Doctor D: 'No.'

Me: 'If you are going to relieve only half the pain, dizziness, breathlessness or immobility in your patient's chronic disease, most of your patients would not come back to see you.'

This discussion is unsurprising because commonplace medical training and the literature often expound on the process rather than the outcome. Poor reasoners tend to focus on the process instead of the outcome, partly because they dare not mention their (poor) outcomes.

This discussion is alarming, because if doctors are not thinking about outcomes when they train, what are they training to do? If they do not think and are merely following processes, robots can follow the same processes better and get better outcomes than these doctors.

Unilaterally and prematurely deciding to aim for less than 100% is not something any patient — including you, because one day you, my dear reader, will be a patient! — would accept in your doctor.

Though doctors cannot always achieve 100% cure or control, there is a huge difference between unilaterally deciding to aim lower and let the patient suffer, versus discussing the barriers to the ideal outcome with the patient.

Frequent discussions like this, raise more questions:

- Are medical schools covering so much knowledge, that they have failed to adequately teach the aim of healthcare? Are schools and medical students missing the forest for the trees?

- What are senior doctors (including parents of these unthinking doctors, who are doctors themselves) doing and teaching their juniors, such that junior doctors struggle to realise that 'the patient is better' is not always the same as 'this is good enough'?

- Since aiming for 100% cure or control is usually intuitive for doctors who have empathy, is empathy being selected for or encouraged in medical students?

The mistake of 'the patient is better' being equated to 'this is good enough' is particularly dangerous when the doctor assumes that if the patient improves, the treatment is *ample*...and the doctor then reduces the treatment intensity.

Consider this example. A patient has congestive cardiac failure, due to an acute myocardial infarction. The doctor treats this patient with diuretics. The patient improves partially, with the breathlessness and hypoxia improving but still present. Upon seeing the partial improvement with diuretics, the doctor assumes the diuretics may be excessive, and then reduces the diuretic dose. The patient's breathlessness and hypoxia worsen afterwards.

Some of these situations result in the patient who had just left the Intensive Care Unit (ICU), returning to the ICU. The doctor who prematurely reduces the treatment intensity can be the doctor in the general ward. Sometimes, the doctor who made this mistake is the ICU doctor, who reduced the treatment immediately before sending the patient out to the general ward.

Another example is a patient with a moderate asthma exacerbation, who improves after initial treatment in the Emergency Department. However, the patient is not well enough to be discharged. The doctors then reduce the treatment intensity — either while the patient is in the Emergency Department or the general ward — because 'the patient is better'.

Over the next few hours, the patient gradually worsens again. The next doctor sees the patient and intensifies the bronchodilator regime. The transiently intensified bronchodilator regime makes the patient feel better, though it is insufficient for breaking the asthma exacerbation. At the subsequent review hours later, the patient is deemed to be better and this is 'good enough', so the treatment intensity is reduced once more. The patient gets worse again.

The patient is now going through the 'asthma cycle' of waxing and waning symptoms and signs. The manifestations of this asthma cycle are being amplified because the doctors are bouncing between half-treatment and far-too-little treatment, leading to oscillations in the disease activity as per the universal equation. The patient may be hospitalised for days.

The most lethal form of this mistake is seen when a sick patient with a severe disease is admitted to the ICU. Initial intensive therapy has been commenced in the Emergency Department. The patient looks better upon arrival in the ICU. If the ICU doctors decide 'the patient looks better, the treatment was good enough', they may maintain or even reduce the treatment intensity. Soon afterwards, some of these patients collapse or die because of the grossly inadequate treatment intensity. The doctors wonder whether the cause of the disaster was insufficient testing or the wrong disease, instead of realising that they had conflated 'the patient is better' with 'this is good enough'.

Capsule summary

- Common mistakes in treatment are part of the disastrous chain of dominoes.
- These mistakes are often copied unthinkingly from other poor reasoners.

QUIZ: TREATMENT

Q1: When dealing with acute appendicitis, how does the universal equation explain the general preference for an appendectomy over intravenous antibiotics?

Q2: You are the anaesthetist counselling a patient regarding general anaesthesia for an upcoming operation. The patient seems anxious and keeps pressing you for the worst thing that can go wrong. This patient also keeps asking you what would be done if something went wrong. The patient keeps saying they do not want general anaesthesia. What are the additional elements you must cover in your discussion?

SECTION 4

Monitoring

This section covers follow-up and the approach to patients with chronic disease.

FOLLOW-UP

Follow-up refers to the process of reviewing the patient clinically, sometimes with the aid of tests. This review allows you to:

- Ascertain if the patient is recovering as expected
- Obtain new information which may change your diagnosis
- Rescue the situation, if surprises arise
- Learn when you were right, thereby reinforcing your correct thought processes
- Learn when you were wrong, thereby giving you an opportunity to recheck and correct your erroneous thought processes
- Learn the final diagnosis, so that you can accurately add information to your illness script for that disease
- Add more information to your illness script for that disease.

Follow-up can take place in the inpatient and outpatient settings.

Any surprises during the follow-up, can imply your diagnosis could be wrong. Since the mainstay of the correct diagnosis is the clinical approach and reasoning, restart at step one. Recheck the history and examination, and analyse the patient's information anew. When you have been surprised, even previously known, reassuring-looking test results may not be reassuring because you may have seen what you wanted to see, instead of what you should have seen.

If you consistently follow up on all your patients, you will discover how frequently doctors are wrong. You will discover the dismal numbers reported in the literature about doctors' accuracy, as I did long ago before I ever read any of the literature. You will realise the huge difference that consistent follow-up makes to your competence, because you have given yourself the chance to learn from reality's lessons. Everyone else who does not consistently follow up on all their patients, is unlikely to learn these lessons.

This follow-up is crucial to ensure your anonymised patient logs have the patients' information accurately assigned to each disease. Accurate and detailed information for each disease will allow you to:

1. Identify the Universal and Secondary Specific clinical features for each disease,

2. Recognise the tests that do not differentiate between the diseases, and

3. Learn how to interpret the test results of tests that do differentiate between the diseases, sometimes even more accurately than the existing literature suggests.

Trying to follow up on the patients who do not show up for their follow-up visits, is important. It is erroneous to believe that if the patient does not (come back to) complain, your diagnosis was correct.

Many patients do not return to see the same doctor because the doctor's diagnosis, predictions and treatment were proven to be wrong.

The doctor who never admits or tries to find out if they were wrong, will not improve much even if they worked for 1,000 years.

It is easier not to follow up on patients than to put in the effort to find out if you were right or wrong. However, since reality is the most accurate judge and teacher, there is no viable alternative to mastering clinical reasoning and attaining expert competence.

Inpatient follow-up

Healthcare

In this setting, the patient is hospitalised. How often do you need to check on the patient?

The answer depends on 3 factors:

1. The certainty and severity of the most likely diagnosis
2. Speed of progression of the disease
3. Duration of symptoms before admission

1. The certainty and severity of the most likely diagnosis

This is the most important of the 3 factors. If you are certain of the most likely diagnosis, the frequency of your follow-up depends on the disease severity. Patients with a more severe disease are in greater danger than those with a milder disease.

A patient with a 'benign' disease requires less frequent reviews than a patient with a more severe or dangerous disease. For example, a patient admitted for acute, symptomatic hyponatremia due to severe gastroenteritis, would require aggressive treatment. The doctor reviews this patient within the next 2 to 4 hours to check for clinical response, additional fluid losses and perhaps the serum sodium level.

If the diagnosis is uncertain, get help. Meanwhile, the patient should be reviewed frequently: at least once every few hours initially, and at least thrice every 24 hours.

2. Speed of progression of the disease

Consider the apparent speed at which the patient's symptoms and functional status (energy levels, appetite) are worsening. More severe disease tends to progress more rapidly, thereby requiring more frequent reviews of the patient.

If the clinical diagnosis was already made but the patient deteriorates surprisingly quickly (i.e. the speed of progression is inconsistent with the clinical diagnosis), this surprise requires re-starting the clinical evaluation and re-checking the clinical diagnosis.

If the diagnosis is unknown, the speed of progression of the patient's symptoms and the decline in function, are useful clues as to the likely disease trajectory. Being uncertain of the patient's disease makes it difficult to accurately predict the subsequent events and potential disasters. The inability to gauge the disease trajectory, makes these predictions even more difficult.

A patient may have non-progressive symptoms spanning several days to weeks, with virtually no deterioration in their function. This patient is unlikely to collapse within the next 6 hours. This reassurance does not mean you can lounge around; you must strive to get the correct diagnosis, because deducing the correct diagnosis facilitates optimal decision-making.

3. Duration of symptoms before admission

Assessing the speed of progression of the disease, is limited by the duration of the symptoms before admission. A history of a few hours or less of symptoms, makes it harder to predict the trajectory of potential deterioration over the next 24 hours than a patient who has had symptoms for days or weeks.

In patients with a short duration of symptoms, review them within the next few hours to get a better sense of the disease trajectory. If the underlying disease is unclear, the patient should be reviewed at least once every few hours for at least 24 hours or until the disease is recognised, whichever comes first. This frequent review has 2 aims: to get more clinical information to gauge the degree of danger more accurately, and to 'catch' any signs of imminent collapse early enough to save the patient.

One example would be the patient with fever and vomiting 4 times in 4 hours, with no other symptoms. Even if the patient looks 'clinically well', the robust reasoner knows that the illness has only just begun. It is premature to assume the patient will be okay. If this doctor does not know what the disease is, they immediately get help. Until the disease is known, this doctor reviews the patient frequently. If the doctor cannot get any help, they rely upon the evolution of the clinical features, including the appearance of new clinical features, to clinch the diagnosis.

Learning

Each disease uniquely manifests over time. Each disease also uniquely resolves, either spontaneously or with appropriate treatment, over time. These time-based patterns differ between specific diseases and between categories of disease. Examples of categories include infectious diseases versus rheumatological diseases versus cancers, diseases in these categories being the usual considerations in a patient with prolonged fever or 'pyrexia of unknown origin'.

Learning these time-based patterns comes through follow-up. You must review the current symptoms, ask for new symptoms, and re-examine the patient periodically, preferably at least twice a day. You must know the patient's final diagnosis, to assign the information you obtained to that disease and that category.

These clues add the dimension of time to your illness scripts. Time-based illness scripts are more advanced than the basic illness scripts described earlier in this book. When wielded properly, time-based illness scripts confer superior speed and accuracy over basic illness scripts. Knowing how each disease and category of disease manifests over time, including their response to treatment, allows this doctor to recognise the disease where other doctors would not.

The greater potency of these time-based scripts over basic scripts, is demonstrated in Conversation #11 in the chapter 'Theoretical disease approaches'.

Outpatient follow-up

Healthcare

The patient comes to the clinic/office for follow-up.

The interval for follow-up depends on 3 factors:

1. Danger level of the patient's diagnosis
2. Estimated ability of the patient to cooperate with healthcare
3. The next decision point

1. Danger level of the patient's diagnosis

The danger level is based on the disease and its severity. A patient whose disease may swiftly impair the patient or cause grave injury, requires a follow-up visit sooner than a patient with a benign disease. Examples of high danger levels include the patient with myocarditis who was just discharged from the Intensive Care Unit, and the patient with uncontrolled lupus with Class IV nephritis.

2. Estimated ability of the patient to cooperate with healthcare

If the doctor has good reason to expect non-compliance, such as the patient and their caregivers seeming unconvinced about the treatment, an early follow-up is important. This follow-up helps to 'catch' struggling and non-compliant patients much earlier. The doctor can plug gaps in the patient's understanding and get help for previously unknown social or financial difficulties.

3. The next decision point

To make sensible changes to treatment, enough time must elapse for the effect of treatment to prove its adequacy in meeting the goal of treatment.

For example, a patient who has uncontrolled asthma is commenced on controller therapy, and then reviewed 2 months after commencement. At the follow-up visit, there has been zero disease activity for the past 2 months. Though the weekly symptoms are gone, the patient also has an average of 1 hospitalisation every 4 months for a moderate asthma exacerbation. Thus the doctor decides the patient needs a total of 6 months of perfect control before weaning of the inhaled corticosteroids can be considered. This means 4 more months of perfect control after the follow-up visit. Thus, the next follow-up visit is scheduled in 4 months.

Sometimes, waiting until the next formal visit may be imprudent. In the patients most at risk of developing problems, 1 solution is to offer a follow-up phone call or teleconsultation within the next few days.

Learning

Outpatient care makes it harder for the doctor to study the changes in the patient's symptoms and signs each day. At the follow-up consultation, I recommend requesting brief descriptions of the changes in the symptoms over the preceding days to weeks.

Some patients do not require a formal follow-up visit, or do not turn up for their scheduled follow-up visit. It is unjustifiable to require patients who do not need a formal follow-up visit for their healthcare, to come back to your clinic anyway so that you can learn from them. For these patients and the patients who do not turn up for the scheduled follow-up visit, a telephone call is recommended. This phone call helps you to check in with them as well as to learn how their symptoms changed over time. Most diseases, if missed, become more obvious within 2 weeks from the last visit or within 2 weeks after the last day of treatment (the treatment masked their disease activity). Thus, I recommend the last follow-up call be at this 2-week mark or later.

Uninvited phone calls, messages or emails may be disturbing. A phone call at the wrong time such as in the middle of a nap or business meeting, is inconvenient. Even the notification sound from a message can wake a sleeper. Thus, the doctor should ask themselves what the patient is probably doing at that time before they attempt any messages, emails or phone calls. Some patients do not want to be contacted for anything unless they have personally requested such contact beforehand.

To get permission to re-contact the patient outside of formal consultations, ask the patient at the end of the consultation or provide the option at the end of the clinic/hospital registration form. This request or form should state your purpose: follow-up, informing them of test results, new information that may be relevant to their treatment, and so on. If they agree, ascertain how and when they wish to be contacted.

If you are calling the patient and someone picks up the telephone call, ensure it is the right person and the right time to talk. Verify the patient's identity and confirm this is a convenient time for the patient before you begin the discussion.

What happens if you do not follow up on patients?

Though you could adopt the throwaway attitude that 'it is entirely up to the patient to choose another doctor', this attitude does not change reality: failure to follow up means depriving yourself of the chance to learn if you were wrong.

Often, patients who are unhappy with their doctor will seek out another doctor, instead of spending more time and energy to return to the doctor who disappointed them. Thus, a timely phone call to these patients, where you learn that you were wrong, gives you the chance to rescue the situation by reviewing the patient again and correcting your mistakes.

If you do not follow up on patients who fail to turn up at the follow-up visit, your first warning that you were wrong, may be an official complaint.

For learning purposes, experience from seeing patients is virtually useless if you do not learn anything useful from that experience. It is okay to see the patient only once in their lifetime (provided they only need one healthcare visit), but if you do not try to follow up or teach yourself afterwards, then you are unlikely to learn from your experience.

If a doctor chooses not to learn whether they were right or wrong over many years and hundreds of patients, they often repeat the same mistakes over and over, not improving even after decades of practice. Eventually, the disastrous chain of dominoes can be so tragic that these 'experienced' doctors face, and lose, a lawsuit for medical negligence.

If you want to minimise mistakes, complaints and the chance of being sued, you should follow up and learn from as many of your patients as possible.

Capsule summary

- The interval for follow-up of patients in the inpatient and outpatient setting, is primarily decided by the degree of uncertainty and danger.
- Follow-up provides the opportunity to intervene in time for your patients, and to learn.
- Failure to follow up can be lethal for the patient, and the doctor's career.

TACKLING THE CHRONIC DISEASE

Chronic diseases can be categorised in many ways, and categories can overlap. Examples of categories include:

- Diseases of affluence: e.g. coronary heart disease, diabetes mellitus
- Atopic disorders: e.g. asthma, allergic rhinitis, eczema
- Gastrointestinal disorders: e.g. chronic gastritis, gastrointestinal reflux disease
- Renal diseases
- Rheumatological diseases
- Psychiatric diseases
- Diseases pre- and post-organ transplantation,

and so on.

This chapter applies to the assessment of the status of known chronic diseases.

At the start of the assessment, ask the patient for their disease diary. Many patients with chronic diseases are given or encouraged to keep a detailed diary that can include symptoms, results of home monitoring and treatment taken. The information in this diary can save a lot of time in history-taking.

There are 2 types of assessment:

1. The quick assessment
2. The follow-up-focused assessment

Both types of assessment will be discussed, followed by the physical examination.

1. The quick assessment

The quick assessment covers the essentials of clinical evaluation whilst briefly screening for prominent concerns.

This assessment takes 6 to 10 minutes to complete. This time requirement may decrease as you become more proficient.

This assessment is ideal for opportunistic care. In opportunistic care, the doctor is handling another primary problem and then takes this brief time to assess a known, co-morbid chronic illness.

The data points to cover are listed chronologically:

1. The duration of the chronic illness
2. How the patient is in an average period
3. The most recent chronic illness-related test results, if any
4. Checkpoint (if disease activity is prominent or has increased)
5. The usual, chronic control therapy that was used
6. Relevant physical examination
7. Is the patient facing any difficulties coping with the illness, which were not mentioned earlier?

Point #6, the relevant physical examination, is covered at the end of this chapter.

The duration of the chronic illness

The duration of the illness can indirectly point to the patient's burdens from the disease and its treatment.

These burdens may leave the patient weary, may contribute to non-compliance, or can be powerful motivators for compliance with a new treatment plan.

As complications of disease tend to arise when the disease is uncontrolled for a sufficiently long duration, the duration of the chronic illness alerts you to the need to look for potential complications. Examples include peripheral neuropathy in someone with diabetes mellitus, and chronic sinusitis in someone with allergic rhinitis.

Checking for these complications is not one of the 7 data points, and should be tackled after completing the quick assessment if time allows.

How the patient is in an average period

This information recognises the Law of Central Tendency (described in Section 3). Thus, all indicators of disease activity (such as intermittent symptoms, crisis points, firefighter medication use and functional impact) are determined over the average week, month, or past 6-month period:

Points to cover	What these are	Examples
Intermittent symptoms	Regular symptoms, often present at least once a week. Ask for the frequency and severity of these symptoms in an 'average' week.	Asthma: the 4 symptoms of cough, wheezing, chest tightness, and breathlessness Migraine: headaches in an average week
Crisis points	Short periods of continuous symptoms that are worse than the intermittent symptoms. Often called 'flares/attacks/exacerbations'. Ask for the frequency and severity of these, every 1 to 6 months.	Asthma: asthma exacerbations Inflammatory bowel disease: flares of disease

(Continued)

(Continued)

Points to cover	What these are	Examples
'Firefighter medication' use	Medication is often used to deal with crisis points and troublesome symptoms. Firefighter medication use is akin to using water to fight a fire. Frequent use will point to problems with control and/or disease understanding.	Asthma: Bronchodilators Migraine: Analgesia
Impact of the disease on daily activities and lifestyle	This is additional information on disease activity. This is also a major motivation for compliance with treatment.	Disruption to normal activities like sleep and socialising Absenteeism from school or work

In some diseases, some symptoms may point to over-treatment. For example, in patients with diabetes mellitus, excessive doses of insulin relative to the patient's usual dietary intake and disease severity, may lead to hypoglycemia. This hypoglycemia can manifest as dizziness, accompanied by a low hypocount reading.

The most recent chronic illness-related test results, if any

The activity of many chronic diseases is tracked through tests. These tests can be performed at home or in the clinic.

Examples of home monitoring include blood pressure readings in hypertension, and glucose hypocounts in diabetes mellitus.

Examples of clinic monitoring include renal function and retinal pictures in hypertension, and HbA1c in diabetes mellitus.

Some patients undergo an invasive test, whose result alters the treatment of their disease. If you are going to enquire about the result of an invasive test in diseases where the test is not always required, preface your question by stating the name of the test, and then stating that not all patients require the test. This helps the patient understand the context of your question. If the patient did not undergo that test, this preface also avoids giving them the mistaken impression that their previous doctor forgot to order a crucial test.

An example would be a patient with nephrotic syndrome who underwent a renal biopsy to determine the underlying pathology. Name the renal biopsy, providing a short description of it if needed, and state that not all patients require the biopsy. Then ask the patient if they underwent this test. If they say 'yes', enquire politely about the result.

Checkpoint (if disease activity is prominent or has increased)

If the information thus far suggests prominent or increased disease activity in recent months, this checkpoint is used. Ask the patient: what do they suspect is the reason for the disease activity?

If you are not the primary doctor managing that chronic disease, ask the patient what their primary doctor suggested as the reason.

In addition, the universal equation of disease severity, disease activity and treatment intensity must be considered. Discern the answer to these questions:

- Has the treatment been changed or the doses decreased, either by the patient (or their primary doctor, if you are not the primary doctor)?
- Have there been any triggers?

Ask if there are any new symptoms. The patient may have another disease that mimics the current (wrong) diagnosis. Failure to make the correct diagnosis can manifest as failure to respond to treatment for the current diagnosis or the appearance of new clinical features (or both).

The usual, chronic control therapy that was used

Since disease activity can be masked by treatment, the information you have already gathered on the recent, average disease activity should be matched to the treatment during that period. Treatment includes drugs, lifestyle measures, procedures, and all other steps taken to control the disease.

You should ask the patient what they have used, not what they were instructed to use. If you only ask the patient what they were instructed to use, the patient can merrily describe the treatment regime they were instructed to follow, whilst failing to mention that they were non-compliant.

These questions on treatment are customised based on the reported disease activity:

- If the disease seems perfectly controlled, weaning down or stopping one or more components of treatment becomes the focus of the questions. For weaning purposes, focus on the smallest contributors to treatment intensity and the components causing the patient the most problems (such as side effects). Ascertaining the doses of these components helps you to decide whether to reduce these doses or stop these components entirely. Getting this decision right, requires you to accurately estimate the proportion of treatment intensity that this component contributes to the overall treatment intensity of the entire treatment regime.

- Conversely, active disease points to the need to increase the intensity of control therapy. The focus shifts to the treatments that require intensification, especially if the disease has many aspects. Examples of multi-aspect diseases include eczema and end-stage renal failure.

For example, in a patient with diabetes mellitus, which is perfectly controlled through a combination of dietary measures and insulin injections, weaning of the insulin regime is a consideration. If the patient has episodes of hypoglycemia, reduction of parts of the insulin regime becomes a priority.

If this patient instead had poorly controlled diabetes mellitus, the dietary history and exact insulin regime are correlated with the timing of the high hypocount readings. This correlation provides insight into the treatment areas requiring intensification.

Is the patient facing any difficulties coping with the illness, which were not mentioned earlier?

This is a screening question meant to catch any concerns the patient may not have volunteered so far, such as side effects or difficulty paying for the treatment. Any information volunteered here must be addressed in the subsequent management plan.

2. The follow-up-focused assessment

The follow-up-focused assessment covers all data points in the quick assessment, and additional minor points of lesser, but still significant, importance.

This is a thorough assessment of the disease and all relevant information that can affect the management plan.

For undergraduate and postgraduate medical exams, this template should suffice to ace the station if you can complete it within the allotted time. If you do not think you can complete this assessment within the allotted time for the station, use the quick assessment instead.

This assessment takes 12 to 20 minutes to complete.

The additional data points on top of the quick assessment, are highlighted in purple. Go through the data points in chronological order:

1. The duration of the chronic illness
2. How the illness began
3. How the patient is in an average period
4. The most recent chronic illness-related test results, if any
5. Checkpoint (if disease activity is prominent or has increased)

How the illness began

At the beginning of the disease, effective treatment has not begun. Thus, the symptoms and necessary healthcare to 'firefight' the disease provide an accurate estimate of the true disease severity.

This information about disease severity influences your monitoring and treatment plans. This influence extends to the weaning of controller therapy, even if you deem the disease controlled.

Let us illustrate how this initial information about the disease severity can alter the weaning of seemingly controlled disease, using 2 hypothetical patients with asthma.

Patient #1's initial manifestation of asthma was a moderate exacerbation of asthma, followed by another similar exacerbation 3 months later. Both exacerbations required brief hospitalisation without needing Intensive Care. In the subsequent year, the asthma has been perfectly controlled. Weaning controller therapy is straightforward.

Patient #2 required admission to the Intensive Care Unit twice for severe exacerbations of asthma in the first 4 months of the disease. This points to underlying, severe asthma. Patient #2 requires more frequent follow-up and more intensive controller therapy than Patient #1. Patient #2 has a much greater danger of a life-threatening asthma attack than

Patient #1. Thus, Patient #2's controller therapy should be weaned much more slowly and carefully than for Patient #1.

Complications of the chronic illness

Complications have 3 elements:

1. They are separate, often pathologically definable diseases instead of being part of the original disease.

2. Being separate diseases, complications often require management that differs from that of the original disease.

3. Complications tend to occur when the original disease has been inadequately treated or is uncontrolled for a sufficiently long duration.

Search for the clinical features pointing to these complications. Patients may have been referred to specialists for review for these complications. For example, a patient with diabetes mellitus may have been referred to Ophthalmology for eye checks.

If complications are present, briefly ask about their severity and treatment.

Armed with the knowledge of the chronic disease's activity and the complications, your subsequent exploration of the treatment regime can expand to encompass the treatment of these complications.

You should be attentive to the complications. However, if you are constrained for time, your main priority should be control of the original disease. The presence of complications compels you to strive for perfect control of the original disease. It is illogical to treat a complication whilst ignoring the uncontrolled original disease. If you make this mistake, the patient often develops more complications that could have been avoided by controlling the original disease, which you had neglected.

This awareness helps you formulate a holistic treatment plan that addresses both the original disease and the complications simultaneously.

Changes in the control therapy in the past 6–12 months

This question assesses changes in control therapy and their effect on disease activity over a long period, instead of relying only on the 'average' therapy the patient was using.

Ascertain the reason for each change in treatment. Was the change ordered by the primary doctor, or initiated by the patient? And if so, why? Then check for changes in disease activity as a result of the change in treatment.

This information provides a detailed picture of the disease activity in relation to changes in treatment intensity, and may yield insights into the patient's perspective.

Side effects and concerns over the control therapy

This question deliberately checks for problems posed by the controller therapy, such as financial difficulties and side effects.

You may discover the patient is using other treatments, such as complementary treatment or unvalidated treatments for the disease.

Social setup and other information for management

These questions assess the patient's situation to gather information for management. This task was covered in detail in the chapter 'Gathering additional information to manage patients'.

Undertake a detailed exploration of the psychological impact of the disease on the patient, the disease's impact on their relationships, and their support.

The following table demonstrates 1 area of support: the patient's caregivers.

Assessing Caregivers: areas to explore	Sample Question(s) for the area	Why it matters
Who is/are the caregiver(s)?	Who helps to provide care for the patient?	Identify the caregiver(s), as they may be needed to help with the care of this patient.
Is the caregiver able to provide the necessary care, every day and week?	Ask the caregiver: For each day, what are the times you are available to help with the care?	Compliance with your treatment plan requires the caregiver to be available. A problem in this area may require looking for alternative caregivers.
Does the caregiver have to care for anyone else in the family?	Ask the caregiver: Do you have other children? Is there anyone else in the family that you are caring for?	The caregiver's existing burden must be understood before you attempt to give them more work. A problem here may require exploring other areas of support for the caregiver.

The physical examination

The physical examination has 4 aims:

1. Detect signs of chronic, uncontrolled disease
2. Look for side effects of the treatment
3. Detect signs pointing to another diagnosis (especially if the disease you were managing seems difficult to control)
4. Detect complications

The physical examination is often near the end of the chronic disease assessment.

If you are running out of time, focus on the first 3 aims. The 4th aim is important, but proper execution of the quick assessment and tackling the first 3 aims of the physical examination, often gives you enough information to decide the immediate priorities of management. In someone with an uncontrolled chronic disease that has led to a complication, you must control the original disease.

1. Detect signs of chronic, uncontrolled disease

These signs point to uncontrolled disease for prolonged periods.

One example in young children with uncontrolled asthma, is Harrison's sulci. These sulci occur when the child has increased work of breathing over prolonged periods at a young age, suggesting uncontrolled asthma for prolonged periods.

One example in patients with eczema, is skin lichenification. This sign points to prolonged and intense scratching over that area of skin.

2. Look for side effects of the treatment

These signs warrant reconsideration of the treatment and/or a review of the method of administration.

Examples include lipodystrophy from insulin injections, and hypertension and Cushingoid features from chronic use of systemic steroids.

3. Detect signs pointing to another diagnosis (especially if the disease you were managing seems difficult to control)

Treating the wrong disease can explain the failure of treatment.

Detecting signs that help you realise that the current diagnosis is wrong, and that the patient has another disease, allows you to 'rescue' the situation.

Examples include:

- 'Difficult to control asthma': you detect clubbing, realise the patient probably has bronchiectasis instead, and then re-evaluate the patient for bronchiectasis and the underlying disease causing the bronchiectasis.

- 'Difficult to control essential hypertension': you detect a renal bruit, realise the patient may have renal artery stenosis instead as the cause of the high blood pressure, and proceed to evaluate the patient for renal artery stenosis.

4. Detect complications

When diseases are uncontrolled for a sufficiently long period, complications are more likely. As complications are usually symptomatic, their presence in the clinical history should prompt you to look deliberately for these complications in the physical examination. Examples include neuropathy and kidney disease in patients with diabetes mellitus, and impetiginisation in patients with eczema.

Capsule summary

- When assessing the status of a known chronic disease, ask for the disease diary.
- There are 2 types of assessment. Pick the type that suits the consultation (or exam station).
- The physical examination is usually near the end of the assessment.

Frequently asked questions

Q: Why don't you check for complications during the quick assessment (except at the end, and then only 'maybe')?

A: Completing the evaluation of this chronic disease is your main task. Having to use the quick assessment instead of the follow-up-focused assessment usually means you are short of time. Thus, complications are left to the end.

If you split your time between both the original chronic disease and its complications equally, you may fail to gather enough information to manage any of the diseases appropriately. It is often better to do 1 job well than to do 2 jobs badly.

Complications tend to arise when the original chronic disease is uncontrolled for a sufficiently long duration. Thus, the original disease must be managed properly. It would be silly to address the complication during the visit whilst ignoring the uncontrolled original disease, and then discover at the next visit that the patient developed 2 more disastrous complications because you neglected the control of the original disease. You can provide some treatment for the complication, but you must get your priorities right.

If you need another clinic visit to address complications fully, schedule the next visit within a few days.

SECTION 5

Clinical Reasoning, Ignored

This section discusses real-world performance, its correlation with clinical reasoning, and the behavioural indicators of reasoning. Like the crescendo of a song, this section delivers lessons of greater scope and import than the preceding sections.

Here, the book comes full circle, demonstrating the wider ramifications of Section 1 and the chains of dominoes.

DECEIT

Doctors can misleadingly use words. This misleading use of words can be unintentional: the doctor did not reason properly for themselves and their audience, without consciously intending to deceive others.

Deceit can be deliberate, as evidenced by the clear intent to benefit oneself at the expense of others.

This chapter will cover potentially unintentional deceit and deliberate deceit.

Potentially unintentional deceit

It takes effort to be empathetic, logical and knowledgeable about the patient. This effort manifests as proper clinical evaluation and reasoning.

Doctors are busy. Thus, it may be tempting to skip the effort to be empathetic, logical and knowledgeable about the patient.

Doctors, like all humans, have fears. These fears include fear of missing dangerous diagnoses, fear of being embarrassed, and fear of change.

To have fear, is human.

To give in to fear and allow it to dictate your actions, is cowardice.

The combination of being busy and afraid can tempt anyone to skimp on the clinical evaluation, abandon logic, and instead perform actions that seem superficially useful (such as treating numbers).

Fear-crazed behaviour can be questioned by patients, medical students and peers. When questioned, it is often difficult to admit giving in to fear. It is rare for someone who has given in to fear, to have the courage to admit to their cowardice. Instead, the usual response is to ignore, attack, or run away from the questioner.

Some common phrases that are widely used for general purposes by laypeople, are misused when a doctor is trying to justify their unacceptable behaviour toward others. This misuse may not be deliberate. Since clinical reasoning derives from overall reasoning, a doctor who lacks reasoning tends to behave illogically, tends to get challenged as a result of their behaviour, and tends to misuse phrases because they also lacked the overall reasoning to use these phrases correctly.

The speaker's words deceive themselves and their challengers. Like misuse, deception is not always deliberate. Unfortunately, deliberate or not, these actions come at the expense of themselves and others around them, such as their colleagues and the patient.

The speaker chooses their words and actions and thus, is fully responsible for their words and actions. For example, the speaker could have chosen to check the truth of an assertion in the preceding days, months or years before they declared their assertion aloud. Instead, they did not check for the truth. If they lie about this failure to check, such as pretending the assertion is true instead of admitting 'I do not know', they are engaging in deliberate deceit.

Thus the choice to deceive, intentional or not, was made by the speaker:

- Pretending that something you believe must be true because you never bothered to think or check, does not change the self-deception.

- If the speaker does not check the truth of a falsehood they tell the listener (colleague, student or patient), they are still telling a falsehood.

Throwing words versus throwing bricks

Words have power. Words are choices. Choices lead to consequences. The speaker of those words has some, if not most, of the responsibility for those consequences.

Thinking is a choice, and mindfulness is a choice. Failing to think or care about other people, comes from choosing to do so, with the attendant personal responsibility for the consequences.

Speakers who care enough about their listeners would consider the consequences of their words and actions. By extension, a speaker who did not care enough about the listeners to think of the consequences of their words and actions, will often prove this in their words.

Once you consider the impression the speaker gives to others and the inevitable harm they inflict on the patient, the distinction between deliberate and inadvertent deceit becomes academic.

Unthinkingly throwing bricks out of the window of a high-rise building, which harm or kill passers-by, is a crime. It means nothing to the deceased to hear their killer's apology.

Likewise, deceiving colleagues and harming patients in a profession that requires thinking and caring, cannot be excused by a failure to think or care.

It is often no comfort to the victim (who may be a colleague, not a patient) after the disaster these doctors inflict upon them, to hear 'I did not intend this to happen' or 'at least you are not dead'.

Imagine a pedestrian is walking on the street, near a high-rise building. A brick is unthinkingly thrown out of a window of the high-rise building. This brick strikes the pedestrian and breaks the pedestrian's arm. Would this pedestrian be happy with the brick-thrower saying to them: 'I did not intend this to happen' or 'At least you are not dead'?

By saying 'I did not intend this to happen', the speaker's behaviour demonstrates the full sentence is 'I did not intend this to happen *because I was not thinking or caring enough about you anyway*', but they dare not say the last few italicised words.

By saying 'At least you are not dead', the speaker's behaviour demonstrates the full sentence is 'At least you are not dead *because I could have done worse to you*', but they dare not say the last few italicised words.

In both situations, it matters little if the speaker is a doctor or a brick thrower.

When doctors see and hear other doctors, especially senior doctors, misuse words and get away with it, this can embolden them to do the same: 'Hey, a doctor is showing there is no need to care, think, or tell the truth. I can do the same.'

An objective listener who can reason well, 'sees through' the veneer of the words and realises the speaker is unable and unwilling to admit the truth to themselves and others. This listener realises self-deception and deception of others are occurring, intentional or not.

Even if the listener wants to give the speaker the benefit of the doubt and assumes the deception is not intentional, prudence compels the listener to treat the speaker as self-serving and untrustworthy.

Intent matters little if the outcome (intentional or not) is uniformly disastrous.

Some of the common phrases used for both intentional and unintentional deceit, are:

1. Anything is possible
2. This is multifactorial
3. This is (quote authority or document that apparently condoned the behaviour)

1. *'Anything is possible'*

'Anything is possible' (or 'never say never', or 'you never know') is useful for trying to inspire oneself or others to greater achievements, and as a reminder to prepare for contingencies.

Factually, this phrase is not 100% correct. Anything is *not* possible in you, me, or the patients. I do not use this phrase. If I try to inspire or warn people, there are other words that are less misleading and more useful than this phrase.

To succeed in reality, one must accept reality. Therefore, excellent decisions are not based on 'anything is possible'. There are limits to time, energy and money.

Excellent decision-making recognises these limits and thus, prioritises the best choices.

The most likely diagnosis must be decided, as this diagnosis drives most of the optimal decisions. Less likely differentials must also be decided, as these differentials may also drive optimal decisions. Certainty must be compared to decision thresholds.

'Anything is possible' is often used by poor reasoners to convince themselves and others, that logic and reasoning are unimportant. Some manifestations include:

- Anything the patient says may be subjective, and subjective can be the same as unreliable. Therefore, I will believe what I want to believe.

- Any diagnosis is possible in the patient, therefore there is no point in trying to figure out the diagnosis or decide on probabilities.

- Any disease I fear can occur, so I should always check for those diseases.

- Any fever can be due to bacterial infection, so I should always give antibiotics.

- Any test may help, so I should do all the tests I want.

- Any test can be wrong, so I can choose to believe whatever result I want.

- Anything is possible, so any patient who is on antibiotics must finish all antibiotic courses in case there is a bacterial infection.

- Anything can be causing that abnormal number, so spending effort to figure out the cause is wasteful.

- Any abnormal number can be dangerous, so I should correct it.

- Anything is possible, so I can say anything I want to the patient.

Combinations of these manifestations are common. For example, a patient with fever, sore throat, cough and rhinorrhea of 2 days' duration sees a doctor. Their drinking ability is unchanged. The vital signs are normal. The physical examination is unremarkable.

The doctor decides 'any fever can be due to bacterial infection so I should always give antibiotics'. Simultaneously, viral swabs and bacterial cultures are performed because 'any test can help'. After the cultures return negative and a viral swab returns positive, the doctor decides the cultures are inaccurate and thus, their results cannot be trusted. The doctor tells the patient that they have the viral flu (which was clinically obvious anyway) because the swab result was positive. The doctor then insists the patient must finish the antibiotic course anyway.

The doctor believes 'anything is possible', so they hope all of their patients will never notice their lack of logic, indiscriminate prescription of antibiotics, and failure to apologise for mistakes.

The speaker who uses 'anything is possible' can be challenged with their own words: 'You say anything is possible. Why don't you also test and treat for (insert the correct diagnosis)?'

The speaker's response often contradicts their previous words. The speaker argues that the most common or most dangerous diseases in the speaker's mind are the only possibilities to consider.

This self-contradiction — claiming anything is possible, then proceeding to ignore other possibilities that are suggested — reveals the truth about the speaker: reasoning and logic have been abandoned.

2. 'This is multifactorial'

Patients can suffer from debilitating problems, with multiple factors that contribute to the problem. This situation tends to occur in complex diseases, elderly patients, and patients with multiple uncontrolled co-morbidities.

For example, an old lady may be prone to falls because of impaired balance, eyesight, bouts of dizziness and joint pains. The caring, effective doctor recognises the multi-factorial nature of the debilitation, and puts in the effort to systematically assess and address all the contributing factors to restore the lady's function as much as feasible.

Instead of engaging in batteries of unfocused tests and treatments, this doctor targets and assesses each factor, using clinical reasoning to ensure that all chosen tests and treatments are necessary. If additional help is needed, such as referring to an ophthalmologist or rheumatologist, this doctor discusses the referral with the patient.

Unfortunately, the phrase 'this is multifactorial' is often misused to suggest: This problem is multifactorial. Since there are multiple factors, it is too much work to figure out what to do about these factors. Therefore, nothing should be done about these factors.

Thus, this phrase is often misused to justify apathy and inaction.

This inaction is most obvious when a semi-decent reasoner who can make the correct diagnosis and suggest optimal decisions for the patient, witnesses their senior colleague use this phrase when discussing the same patient. The senior colleague then refuses to think or take more than superficial action about the 'multiple factors'.

To quote 1 student: 'When the doctor tells you "this is multifactorial", sometimes there is clearly a single disease, or the patient has 1 obvious, major, treatable contributing factor to the disease out of the multiple theoretically possible factors. If this doctor then walks away without trying, the truth is that they have no idea what the patient has, do not want to try to figure it out, do not know what to do, and lack the courage to admit it.'

If more than 1 doctor is involved in the patient's care, this inaction leaves colleagues to do the work that the doctor who spoke the phrase 'This is multifactorial' was supposed to do. Though the speaker may not have intended to give their colleagues more work (because the speaker did not think or care), the presence or absence of such intent does not change the work their colleagues now have to do. Even if the speaker did not intend to abandon the patient and their colleagues, their inaction makes it hard to argue that they are not abandoning the patient and their colleagues.

Once you recall the disastrous chain of dominoes, abandonment (intentional or not) by the speaker is not always a bad thing. Poor reasoners can be more harmful than helpful when they participate in patient care.

This phrase is also misused to avoid thinking about cause and effect for worrisome data, such as the correlation of the prevalence of defensive behaviour with allegations of medical malpractice. For example, one could ask themselves:

- Do the disastrous consequences of defensive behaviour drive frequent allegations of medical malpractice?

- Do the frequent allegations of medical malpractice drive defensive behaviour?

- Do other factors drive both worrisome manifestations?

Even though the answers would be valuable, the speaker has decided that the information is not worth the effort to question or understand.

Sometimes, the speaker uses this phrase to run away from disturbing conclusions. They can say 'this is multifactorial' instead of admitting, 'I do not want to hear this because I do not want to change what I am doing. What you are telling me is making me uncomfortable.'

3. *This is (quote authority or document that apparently condoned the behaviour)*

This phrase is often used as a last resort when the doctor is being challenged by a peer of equal or greater rank. The speaker cannot use phrases like 'I am your teacher/senior, so you must obey me' to silence the challenger. Instead, the speaker claims that a hospital policy, guideline, or authority supports their behaviour.

The speaker's response to the challenger is often vague, using this exact phrase and then failing to elaborate on what the policy, guideline or authority says. The exact policy, guideline or other reference is not specified. The 'hospital policy', guideline or authority may not truly support the speaker's behaviour, or may not even exist.

What is *not* said is even more revealing than what is said:

- If the speaker's behaviour was for the patient's good, they could have said so and easily justified their behaviour with a logical, patient-centred reason. They cannot.

- If the speaker truly knew the reference, they could tell you the specific reference or will show it to you. They do not, because they cannot. They cannot, because they either did not read the reference or the reference does not exist.

The vague response (intentionally or unintentionally) serves the speaker's interests, because the absence of specifics would burden the challenger with checking multiple long documents, or locating and contacting a specific authority.

The challenger can try to turn the tables by asking the speaker to provide the specific name of the reference or send them the referenced document. This shifts the burden of proof back on the speaker. The speaker then either says they:

- Are too busy to check, or

- Cannot remember the name of the reference, or

- Will send the challenger the reference later, and then 'forgets' to do so and hopes the challenger gives up. Some challengers keep reminding the speaker to send the reference over, who keeps replying that they will send the reference to the challenger and then 'forgetting' to do so. The challenger eventually realises after 3, 5 or 10 reminders (and several months later) that the speaker is stonewalling them; the speaker either never bothered to look for the reference or the reference does not exist (or both).

Sometimes, the speaker names a specific document, but they misquote or misuse it. For example, they insist on a battery of tests and treatments 'to cover for sepsis' in a well-looking baby with an obvious viral flu. They say 'the guideline says I must do this in all babies with fever'. The challenger knows the guideline says, 'For babies with fever *with no obvious source*'. The guideline does not apply to the patient. Either the speaker:

- Did not read the document properly (and if so, cannot be trusted to execute its steps properly anyway), or

- Knows the document does not apply to the patient, but is trying to conceal their inability to recognise bacterial infections.

In very rare situations, the speaker names a specific document and does not misquote it. They are quoting a flawed defensive document that makes poor recommendations. The speaker is not reasoning, so they are unaware of the quality of the recommendations.

Deliberate deception

Healthcare, like any other profession, has its black sheep.

Sometimes, words are used to deceive the listener intentionally. The speaker is trying to get the listener to agree to their recommendations. The speaker deliberately impugns the reputation and words of others. The listener cannot trust the speaker and should end the encounter as soon as possible.

Deliberate deception alone, is bad. Deliberate deception to serve the speaker's interests, is worse. Deliberate deception that is likely to harm the patient and the profession, is a deliberate betrayal of all these parties.

Examples include:

1. 'This is different from medical school, just follow my orders.'
2. 'You should listen to me. (Obey my orders.)'
3. 'You should listen to me. The other doctor is (insert illogical reason).'

1. *'This is different from medical school, just follow my orders.'*

The speaker is senior to the listener. The speaker orders the listener to perform an action or procedure that is contraindicated, such as administering antibiotics to which the patient is allergic. If challenged, the speaker can reply: 'How do you know the patient is really allergic? Besides, they need this antibiotic to get better.'

The speaker is careful not to leave written proof that can incriminate them.

If the order is executed and the patient suffers an adverse outcome, which then prompts a complaint or official enquiry, the speaker pretends they never gave the order and points the finger at their dupe: the junior colleague who executed their orders. This becomes a situation of 'my word against yours'.

The junior colleague realises that the speaker had used and then abandoned them. Even when other junior doctors or medical students were present and heard the same order, they often remain silent because they are afraid of being punished by the speaker.

The speaker is behaving exactly like the gang leader who orders a gangster to commit a crime, and then disavows this gangster if this gangster is caught.

Such orders are often so blatantly dangerous that only the poorest reasoners obey them. The speaker is inadvertently exposed as a poor reasoner, because it is foolish to treat a colleague as a mindless and suicidal drone, and then hope that nobody suspects the truth after disaster has struck.

Instead of obeying dangerous orders, the horrified listener often asks other colleagues and seniors for advice.

The listener cannot obey such orders. They always have the choice to refuse and then escalate the matter above the speaker's level. Because the speaker often leaves no written proof that can incriminate them, and other doctors are reluctant to confront the speaker even if there is proof, the speaker is often left untouched.

Can the speaker be correct? In rare situations, yes. However, if the speaker is correct, they would explain the reasoning to the listener and willingly document their orders. There are often experts or literature backing up the speaker's explanation.

Thus, the listener should insist that the speaker provide an explanation and a written order naming the speaker. A speaker who is intentionally deceiving the listener, cannot give a logical explanation (because there is no logic) and will refuse to give the listener proof of the specifically worded order naming the speaker. This response confirms the listener's suspicions.

2. 'You should listen to me. (Obey my orders.)'

The speaker wants the patient to undergo a treatment or procedure that serves the speaker's interests.

The treatment/procedure is expensive, or is part of an experimental study in which the speaker has a vested interest.

There are commonly available alternatives that would suffice for that patient's disease. The treatment/procedure the speaker recommends is unnecessary.

Though the alternative options are viable, the speaker may refuse to mention them, or dismisses them with statements such as 'other treatment will not work for you'.

The speaker may be pushy and employ fearmongering: 'If you do not do as I say, your health will suffer. You cannot delay making this decision. Do what I say.'

These tactics mislead the patient into thinking the only viable choice is to agree to the speaker's recommendation.

The wise patient recognises such tactics, ends the encounter, and then consults another doctor.

3. 'You should listen to me. The other doctor is (insert illogical reason).'

The speaker is trying to convince the patient to stop a treatment given by a previous doctor, and try the (usually expensive) unnecessary treatment the speaker is recommending. Sometimes, there is no relationship between the previous treatment and the speaker's recommended treatment.

For example, the patient who is being treated for an allergy-related disease by a specialist in allergy, consults an endocrinologist for an unrelated concern. The endocrinologist recommends expensive hormonal injections, which have no relationship to the allergy treatment. Neither of the treatments interferes with the other.

The endocrinologist tells the patient to stop seeing the previous doctor and stop the previous treatment for the allergy.

The endocrinologist ignores the allergy-related disease. If the patient suffers as a result of the endocrinologist's advice, the endocrinologist is not the sufferer and thus does not care.

If the previous doctor was a robust reasoner and explained the logic behind their plans clearly to the patient, that contrast between the previous doctor's empathy and logic, and the current speaker's lack of empathy and logic, leaves the patient suspicious of the speaker.

If the previous treatment was making the patient better, the recommendation to stop the previous treatment is puzzling. The patient's suspicions are heightened by the speaker's 'explanation', which is often vague and impugns the words or reputation of the previous doctor.

No logic is provided because there is none to provide. The speaker knows this and therefore resorts to raising doubts about the previous doctor instead.

As a wise saying goes: 'What you say about others may reveal more about you than those others.' Examples of deliberate impugning can include:

- 'The other doctor is younger than me.' (Competence and morality are more important than age, which the speaker proves through their behaviour.)

- 'The other doctor has not done research but I did.' (The speaker is usually guessing wildly about the other doctor, and hopes the listener does not realise this.)

- 'The other doctor does not know what they are doing.' The speaker then fails to elaborate, because they cannot go on without further incriminating themselves.

If the patient suggests that the speaker discuss their opinion with the previous doctor, the speaker refuses, citing excuses such as 'I am too busy'. The speaker dares not speak to the previous doctor because they fear their attempt at deceit will be exposed.

The classic line that confirms the patient's suspicions is the speaker ending the encounter with: 'Do not tell anyone else what I said. Do not see other doctors.'

If the speaker was correct, they should not fear their colleagues hearing their words. By extension, wanting to conceal their opinion from others reveals their fear of being caught.

At this point, a perceptive patient will realise that the puzzling recommendation to stop all other treatment, has nothing to do with the speaker's new and expensive treatment. Instead, by telling the patient to stop all other (unrelated) treatments, the speaker is trying to dissuade the patient from consulting any other doctor, who might then expose the speaker's deceit.

The suspicious patient ends the encounter and seeks another opinion, often checking with the previous doctor who was treating them.

Knowledge of the unhappy encounter often saddens and annoys other doctors, because mistrust of the healthcare profession is driven by doctors who are perceived to be self-serving and deceitful.

Even if the other doctors want to disbelieve the patient's account, the patient often gives a convincing account that matches the speaker's specific speaking style. When the patient then asks if they should stop their previous treatment and follow the speaker's recommendations, this reveals the patient is trying to get wise advice instead of trying to get the speaker into trouble. Thus, the patient is probably telling the truth, because they cannot get wise advice if they are lying!

When my patients report these (thankfully, rare) accounts to me, they are always angry and disappointed at the speaker. I check the patient's understanding and try to see the reasoning behind the other doctor's words.

It saddens me that some doctors pretend to be friendly when facing these colleagues, but readily denigrate them behind their backs, purely for self-gain. I know the patient has enough reasoning to make the right decision.

When the speaker tried to impugn my words or reputation, I tell my patients to consider my words and conduct, then consider the words and conduct of the doctor they suspect, and then decide whom to believe.

I also suggest that whomever they decide to disbelieve, is not someone they should trust or ever see again. By extension, I readily point out that if I am not getting them the results I predicted at the consultation, they should seek a better doctor. 'Reputation' is best decided by the results obtained, not age, title, self-declaration, misleading advertising, or anything else unrelated to outcomes.

I do not insist that my patients blindly believe me over the speaker, because this is basic respect for all human beings. The patient should be treated as a human who can make informed decisions based on the truth. The speaker did not show the patient this basic respect.

Actions and outcomes, sustained over time, speak louder than words.

Deceit without words

Can doctors deceive their patients and colleagues by withholding information? Yes.

When doctors deliberately withhold critical information that they are reasonably expected to share, this omission can predictably mislead the listener. During a handover, if the doctor withholds crucial information about a patient that they knew was deteriorating, their colleague often gets a rude shock afterwards upon seeing the patient. One example was described in the chapter 'Interpreting test results': The day team knew the patient had worsened. The day team was providing more supportive care in response to the deterioration, yet withheld this information during the handover. Doctor R got a rude shock upon discovering the patient was near collapse.

When doctors deliberately withhold important information from the patient during counselling, this is intentional abandonment of their responsibility to the patient. An analogy was described in the chapter 'Treatment decisions': Ken knew what his mother was doing, knew that his mother knew his occupation, and knew how to avoid the injury. However, he said nothing useful or specific initially, which misled her into thinking that he had no advice to offer. After she was injured, Ken told her he was not responsible for his behaviour and his omission of advice.

Doctors who indulge in this behaviour seem to have no shame or remorse for the victims, giving others the impression that they do not truly care about anyone else.

Capsule summary

- Misused phrases are often used to deceive oneself as well as others.

- Beware those who use these phrases in healthcare. Pay attention to their actions and outcomes. Actions and outcomes speak louder than words.

- Omission of expected words is also a form of deceit. Deliberately withholding important information when such information is predictably expected to be shared, is a form of deliberate deceit.

TIERS OF PERFORMANCE

Based on my observations, a doctor's sustained behaviour corresponds well with their outcomes. This chapter discusses my observations and estimates as of the end of 2022.

The spectrum of performance looks like this:

Tiers of performance (from best to worst, moving down)
Expert generalist
Expert diagnostician within the field
Good
Common
Fresh graduate of medical school
Medical student who is not defensiveness-obsessed
Defensiveness-obsessed
Apathetic

Apathetic refers to doctors who seem uncaring about the fate of others. Hallmarks of these doctors include:

- Apparent modus operandi: 'I just want to do what I want. Someone else can help the patient or help my colleagues.'

- Making every mistake in this book

- Rarely admitting to or apologising for their mistakes, even when under legal or professional pressure
- No apparent interest or effort put into improving
- Regularly engaging in deceit.

The form (outward appearance) of the doctor can be misleading. Apathetic doctors can be very polite and well-dressed. Being charming and well-dressed helps to convince some patients to keep seeing this doctor, though wiser patients rapidly realise that actions and poor outcomes speak louder than words and appearances.

Apathetic doctors can loudly denounce wrongdoing whilst engaging in similar (or worse) acts in healthcare. This denunciation can mislead others into thinking the speaker has high standards. Diverting attention to others is a tactic used by wrongdoers.

You may ask: how do apathetic doctors even get promoted? Sometimes, doctors are promoted based on age or connections, not merit. Sometimes, the doctor works hard only for as long as it takes to reach their desired rank and salary, and then stops putting in effort. Their colleague muses sadly: 'This doctor previously seemed to care somewhat. Once he/she reached this position, their behaviour totally changed. They revealed their true colours.'

Some of these doctors engage in fraud, such as peddling unnecessary treatments, anti-vaccine myths and fake 'cures'.

Defensiveness-obsessed refers to doctors who indulge in ruling out OAF.

Hallmarks include:
- Modus operandi: Often ruling out OAF
- Being described as 'does a lot of tests and treatment, often unnecessarily' and 'they appear to listen to the patient, but their decisions suggest otherwise'
- Making almost every mistake in this book regularly
- Reluctance in admitting to their mistakes
- Regularly engaging in deceit.

This tier overlaps with the 'apathetic' tier. Frequently ruling out OAF accompanies deliberate inattention, deceit, and callousness to patients, all of which can suggest apathy towards the patients and to oneself. However, some defensiveness-obsessed doctors are not apathetic.

If even a minority of doctors rule out OAF, this behaviour translates into a massive, unnecessary expenditure of resources, and can strain healthcare resources at regional and national levels.

Medical student who is not defensiveness-obsessed is a young adult who enters medical school, aiming to be a safe and competent doctor.

This is the crucial stage of malleability where ethics, professionalism, empathy and clinical reasoning must be woven throughout their training, and taught both implicitly and explicitly.

Once this window of maximum opportunity has passed, inculcating clinical reasoning is much harder.

Some of the most robustly reasoning medical students outperform many of their seniors.

Fresh graduate of medical school refers to the doctor who has been working for less than 2 months after their graduation. Their competence reflects their learning in medical school.

At this stage, the window of maximum opportunity for embedding clinical reasoning, is closing. They are now trying to cope with daily work, handling other adult-level duties simultaneously such as family, budgeting, handling salary and paying bills, and so on. With less free time and energy, many may not pursue clinical reasoning if they never realised its importance.

Common refers to most of the doctors who have worked for at least 1 year. These doctors are often using conventional tests, guidelines, and protocols without fully understanding the role of these tools. There is a small chance of mishaps and patient complaints. Hallmarks include:

- The mistakes described in this book are committed regularly
- Clinical competence is variable. Their performance is described in the literature
- They may fail to make appropriate or timely referrals
- They are uncomfortable with uncertainty
- They are often reluctant to voluntarily admit their past mistakes or weaknesses to peers, patients and students
- When challenged with a question they cannot answer, inconsistent effort is put in to find the answer.

Good refers to doctors who consistently make correct clinical diagnoses and excellent decisions. These doctors reason well most of the time. As of the end of 2022, I estimate their prevalence at less than 2% of all doctors. Hallmarks include:

- Their performance matches or exceeds the upper limits of doctors' performance described in the literature as of the end of 2022
- If they are the best doctors in their region or country, patients and other doctors tend to recommend them over and above other doctors
- They are humble enough to ask their peers for help with some patients, while simultaneously admitting their inability to handle those patients. They virtually never fail to make a timely or appropriate referral.
- When challenged with a question they cannot answer, they usually try to find the answer
- Moral courage and transparency: when in comfortable company (people they trust), they are willing to admit their mistakes. Doing the same with strangers, such as medical students and patients, is sometimes difficult.

Expert diagnostician within the field refers to the top medical experts within a particular speciality or setting in the world. These experts are superb at clinical evaluation, clinical diagnosis and decision-making. This expertise is limited to their particular niche.

Given that the upper limits of performance of hundreds of experienced doctors in the literature are far below the performance of this group of experts, I estimate the prevalence of these experts at less than 0.01% of all doctors.

Some of these doctors are not well-known academics, and have no titles beyond 'Doctor'. If you searched only among the doctors with lofty-sounding titles such as 'Professor', you would miss some of these experts. They have devoted themselves almost entirely to honing their clinical performance.

Their renown, which comes from their track record in patient care, is such that they do not need to advertise themselves. Others, including patients and prominent doctors, recommend them overwhelmingly over every other doctor. Thus, they are often very busy.

Hallmarks include:

- An unrelenting dedication to clinical diagnostic skill and decision-making
- Renown within their speciality, often at the national or international level
- Fluid, patient-centred approaches that 'flow' with the patient's responses and information. Their approaches often employ questions and examination steps that are not found in textbooks or literature
- Diagnostic accuracy rates of at least 90% clinically at the first patient encounter, which drops to 50% (at the lowest) when facing significant diagnostic puzzles
- Proficiency in managing patients outside conventional norms, including using medications and procedures outside of standard regimes
- Humility and curiosity: When asked about something they are ignorant or uncertain about, they readily admit this to their patient

and their students. They then aggressively pursue the answer, sometimes in partnership with their patient and students

- When a problem falls outside their expertise, they readily refer the patient to the appropriate expert to handle that area

- Moral courage and transparency: willingness to admit their mistakes and teach others to avoid making the same mistakes.

Expert generalist refers to the expert who seems to possess encyclopaedic knowledge of diseases across multiple healthcare professions and speciality fields, uncanny proficiency in pathophysiology and the basic sciences, and extremely robust reasoning.

Combining all these advantages and using them synergistically, allows clinical diagnosis and decision-making as well as (or better than) the expert diagnostician within the field, without the limitation of being restricted only to 1 field or speciality. The expert generalist can often handle at least 3 other speciality fields outside their official speciality appointment, at the expert-tier level.

When faced with puzzling patients, they perform even more superlatively than the expert diagnostician limited to 1 field, because they readily recognise and handle multiple diseases across multiple fields.

They share the hallmarks of the expert diagnostician within a field, sometimes being even more so. In addition, they seem to have 2 more traits.

The first trait is that they seem extremely introverted and introspective, so much so that they appear reclusive to almost everyone else. This reclusiveness is unsurprising, given the behaviours linked to introversion. Research has shown the association between introversion and positive traits such as creativity, innovation, perseverance and self-reflection. Since these experts are reclusive, it is difficult to identify them using cursory means. For example, if you opened an Internet search engine and did a cursory search using words like 'best doctor in…', you would often get sponsored self-advertisements and misleading lists of names, instead of the truth.

The second trait is zero tolerance for disrespectful behaviour in any form. Generalists tend to be polite, but firm and no-nonsense. I surmise this to be a consequence of their learning journey, which embodies respect for themselves and others: they have attained their expertise through recognising mistakes and weaknesses in themselves, and aggressively fixing these. This zero-tolerance-for-disrespect also reflects their respect for others; allowing others to disrespect people, is to condone disrespect to themselves and to other people in general. This zero-tolerance policy often offends other people who indulge in disrespectful behaviour or cannot recognise disrespect.

One example of this zero-tolerance policy is punctuality. An expert generalist is almost always punctual. If they are unexpectedly delayed, they respect the time of others: they do their best to inform the people who are waiting for them, and do so in advance where possible. They expect the same of others who want their help. When teaching a group of students, they respect the effort and time of the attendees who are punctual, and will thus start the lesson on time. If there are latecomers or absentees, the generalist does not bend over backwards to compensate for their lateness or absence.

This 'I will respect your choice, but do not expect me to bend over backwards because of your choice; you must respect me too' behaviour offends some students, and others whom the generalist is helping.

The latecomers to the lesson may wonder why this teacher does not wait for them to arrive before starting the lesson. The absentees can claim: 'If this lesson was *really* important, you should have said so previously. Or you will conduct a make-up lesson for us.'

These latecomers and absentees inadvertently fail to realise that their thoughts derive from a self-defeating entitled mindset, arrogance and disrespect for the efforts of others. They fail to realise they are disrespecting *themselves:* a self-respecting learner respects their potential for learning and their future, and thus maximises their opportunities to learn, such as being punctual for important lessons. Habitual latecomers and absentees demonstrate the lack of this respect for themselves.

The generalist embodies ownership of their choices. The latecomers and absentees demonstrate denial of ownership of their choices; they want to escape the consequences of their choices by wanting to own other people's choices, such as 'you must do more for me, so I do not have to face the consequences of lateness or absenteeism'. The generalist's behaviour does not allow latecomers and absentees to escape the consequences, thus teaching them ownership: make a choice, and then live with it.

This zero-tolerance policy encourages positive behaviour. Thus, generalists are often the best teachers alive, because they teach more than just healthcare. They embody and teach positive qualities too.

The generalists are often aware of the ripple effects of their zero-tolerance policy, such as encouraging their students to develop positive qualities, but say nothing unless directly asked about their policy.

If the expert diagnostician within a field is rare, the expert generalist is even more so. I estimate their prevalence at less than 0.001% of all doctors. I consider it a great honour and privilege to meet one of them.

When 2 expert generalists meet (which is an extremely rare event) and start talking to each other, they recognise the truth of the other person instantly. The recognition signal is the robust, and often advanced-level, reasoning they wield when discussing healthcare. Since they do not need to simplify their explanations to each other, they can leap 5 mental steps or more with each sentence, their words demonstrating reasoning that is often beyond the basics described in this book.

Though their discussion is a marvel to behold, everyone else who is listening to the discussion lacks their mastery of clinical reasoning. Thus, everyone else cannot understand the discussion and wonders how the generalists make those mental leaps, and leap so quickly through so many specialities and settings and areas of healthcare. Even expert diagnosticians limited to 1 field (the tier of performance directly below the expert generalist) are left with a vague awareness of the essence of the discussion.

--

The aim of describing these tiers, is to demonstrate the global necessity of embedding clinical reasoning.

Conventional teaching and unaudited practice as of the end of 2022, explain much of the current tiers and their prevalence. I hypothesise that if robust clinical reasoning was a central tenet systematically enshrined in healthcare teaching, documentation and assessments, the widespread improvement in performance would lead to superior outcomes, higher productivity and less wastage of resources. These benefits would be obtained without needing vast improvement in technology or increased monetary expenditure.

It is my hope that after this book is published, many more doctors will reach the Good tier and above.

Capsule summary

- The tiers of performance mirror the underlying proficiency of clinical reasoning, and reflect the behaviours that accompany the doctor's reasoning.

- To 'up-skill' large proportions of doctors, clinical reasoning must be systematically embedded and taught during medical school, then encouraged (or even explicitly required) in the workplace.

Frequently asked questions

Q: Journeys can have milestones to mark the distance that has been travelled. These milestones measure the progress of the traveller. For the learning journey of this Universal Clinical Reasoning Method, what are your milestones?

A: This book describes the basics of the Universal Clinical Reasoning Method in detail. For these basics, there are 2 milestones:

1. Proficiency in the basics, and
2. Mastery of the basics.

Like the tiers of performance described in this chapter, the 2 milestones are distinguished by their outcomes.

Some learners will take longer than others to attain these milestones. What you get out of the journey, depends on the effort you put into it. Use your regular performance to gauge your progress.

Proficiency in the basics is the first major milestone. This milestone is roughly equivalent to the Good tier of performance, with the same hallmarks in behaviour, generally excellent outcomes in most patients, and few mistakes in clinical reasoning. I estimate a practitioner who has reached this milestone, consistently makes 5 reasoning mistakes or less out of every 100 patients they see.

Clinical accuracy is not dictated by the number of reasoning mistakes alone; the detail of one's illness scripts also drives outcomes. Thus, it would be inaccurate to assume that someone who makes reasoning mistakes in 5 out of 100 patients, has an accuracy of $(100-5)\% = 95\%$. Even when no reasoning mistakes are made, the doctor still needs their detailed illness scripts to consistently deduce the correct clinical diagnosis.

For doctors, I estimate a minimum of 3 years of dedication is needed to attain this first milestone.

Since this milestone requires detailed illness scripts, even a dedicated medical student who trains themselves to make virtually no reasoning mistakes, will need more than 3 years to develop the necessary illness scripts. If starting in medical school, I estimate a minimum of 5 years.

This practitioner may begin to develop awareness of advanced-level reasoning (which is not discussed in detail in this book). If they choose to use advanced-level reasoning, they must be cautious and do so in a limited fashion.

Mastery of the basics is the second milestone. The main difference between proficiency and mastery, lies in the detail and potency of your illness scripts. A master of the basics will have detailed illness scripts that often eclipse the information on those diseases in the subspecialty textbooks and literature. This practitioner will also have followed up on enough patients to acquire a sense of the advanced illness scripts. Combined with their increasing awareness of advanced-level reasoning, this practitioner can wield advanced-level reasoning with some proficiency. Through fierce dedication, this practitioner will also have weeded out the temptation to make any reasoning mistakes: I estimate they might make 1 reasoning mistake *at most* out of every 100 patients they see.

If you aim to reach the tier of 'Expert diagnostician within the field', mastery of the basics is almost certainly a requirement, and should bring you to (or near to) this tier.

For doctors, I estimate a minimum of 6 years of dedication is needed to attain this second milestone.

If starting in medical school, I estimate a minimum of 8 years.

These minimum estimates may seem overly optimistic and aimed at the most brilliant, open-minded and self-disciplined learners. A more conservative estimate (which still requires intense dedication and adhering to the learning journey described in this book) for the <u>expected</u> time taken to attain either milestone, would be twice the minimum number of years.

Though my estimates of the duration of dedicated effort needed to reach either milestone may seem disheartening, here is another observation of mine: before 2023, the doctors who reached those tiers of performance through trial-and-error, with no instruction manual to guide them, often needed *decades*. This book can serve as the instruction manual to reach the milestones. This book removes much of the painful trial-and-error, and can greatly accelerate the journey towards excellence.

Reaching the second milestone requires continued effort at self-improvement, even after reaching the first milestone. Thus, someone who has attained the first milestone and does not keep driving themselves to keep improving, is unlikely to attain the second milestone even if they worked for 30 more years.

If you attain the 1st milestone and then decide not to keep pushing to attain the second milestone, this is okay. Attaining the first milestone is already a major achievement.

The third milestone of the learning journey focuses on advanced-level reasoning and is the hallmark of the expert generalist. Since this book is devoted to the basics, the third milestone will not be discussed in detail in this book.

Q: Would an apprenticeship to a master of clinical reasoning, be of great help in my learning?

A: Perhaps.

Some learners pursuing proficiency in a skill, apprentice themselves to masters of that skill. Apprentices observe and help the master in their work, whilst expecting to learn in return. Direct observation can accelerate learning. However, there are 2 caveats to an apprenticeship.

The first caveat is the need for open-mindedness when observing a master. Masters can make mistakes. The apprentice who aims to match or exceed the master's skill should question the master about actions they cannot understand, or perceive as mistaken.

The second caveat is the necessity of dedicated effort for attaining mastery. The apprentice who thinks that they do not need to constantly put in the effort to hone the skill themselves during apprenticeship, often emerges from their apprenticeship with a half-baked idea of the skill. A genuine master has high standards and often, no patience for apprentices who waste their time; such an apprentice may be told to leave soon after beginning their apprenticeship.

These 2 caveats demonstrate why many learners who apprentice themselves to a teacher in any profession, emerge with little to show (other than a certificate of attendance, which is sometimes used as a misleading-seeming qualification to apply for a competitive position) for their apprenticeship. This outcome explains the recurring pattern of problems and scandals in many industries, where people with seemingly impressive paper qualifications/certificates are hired more on the basis of their paper credentials instead of genuine proof of competence. These people proceed to demonstrate gross incompetence.

Most of the results the learner gets, comes from the learner's efforts. This book has described the learning journey. Apprenticeship to a master can accelerate this journey somewhat, but is not a substitute for a full understanding (through constant practice and reflection) of the basics of this technique.

If you intend to petition a master of clinical reasoning for an apprenticeship, there is a third caveat: a genuine master of reasoning will be extremely mindful, perceptive, and know the caveats I have cited above. They will also be very busy people. Thus, these masters will not be deceived by half-hearted attempts at learning, and may require proof of at least a decent level of reasoning and dedication, before even considering the petitioner's request.

MISTAKES: WHAT TO DO

Every doctor will make mistakes in their learning and patient care.

Doctors who make 1 mistake when handling a patient, often make other mistakes while handling the same patient. By the time someone notices that something is amiss, the attending doctor has usually made multiple mistakes in their clinical reasoning and decision-making.

The best doctors make mistakes too. The difference between them and everyone else is the best doctors:

- Always try to do the right thing, instead of taking the easy way out
- Readily admit to and learn from mistakes, no matter how minor.

Doing the right thing

'Doing the right thing' means performing a proper clinical evaluation, obeying the basic diagnostic reasoning requirement, generating and prioritising the most likely clinical diagnosis and differentials, making logical plans, asking for help when help is required, and following up on patients.

In trying to 'do the right thing', you are reducing the chance of mistakes. In practising your reasoning process and tracking the outcome, you give yourself the chance to discover if you were right or wrong, which then gives you the chance to fix your mental processes. If you were making mistakes, attentiveness and reasoning allow you to rescue the situation and stop you from making any further mistakes.

If you do not 'do the right thing', you are usually disregarding the entirety of each patient and then making seemingly logical decisions, which, on deeper scrutiny, are just wild guesses. Not following up on the patient deprives you of the opportunity to improve.

Readily discovering and learning from mistakes

To effectively discover and learn from mistakes, 4 steps must be followed:

1. Put in the effort to discover mistakes (such as following up on patients), then

2. Have the humility to admit these mistakes, then

3. Search your heart and mind for the weaknesses that led to your making the mistakes, and then

4. Take effective action to fix all the underlying weaknesses that led to these mistakes.

When mistakes occur, there are usually multiple mistakes. Multiple mistakes point to multiple underlying weaknesses.

Without discovery, one cannot fix one's weaknesses.

Even after discovery, refusal to admit mistakes often leads to a refusal to learn from them. Even if one discovers and admits mistakes, the subsequent corrective action must be to reflect, recognise and then take effective action to fix the weaknesses.

Categories of mistakes

There are 2 categories of mistakes:

1. Unavoidable mistakes
2. Unnecessary mistakes

Unavoidable mistakes are those that occur during your learning and professional journey. Each of us has weaknesses in our knowledge, qualities, and skills. These weaknesses predispose us to make unavoidable mistakes. Fixing the weaknesses prevents future mistakes.

Will you step up and use these mistakes as learning opportunities?

If you want to be excellent, you must search inside yourself, promptly admit your mistakes and your underlying weaknesses, and then undertake the sustained effort to permanently fix the weaknesses.

When the best doctors make these mistakes, they take corrective action to rapidly reduce or prevent the repetition of these mistakes.

Unnecessary mistakes are actions that you know are mistakes, but you perform these actions anyway.

By the time you finish reading this book, all the mistakes in this book would fall into this category. An example is an illogical 'rule of thumb' such as 'perform this test and/or treatment for every patient with (insert symptom or sign)'. These rules of thumb usually ignore the patient's entirety.

Knowingly making mistakes, reveals even greater weaknesses in yourself.

At best, unnecessary mistakes represent conscious, deliberate actions taken for the sake of the doctor's convenience and insecurity.

At worst, such mistakes reveal apathy, greed or worse.

If you find yourself making an unnecessary mistake, face the truth of your character. And then fix the weaknesses.

Failure to follow all 4 of the earlier steps when making an unavoidable mistake, transforms repetitions of unavoidable mistakes into unnecessary mistakes. You have chosen to run away from the truth of yourself.

It is easier not to put in the effort to check the outcomes of your actions. It is uncomfortable to face the truth: the truth of character, and the truth of responsibility. This is why unnecessary mistakes are so common and persistent in humankind.

Many doctors, regardless of age, rank, title or setting, make unnecessary mistakes regularly.

Being wrong, and how to react

Reacting to patients

It is human to err. Patients may be unhappy when a mistake has been made. Their anger is often mitigated by:

- A sincere apology
- Listening to understand the patient better
- Transparency and partnership in decision-making
- A sustained commitment to be better.

Poor reasoners are often inattentive and make mistakes. Inattentiveness makes it harder to notice the mistakes and the consequences until it is too late. Poor reasoning predisposes the doctor to fail to promptly inform the patient of mistakes.

If the patient and their family ask patient-centred questions, the poor reasoner's previous inattentiveness to the patient now leaves them unable to answer. Instead of admitting their inattentiveness to themselves and the patient, the poor reasoner evades the question or fabricates answers. The poor reasoner may try to run away from responsibility or push blame. Many patients can instantly recognise the deceit and cowardice. Their mistrust of the doctor increases, and rightly so.

Once this mistrust has been created, it is very difficult to salvage the situation. The likelihood of an official complaint or lawsuit increases dramatically.

Many people in different professions sometimes suggest: 'If you don't tell them (the customer or patient) what you did wrong, they will not know, right?'

By treating other human beings as inattentive mindless people, this statement radiates arrogance and disrespect to other human beings. The speakers of this statement are poor reasoners. Unsurprisingly, these speakers usually underestimate everyone else, make unnecessary mistakes, refuse to learn from mistakes and ignore advice. Doctors are no exception. Though some patients might not notice when their chronic illness is half-controlled or their acute illness improves very slowly, many patients do notice when something is going wrong. Thus, if you treat patients as inattentive mindless people, there is definitely at least 1 'inattentive mindless person' in the consultation room: you.

Patients often consult another doctor when the outcome is poor. The poor reasoner who hopes they can always get away with continued inattention, evasions, fabrications and concealment, is mistaken.

Reacting to emotions

Doctors sometimes go through an emotional rollercoaster when they make a mistake: anger, guilt, shame and regret.

It is not useful to wish for impossibilities, such as turning back the clock or being perfect.

Instead, use your emotions to fuel the corrective actions for your mistakes and weaknesses. Emotional disturbances should become lessons on self-awareness: 'This is how I reacted when I made this mistake. Instead of being destructive, I should use my emotions to motivate me to do the right thing now, and in the future.'

Taking appropriate action helps to give the distraught doctor a sense of lasting closure as well as security: 'I will probably not make this mistake again, because I have identified the root cause in myself and fixed it.'

In contrast, running away from the mistake leaves a deep-seated, hidden wound and insecurity that can fester and grow over the years. Without facing and dealing properly with one's fear and insecurity, the fear and insecurity can just keep increasing.

Reacting to colleagues

When a colleague becomes alarmed enough to raise a concern about a potential mistake, the wise doctor realises that something is wrong. Many doctors dislike conflict and thus, often ignore the worrisome behaviour of their colleagues. It usually takes more — such as a potentially devastating mistake — to prompt a colleague to raise a concern.

Robust reasoners are open-minded, and thus will pause to consider the concern. Even if the robust reasoner disagrees with their colleague, robust reasoners realise that disagreements are not solely win-lose situations where one party must be right, and the other party must be wrong. Both parties can be right. Both parties can be wrong.

The doctor who is being questioned, may not have made a mistake. Sometimes, the colleague who is raising a concern, is mistaken. The colleague who is raising a concern is more likely to be mistaken if they reason poorly. Poor reasoners may complain about anything unfamiliar to them, because they have assumed that being different from what they want to believe, is automatically the same as being wrong. When there are many poor reasoners in 1 setting, they may question a colleague for not doing the same common thing as the many poorly reasoning colleagues, instead of asking themselves if they are doing the *right* thing.

Different is not the same as wrong. Ignorance of (or refusal to accept) this truth predisposes men to be prejudiced against females, females to be prejudiced against males, humans to denigrate others of different religious beliefs or skin colour or race or occupation, and so on.

When a poor reasoner is challenged or questioned in this manner, the response is often different from that of robust reasoners.

Poor reasoners tend to assume all situations are win-lose situations. Poor reasoners want to win and therefore often believe they must be right; therefore, those who disagree with them must be wrong and must 'lose'.

Thus, the poor reasoner tends to react inappropriately when questioned:

- Common responses include conjuring illogical explanations, pushing blame and attacking the colleague who raised the concern. An example of attacking would be to complain about something subjective and unverifiable, such as that colleague's tone of voice. The poor reasoner resorts to such tactics because they cannot offer a logical, professionally acceptable explanation for the concern their colleague raised.
- If the colleague is senior to them, the poor reasoner can appear to listen and agree, but ignores any advice.

The failure to be open-minded, accept differences and realise that situations are not always win-lose situations, implies a lack of overall reasoning.

This begs the question: why is poor clinical reasoning linked to poor overall reasoning?

Clinical reasoning is the medical application of overall reasoning. Poor clinical reasoners tend to be poor overall reasoners. Overall reasoning is not crucial for survival; thus, being alive is not proof of robust reasoning. Intelligence, knowledge, wealth, and connections can allow people to function somewhat, or get a place in medical school.

Overall reasoning also affects many positive traits such as courage, honesty, humility, open-mindedness, self-security, and gratitude. People who take action on their robust overall reasoning seem to become more observant, accept and adapt to reality, respect and value teamwork, and stand their ground when necessary. These behaviours, repeated over the years, build positive traits such as courage, honesty, humility and gratitude.

Thus, it is no accident that highly successful robust reasoners also possess these positive traits in abundance.

Conversely, a poor overall reasoner tends to lack the positive traits. This lack is demonstrated by the poor reasoner's inappropriate response when a mistake is made. Whilst a robust reasoner tends to demonstrate positive traits in their open-minded, humble and objective response to a challenger, a poor reasoner tends to demonstrate the exact opposite traits in their response. These negative traits may also explain their behaviour towards their patients, which is what precipitated the scenario of the colleague questioning them in the first place.

Reacting inappropriately with (irrational) quick fixes/rules of thumb

When a mistake has been made, it is tempting to go for 'quick fixes' or 'rules of thumb' such as 'in all patients with this symptom or sign, just perform this test and/or treatment'.

These quick fixes often suggest taking an action without thinking, and without paying attention to the entirety of the patient. This combination of lack of thinking and inattentiveness appeals to poor reasoners. Thus, these convenient quick fixes are readily suggested and happily adopted by poor reasoners, who continue to make mistakes in their patients despite using the quick fix.

Ignoring your underlying weaknesses that led to those mistakes, would not make you a better or safer doctor. Learning to react unthinkingly may make you a worse doctor than before.

The following conversation took place in October 2022.

Conversation #10

Colleague: 'I have an elderly lady who presented with breathlessness for a day, with no other respiratory symptoms. No chest pain. She had a history of deep vein thrombosis and atrial fibrillation. She had tachycardia and transient atrial fibrillation soon after admission. Otherwise, the physical examination did not seem remarkable. I sent off the D-dimer and the cardiac enzymes.'

Me: 'I did not hear the differentials. Were your differentials pulmonary embolism and acute myocardial infarction? Your decision implies that those were your differentials. Those differentials seem fair.'

Colleague: 'No. I sent off the cardiac enzymes as an afterthought. I did not really consider myocardial infarction, because I did not expect that a patient with myocardial infarction would not have chest pain. The D-dimer came back slightly elevated. However, the cardiac enzymes were elevated! The electrocardiogram was also consistent with a myocardial infarction, which was the eventual diagnosis. I almost missed a myocardial infarction!'

Me: 'You seem distressed. And scared.'

Colleague: 'I am! She did not have any chest pain. It caught me off guard. I know patients with myocardial infarction do not always have chest pain, but I did not expect this anyway. This was a near miss! How can I learn from this case if I do not know what I did wrong?'

Me (gently): 'You already know what you did wrong. You have just said it. Listen to yourself. Having theory knowledge is not the same as applying it clinically.'

Colleague: 'What are the differentials for isolated breathlessness without other "respiratory" symptoms or signs?'

Me: 'In addition to myocardial infarction and pulmonary embolism, metabolic conditions like diabetic ketoacidosis, anxiety and various psychosomatic disorders are differentials. The relevant differentials for each patient are decided by evaluating each patient clinically.'

Colleague: 'How about anaemia? Then again, that usually causes breathlessness on exertion, first. Should I do an arterial blood gas and cardiac enzymes for everyone with isolated breathlessness?'

Me: 'No. I had previously taught you that my first question for someone presenting with isolated breathlessness without other details, is to indicate the region: nose, throat or chest? The answer dramatically narrows the differentials. You then proceed to clinically evaluate the patient and think logically. Mindlessly performing a battery of tests for each symptom or sign is not the answer, and can lull you into a false sense of security because you stop thinking. Once you stop thinking, you are going to miss many dangerous diseases in your patients because you did not think of that dangerous disease, and therefore did not look for it.'

Colleague: 'Still feel like I want to do cardiac enzymes for everyone with breathlessness.'

Me: 'Stop spouting tests unthinkingly and fearfully! You are supposed to clinically evaluate and think. Everyone is afraid of being wrong. However, when fear of missing the correct diagnosis is accompanied by fear of trusting your thinking, this can easily become fear of *using* your thinking, which in turn leads to *fear of thinking*.'

'It is easier to not think, and blame the tests if a diagnosis was missed. However, you would be running away from the truth and the only safe solution. The tests cannot do your thinking for you. If you did not think of the correct diagnosis, you may not order the correct tests and treatment. This patient encounter shows you have mental weaknesses.'

'Be fair to yourself. You are human. Do not expect to be perfect! Instead, what matters is whether you now admit those weaknesses and fix them, or run away by resorting to mindless testing. Go sleep on it.'

Colleague: 'Okay.'

The next day, this colleague told me: 'I thought about what you said. Not so scared anymore.'

Me: 'You are welcome. Everyone has fears. The question is: do you own your fears, or do you let your fears own you? Owning your fears helps you keep a clear mind, continue doing the right thing, and try to become better. You are in charge, not your fears. This is the essence and the consequence of courage.'

'Conversely, to allow your fears to own you, is to surrender to your fears. This surrender leads to panic, easy but ineffective "solutions", and failure to improve. This is the essence and the consequence of cowardice. These qualities affect your behaviour and thus, your outcomes.'

'Everyone makes this choice about their fears for themselves every day, even if they never admit it or talk about it.'

Transparency in mistakes: the healthcare profession

My former and current students regularly discuss patients across multiple specialities and settings. Some doctors' insistence on ignoring clinical context whilst obsessing with tests, puzzles the stronger medical students. The students become alarmed as they observe these doctors handle patients.

Part of this alarm stems from the frequent demonstration of the disastrous chain of dominoes. Part of this alarm stems from the doctor's refusal to change their belief and behaviour, despite seeing these poor outcomes for themselves.

When students ask me why many doctors make obvious mistakes and refuse to improve, my answer is: old habits die hard. To learn from one's mistake, one must first admit their mistake to themselves. Learning the humility and courage to voluntarily face and admit one's mistakes, is not something our profession teaches or role models well.

Truly objective and systematic discussion of mistakes in healthcare, is uncommon in our profession and culture. Too often, the only mistakes that are discussed, are major mistakes and disasters. These events show up in Morbidity and Mortality rounds, Quality Assurance meetings, Department meetings and lawsuits.

When major mistakes are mentioned at meetings and rounds, many in the audience will have similar weaknesses predisposing to those mistakes, not just the doctors involved in the cases. However, a lack of reasoning and a sense of shame can permeate these sessions, which can hamper the learning of the right lessons:

- Senior doctors can suggest various seemingly logical 'quick fixes' to 'finish this case quickly', and then rush on to the next item in the meeting.

- Superficial or illogical remedies that do not address the underlying weaknesses in the reasoning of the doctors, are unlikely to help the audience become better.

- Seniors may deliberately and loudly suppress any revelation of the mistakes they made, turning the session into a tension-filled demonstration of cover-up behaviour. If such seniors are not stopped, some attendees notice these seniors 'getting away with it' and then copy the same behaviour when they, too, make major mistakes in patient care.

Mistakes that do not 'hit the news' in the hospital or country should also be discussed.

Recall the disastrous chain of dominoes: a mistake is often made alongside many other mistakes in the care of the same patient. A major mistake or disaster is a demonstration of the disastrous chain of dominoes.

Similar mistakes are almost certainly being made during the care of other patients across the country, for years. However, these chains of mistakes were not openly discussed or addressed.

Thus, if we are serious about reducing the frequency and severity of healthcare disasters, open and objective discussion about all mistakes must become a part of the culture of healthcare.

Ownership of mistakes: personal choice and responsibility

Though it is tempting to blame anyone and anything else for mistakes being made, the doctor is responsible for the consequences of their choices.

The healthcare culture often hides shame and denies mistakes. However, any culture arises from the commonly condoned behaviour of its people. A culture of hidden shame points to an abundance of poor reasoning. Unsurprisingly, unthinkingly copying others becomes commonplace in such cultures, because poor reasoning also predisposes to unthinking copying.

The culture does not force you to copy others. Copying is a personal choice. When you copy the mediocre or poor, you are likely to become mediocre or poor. When you copy the behaviour of those who make mistakes and do not improve, you will probably get the same result as them.

The best doctors become the best doctors because they have ownership, think for themselves, and fix themselves, instead of trying to fit in with the crowd of mediocre doctors.

The healthcare culture does not dictate your choices for learning and patient care; if so, the best doctors would not exist. The culture does not force you to make mistakes or pretend mistakes did not occur.

Take responsibility for mistakes, fix them, and fix yourself to prevent their recurrence. Sometimes, 1 person with the right direction, focus and will, can change the culture (this is another reason for this book).

From my observations, the transparency and humility (or lack thereof) of a doctor correlate with their general accuracy and reliability. Just ask the doctor about a potential mistake they made. I did this routinely; their answer told me much about their accuracy and reliability. The apparent intelligence, knowledge and seniority of the doctor did not influence this correlation.

All the best doctors and teachers I met had no difficulty admitting their mistakes. Some of these teachers spontaneously discuss their mistakes with the other doctors and students, thereby teaching others not to make the same mistakes. The more of your mistakes you readily admit to and fix, the faster you learn.

I have never met anyone who was both a great teacher and a terrible learner. A terrible learner is poor at teaching themselves; how can they be expected to excel at teaching others? A great teacher must first be a great learner and teach themselves well, before they can teach others well.

Conversely, denial, pushing of blame and irrational attacking was the classic reaction of the doctors who were widely regarded as poor teachers and terrible doctors.

The 'in-between the best and worst' group of mediocre teachers and doctors would ignore or deny mistakes to varying degrees. If a mistake was acknowledged, corrective action was usually superficial (such as deciding to use a quick fix), instead of addressing their underlying reasoning.

The healthcare culture needs to change.

Be part of that change.

Be part of the solution, not the problem.

Capsule summary

- 'Doing the right thing' helps to prevent mistakes, both present as well as future.
- Mistakes can be split into unavoidable mistakes and unnecessary mistakes.
- Mistakes will occur. React appropriately with the 4 steps.
- Emotional upheaval can be destructive or used constructively. The choice is yours.
- Own your mistakes.

THEORETICAL DISEASE APPROACHES

Hypothetical approaches to patients and diseases are common in textbooks and online websites.

These approaches have 2 common forms:

1. List of questions
2. Algorithm

The comprehensive list of questions can provide 20 questions or more for each symptom, with brief suggestions on the importance of certain answers.

The algorithm often depicts a flowchart describing questions, steps and decisions, each flowchart targeting 1 symptom or scenario.

These approaches may be useful at the start of medical school. All of these hypothetical approaches have significant limitations. Some approaches have major flaws. As these approaches are tools, their use is dependent on the reasoning of their user.

Limitations of the question list

There are dozens of symptoms and thus, dozens of question lists. Memorising all these lists is impossible for most doctors.

In addition, the rigid list of questions for each symptom tells the student what they can ask.

What you can ask, is not the same as what you should ask.

Many question lists cannot be rigidly followed after the first few questions, since the answers to the initial questions should direct the student to the relevant differentials, which in turn decide the subsequent questions and physical examination.

Limitations of algorithms

Algorithms are written to handle the common diseases, and identify some dangerous diseases. Each algorithm often begins with a single symptom or data point, and then provides suggestions on subsequent data to acquire and analyse.

The algorithms are limited by the real-world presentation of patients. Many patients who have 1 symptom fitting an algorithm, often have other symptoms or signs that fit another algorithm.

When more than 1 algorithm applies to the same patient, which algorithm should the doctor use?

The doctor can try to use all the algorithms that apply to that patient. What should the doctor do if two or more algorithms are applied to the same patient, and the suggested diseases and recommended management decisions, are totally different after such application? (The correct answer is not to unthinkingly assume the patient has all of those diseases and carry out all those sets of management decisions.)

Algorithm flowcharts appear to provide 'forking' as if each data point is 100% accurate. However, most data points, including clinical features and test results, do not have 100% accuracy.

In addition, algorithms cannot obey Rule #1 of clinical reasoning: explain all clinical features.

Strictly following an algorithm will automatically mean missing the correct diagnosis in at least a minority of patients.

The basic diagnostic reasoning requirement will override any tool that fails to 'explain all the patient's clinical features'.

It is neither fair nor feasible to expect that the writers of algorithms help the reader 'explain all the clinical features'. Writers cannot be expected to cover all the variations in presentation and all the data points for each of the differentials mentioned in that algorithm. This task would be overwhelming. The limits on words and page space also preclude such descriptions.

Another limitation is the doctor: no one can memorise all the algorithms. Opening your textbook or using your electronic device to look up one or more algorithms in the middle of each consultation, is not viable. Therefore, imperfect recall of the algorithm often means the imperfect application of the steps, which then results in even lower accuracy than the algorithm's true performance.

Should algorithms be modified for use, or even used at all?

If students observe their patients, build up their mental illness scripts and apply clinical reasoning, algorithms rapidly lose their potential usefulness in favour of holistic patient-centred evaluation and analysis.

Is there a way to modify these algorithms to encourage a patient-centred approach? Yes.

If existing algorithms could be rewritten to include the universal and secondary specific clinical features for each differential diagnosis in that algorithm, this rewriting would help the reader tremendously. Rewriting each algorithm would require at least 2 robust reasoners who are also fully versed in universal and secondary specific clinical features for all the relevant differentials for that algorithm.

If such extensive rewriting is not feasible, stating the need to 'explain all clinical features' and seek help if the doctor cannot fulfil Rule #1 of clinical reasoning, is a useful warning to the reader. This warning tells the reader not to ignore the entirety of the patient.

Even then, these measures cannot address the fact that memorising all those algorithms is impossible.

Having begun to employ and refine clinical reasoning early on, I did not find fixed algorithms useful, either for accurate learning or for patient-centred care. Even now (August 2023), the robustly reasoning medical students express the same sentiments about algorithms: 'potentially misleading' and 'waste of time' being 2 common descriptors.

I only use 'initial algorithms' of my own devising. Recall Conversation #10 in the previous chapter 'Mistakes: what to do'. I mentioned teaching my initial question to isolated breathlessness, provided there were no other details about the patient. Essentially, each self-devised algorithm only has 1 or 2 initial questions based on a specific scenario. Rule #1 of clinical reasoning shapes my initial questioning. If a patient presents with isolated breathlessness with any other details that alter the differentials, I may not use the initial question in that Conversation.

The answers to the first 1 or 2 questions in my algorithms can be so varied, that the many forks after those answers to decide the 3rd or 4th question, would fill several A4-size pages.

Thus, I use *fluid* algorithms, which 'fork' depending on the patient's presentation. These patient-adapted mental algorithms are based on detailed illness scripts and the 3 rules of reasoning.

Diagnostic criteria

Diagnostic criteria have existed for decades. These include criteria for rheumatic fever, systemic lupus erythematosus, Kawasaki disease, multisystem inflammatory syndrome, depression, and so on. Each list of criteria is focused on 1 disease. These criteria may include test-based results. As the years pass, more diagnostic criteria and the accompanying scoring systems are created.

Though the list of criteria for each disease is not truly a 'list of questions', some doctors will apply these criteria as a list of questions to ask the patient.

These lists of criteria have 2 major limitations:

1. Waiting to fulfil criteria
2. Other diseases that also fulfil the criteria

1. Waiting to fulfil criteria: Fulfilment of enough criteria on the checklist, often provides sensitivity or specificity of 90% or more for the disease.

The problem is the waiting. Some patients do not fulfil enough criteria at the first presentation of that disease. Without clinical reasoning, many doctors prefer to wait, letting the disease progress until the criteria are fulfilled. However, the literature, patient observation and pathophysiology demonstrate that delaying treatment without compelling reason, is always unhealthy.

2. Other diseases that also fulfil the criteria: Sometimes, other diseases can also fulfil the diagnostic criteria. This unhappy scenario arises when most of the patient's information fulfils the criteria ascribed to 1 disease, but explaining all of the clinical features points to another disease.

In this situation, a decent reasoner can just point out: 'Hey, the patient's entire clinical picture points to another disease. So, shall we ignore the disease that fits the patient, to prioritise this list of criteria you want to use?'

Overcoming the limitations of diagnostic criteria

Robust reasoning can enable a doctor to consistently overcome the limitations of conventional diagnostic criteria. Let us illustrate this with 2 examples.

Example #1: Kawasaki disease

Kawasaki disease is an inflammatory disorder that affects children. The most common and feared complication of this disease is coronary artery injury, which then predisposes to heart attacks and other problems later in life. Adequate and timely treatment minimises the risk of complications. The mainstay of standard treatment is intravenous immunoglobulin (IVIG).

This disease has a list of diagnostic criteria. The usual definition is having a fever for at least 5 days, plus at least four of the other criteria on the list:

- Bilateral conjunctival injection
- Changes in the lips and oral cavity
- Cervical lymphadenopathy
- Extremity changes
- Polymorphous rash

Incomplete Kawasaki disease is suspected Kawasaki disease that does not meet enough of the criteria.

The suspicion of incomplete Kawasaki disease often creates hesitancy and uncertainty. Resources are often expended on diagnostic testing. If there are delays in appropriate treatment, the child is often suffering whilst waiting for the doctor to become more certain of the diagnosis. Delayed treatment also increases the risk of complications.

The secondary specific clinical features of Kawasaki disease

From my observations, there are 4 secondary specific clinical features of Kawasaki disease:

1. (Early) Mucositis
2. Swelling of the hands or feet
3. Inflammatory disease timeline in the clinical features
4. BCG vaccine site inflammation

Most of the children with Kawasaki disease that I have seen over the years, had at least one of these secondary specific features. The secondary specific feature(s) would often be present by the 4th day of illness. Using any of these specific features and fulfilling the basic diagnostic reasoning requirement allows instantaneous clinical diagnosis, rendering the conventional list of criteria unnecessary. Appropriate treatment can be promptly commenced, sometimes before the 5th day of illness. Delays in care and unnecessary testing, are avoided.

Some of these patients present between the 2nd and 4th day of illness. When I make the clinical diagnosis immediately, the inevitable protest from a watching medical student or junior doctor is often: 'The child has not had 5 days of fever yet! Not enough criteria have been fulfilled for Kawasaki disease!'

I acknowledge their concern, and then ask them to suggest another disease that explains the secondary specific clinical feature the patient has demonstrated. My questions include:

- 'Tell me another disease that explains this symptom/sign/pattern.'

- 'How do you explain the red and cracked lips starting on day 1 or 2 of illness? Was the child drinking poorly enough and long enough, to explain the red and cracked lips?'

- 'How do you explain the swelling of the hands/feet? Does congestive cardiac failure, liver failure or kidney failure, regardless of the underlying disease, explain the patient's fever and other symptoms too?'

- 'How do you explain the temporal pattern of the eye redness in relation to the fever? Does Adenovirus conjunctivitis behave like this?'

The clinical assessment reveals the severity of the patient's Kawasaki disease. The single test that may add value to my clinical assessment, is an echocardiogram. The echocardiogram provides information for adjusting treatment intensity and duration. Thus, if I think the disease is severe, I ask for an early echocardiogram.

Poor reasoning applied to the literature, and thus drawing the wrong conclusions

Without robust clinical reasoning, it is easy to draw the wrong conclusions from the literature. Three mistaken conclusions are:

1. It is okay to wait until day 10 of Kawasaki disease, before commencing treatment.

2. Treatment that is given early for Kawasaki disease, is likely to fail because it was given too early.

3. Since elevated inflammatory markers are often seen in patients with Kawasaki disease, inflammatory markers are 100% sensitive/specific for Kawasaki disease.

Studies have shown that the administration of IVIG by day 10 of illness decreases the risk of poor outcomes, compared to the administration of IVIG after day 10 of illness. Unfortunately, some doctors interpret these findings to mean: 'The risk of complications does not change, as long as the treatment is instituted by day 10. Therefore, I can wait until day 8 or day 9 before instituting treatment. Let me treat for bacterial lymphadenitis and see what happens, first. Let me wait for the results of the viral studies. Maybe the patient does not have Kawasaki disease.'

It is a mistake to believe that delaying treatment until days 7, 8 or 9 of illness instead of promptly treating Kawasaki disease, does not increase the risk of complications. Early and appropriate treatment improves outcomes and reduces patient suffering in all diseases. From a pathophysiology perspective, early effective treatment stops the inflammation that potentially damages the coronary vessels. Multiple studies have demonstrated the same concept, showing that the earlier treatment is given, including day 5 or earlier, the better the outcomes in these patients.

Some studies show that starting treatment in patients with Kawasaki disease before day 5 of the disease, is associated with a higher chance of treatment failure. Doctors have cited such literature to argue that earlier treatment of Kawasaki disease had a higher chance of treatment failure because treatment was given too early.

These doctors have conflated association with causation. If a study suggested that earlier treatment was associated with a higher chance of failure, they should have asked themselves: why did the study demonstrate that association? Especially when giving early treatment in any disease, is not expected to increase the chances of treatment failure?

To assume association is equal to causation, is like arguing that the fever seen in febrile seizures is the cause of the seizure, or that the weatherman carrying the umbrella is responsible for the downpour that occurs an hour later.

The 4 universal reasons for treatment failure, cited earlier in this book, do not include 'treatment was given too early'.

The explanation for the association between treatment failure and early treatment of Kawasaki disease, is self-evident by asking yourself: when would doctors be able to start treatment earlier, in any disease?

Doctors can start treatment earlier if they recognise the disease earlier.

So, how are doctors able to recognise any disease earlier in some patients, compared to other patients with that disease?

Because the disease in that patient is more severe than usual and thus, is easier to recognise early on.

Since treatment intensity must match disease severity, the patient whose disease is recognised much earlier than usual, tends to have more severe disease and thus, needs more intensive treatment than other patients with milder disease.

If the doctor does not realise this universal truth and tries standard treatment in patients whose disease was recognised earlier than usual, the treatment is more likely to fail in these patients compared to the 'classic' patients.

Therefore, the real reason for the failure of standard treatment when a disease is recognised earlier than usual, is the failure to match disease severity with treatment intensity. This failure to match the treatment intensity to disease severity occurs because of the failure to recognise the true severity of the disease, *not* 'the treatment was given too early'.

The literature backs up this principle. Li et al. (2018) conducted a meta-analysis on the predictors of IVIG-resistant Kawasaki disease, and then suggested that it was the severity of the disease instead of the earlier treatment, that predisposed to the failure of treatment.

Once we accept that patients with more severe diseases tend to be recognised earlier than those with milder diseases, and that adequate treatment that is instituted earlier in Kawasaki disease seems to reduce the chance of complications, the conclusion is: in children where Kawasaki disease is recognised earlier because the criteria for Kawasaki disease are adequately fulfilled, the treatment must be more aggressive than those who are recognised later on using the same criteria.

This 'diseases recognised earlier tend to be more severe' observation also applies to many other diseases, including onset at a younger age. Applying this observation to Kawasaki disease, explains the literature stating that younger infants with obvious Kawasaki disease are more likely to be resistant to standard treatment than the average patient.

Elevated inflammatory markers, especially ESR and CRP, are often seen in these patients. However, these markers are not specific to Kawasaki disease. It is erroneous to insist that a high ESR and CRP point only to Kawasaki disease. A significant minority of patients with Kawasaki disease have normal or near-normal inflammatory markers, so insisting that the patient cannot have Kawasaki disease based on seemingly normal inflammatory markers, is a mistake.

Example #2: Systemic lupus erythematosus

See the following conversation.

Conversation #11

Doctor M is preparing a patient's case for the 'diagnostic dilemmas' presentation. She decides to 'test' the case on a senior colleague, Doctor G.

Doctor M shows Doctor G the first slide of the Powerpoint slideshow. 'I am preparing a difficult case for the department! This slide describes her first presentation. I know you want the exact duration of each symptom, so I included that.'

> 16-year-old girl
>
> Fever, 4 days
> Left axillary lymph node swelling, 1 day

Doctor M continues: 'She felt some pain over the left armpit on the 4th day of fever, and found a swelling there. The doctor in the clinic checked, and decided the swelling was a lymph node. Shall I go on to the next slide?'

Doctor G: 'Lupus.'

Doctor M blinks. 'What?!?'

Doctor G frowns. 'Was I wrong? I suppose a lymphoma is possible. Less likely than lupus, though.'

Doctor M: 'No. I mean…you are right. It was lupus. How did you figure it out?'

Doctor G: 'The fever began first. There are no other symptoms initially. On the 4th day, the lymph node swelled up on its own. Probably caused pain by stretching the capsule. This points to a systemic inflammatory process before the overt pathological reaction in the lymph node. Given this picture and the absence of other symptoms, only 2 categories of disease are reasonably likely: autoimmune and white cell malignancy.'

Doctor M: 'Sure. That leaves 2 categories. So how did you jump to lupus?'

Doctor G: 'What is the first line on your slide?'

Doctor M: '16-year-old girl.'

Doctor G: 'In a teenage girl, which of the 2 categories of disease is more common: autoimmune, or malignancy?'

Doctor M: 'Autoimmune.'

Doctor G: 'And which autoimmune disease is the most common in a teenage girl? Especially if it explains all the symptoms?'

Doctor M: 'Lupus.'

Doctor G: 'There you go.'

Doctor M: 'Why not bacterial lymphadenitis?'

Doctor G: 'Bacterial lymphadenitis implies that the bacterial infection must come from somewhere. There is no apparent source. Furthermore, the clue is in the time pattern. Let us use bacterial cervical lymphadenitis as an example. Think back to all the patients you have ever seen with bacterial cervical lymphadenitis. When did their swelling or pain begin?'

Doctor M: 'Within 2 days of the onset of other symptoms, such as fever. If the corroborative history was unreliable, that number might vary widely.'

Doctor G: 'Using that observation, how could this be bacterial lymphadenitis? Bacterial lymphadenitis would be very, very unlikely.'

Doctor M: 'Well, the first doctor treated for bacterial lymphadenitis.'

Doctor G: 'And would have failed.'

Doctor M: 'That doctor thought the treatment was working. At the next visit a few days later, the lymph node swelling apparently improved! The fever continued, though.'

Doctor G: 'That is the next clue. In all the infections you have ever seen where the patient had both fever — the systemic feature — and localising clinical features, which clinical feature improved first? The systemic feature, or the localising feature?'

Doctor M: 'The systemic feature. Oops. This child's fever persisted even when the lymph node swelling seemed to improve. So this child did not improve as an infection should have.'

Doctor G: 'Exactly. In this child, the doctor did not recognise the "improvement" for what it truly was. Confirmation bias could have contributed, especially when the doctor did not think of any other diagnosis. The change in the swelling was *not* an improvement. This is the inflammatory disease timeline.'

Doctor M: 'The inflammatory markers were checked at the follow-up visit! The ESR was high at 75 mm/hr and the C-reactive protein was normal, at 5 mg/L. Does that not look like a resolving infection?'

Doctor G: 'When the clinical features disagree with the test results, be careful. Consider other diseases that clinically fit the patient and explain the test results, instead of fixating only on the existing diagnosis. Lupus can give that exact combination of CRP and ESR, too.'

Doctor M: 'The fever continued despite the antibiotics. So, the child was hospitalised. And labelled as pyrexia of unknown origin.'

Doctor G: 'Pyrexia of unknown origin is not a diagnosis. Doctors who use this label usually try a battery of tests. Given this patient's diagnosis, the lupus panel would return positive. Weeks after the initial presentation. With the patient suffering throughout. Hopefully, Rheumatology has seen the child and started treatment.'

Doctor M: 'Er…yes. That's what happened to this patient.'

Doctor G: 'I do not encourage batteries of tests hoping to "get lucky". Relevant clinical evaluation and reasoning, followed by targeted diagnostic tests if necessary, is the way to go.'

Doctor M: 'Would you have performed tests looking for lupus at the first presentation?'

Doctor G: 'Yes, if there was nothing else in the history and the examination. Was there? The skin overlying the lymph node was normal?'

Doctor M: 'There was nothing else. Yes, the patient's skin was normal.'

Doctor G: 'Then the entire clinical picture fits lupus. So, yes, I'd test for lupus at the first consultation. That is the most likely clinical diagnosis. Even if I had not, the clinical evolution by the next visit would have pointed directly at lupus.'

--

Conversation #11 demonstrates the importance of embarking on the learning journey described in Section 1.

That learning journey requires obedience to Rule #1 of clinical reasoning, including the pursuit of knowledge to obey this Rule in every patient you handle.

It is not enough to read a standard textbook entry about a disease just to know something. To know something is not the same as to know *enough*.

Instead, you must pursue knowledge of that disease's clinical features in your patient, to the point that you can obey Rule #1 for that patient. Hence the follow-up, the patient logs, and scouring remote sources of knowledge; all to build up detailed illness scripts. Sufficient knowledge is acquired to distinguish between the most likely disease and its differentials, often from the details of the Presenting Complaint alone. Conversation #11 demonstrates the potency of such detailed knowledge and reasoning, to the point of obviating the need for diagnostic criteria.

When robust clinical reasoning is combined with these supremely detailed illness scripts, you can recognise diseases clinically, instantly, and consistently. You can do this even when the patient has only one, or none, of the diagnostic criteria for diseases listed in guidelines and textbooks worldwide.

The illness scripts allow you to pick out secondary specific clinical features that are not published in the diagnostic criteria. For example, at the first presentation, the patient in Conversation #11 was not known to have any of the 11 criteria used by the American College of Rheumatology (ACR). The ACR criteria recommend a minimum of 4 criteria to be used to diagnose lupus. The ACR criteria are among the most widely used criteria in the world for the diagnosis of lupus. Some of those criteria are clinical; some are test-based.

If the patient had been left to suffer long enough, she might have fulfilled at least 4 out of ACR's 11 criteria eventually. When that patient's lupus panel returned positive, she was referred to the paediatric rheumatologist. Her workup left her fulfilling just 3 of the ACR's 11 criteria. By that point, she had already suffered for several weeks. Thankfully, the rheumatologist did not wait and promptly commenced the proper treatment. The patient improved, as expected.

Conclusions

I and my students have encountered many patients whose disease is instantly and clinically obvious, yet would not have fulfilled 'enough criteria' on conventional checklists. The earlier these patients are treated adequately, the less they suffer, and the lower the chance of developing complications.

Both examples — Kawasaki disease and systemic lupus erythematosus — mentioned the Inflammatory disease timeline.

Many categories of a disease have a timeline of clinical features that is common to diseases within that category. Specific diseases also have timelines specific to themselves.

However, knowing the timeline for 1 disease does not automatically confer the ability to use time-based patterns to clinically differentiate between diseases. For example, knowing the pattern of abdominal pain in acute gastroenteritis may not suffice to allow you to distinguish this diagnosis from other causes of abdominal pain, if you lack the illness scripts of the differentials. This limitation applies to timelines too. One must know the timeline of multiple diseases and figure out the universal and secondary specific equivalents of each disease's timeline. These timelines are essentially advanced illness scripts, which rely on the basic principles in this book to use properly.

The timelines are useful for dealing with diagnostic puzzles. However, even my strongest students (some are the most brilliant doctors that anyone could hope to encounter) could not accurately use the simplest timelines until they were proficient in the fundamentals of the universal clinical reasoning method. Thus, I will not describe this advanced knowledge and technique in full detail in this book.

In conclusion, a sufficiently skilled and knowledgeable reasoner does not need to rely upon diagnostic criteria or wait for patients to suffer long enough to fulfil those criteria. A master of this Universal Clinical Reasoning method possesses disease knowledge far exceeding that of, and undescribed in, textbook entries and diagnostic criteria in guidelines. They also possess the reasoning to wield such knowledge with astonishing (to non-practitioners of this method) speed, power, and accuracy.

Does such proficiency require decades of experience? Not at all. Doctor G in Conversation #11 had worked for less than 10 years.

Diagnostic scoring systems

Diagnostic scoring systems are a numerical version of diagnostic criteria.

Thus, they suffer the same limitations. In addition, if the patient has a high score on the scoring system for a disease, this does not automatically mean that the disease is the most likely diagnosis.

The most likely diagnosis fulfils the basic diagnostic reasoning requirement, which scoring systems cannot match. See the next case.

CASE #28: Kuan

Kuan is a 45-year-old man who presents to the Accident and Emergency Department with severe pain in the right groin radiating to the right thigh. The pain is so severe that he cannot stand straight. This pain is accompanied by 10 episodes of vomiting food and water. All of these symptoms began 12 hours ago.

He had an operation to drain an ischiorectal abscess 6 days ago, and is currently on oral Amoxycillin-clavulanate. He has a background of poorly controlled diabetes mellitus.

On examination, his vital signs are normal. He seems lethargic. There is tenderness over the right iliac fossa and groin, without guarding or rebound. There is tenderness over the right hip on flexion. There is pain over the right anterior superior iliac spine on extension of that hip. A purulent discharge is seen over the wound incision.

Blood tests were performed, which revealed leukocytosis at 20×10^9 cells/litre, with neutrophilia.

--

(*Continued*)

Three doctors are discussing what to do about Kuan.

The first doctor argues: 'This patient has a high Alvarado-appendicitis score of 7 points! Therefore, this must be acute appendicitis!'

The second doctor argues: 'No! The patient has signs on examination of the hip! Therefore, this must be septic arthritis of the right hip!'

The third doctor sighs. 'Just put everything together. All symptoms and signs, including the purulent discharge from the wound. The abscess was not fully cleared.'

The subsequent CT scan proved the third doctor correct.

Even if Kuan had scored the maximum score on the Alvarado scoring system, the scoring system would have failed to explain all of his clinical features, such as the purulent wound surface and the other anomalies on physical examination.

Diagnostic criteria and their numerical equivalents (diagnostic scoring systems) cannot be applied without obeying the basic diagnostic reasoning requirement. To do so is to ignore 'inconvenient clinical features' to insist on target fixation.

Always obey Rule #1 of clinical reasoning, overriding diagnostic criteria if necessary.

Capsule summary

- Theoretical approaches may be useful at the beginning of medical school. If you use them, know their limitations and potential flaws.

- Diagnostic criteria and scoring systems do not overrule Rule #1 of clinical reasoning. Often, it is the other way around: Rule #1 overrules diagnostic criteria and scoring systems.

Frequently asked questions

Q: It is often taught that when a patient presents acutely, you should 'only think of acute/short-term diseases first'. What do you think?

A: 'Acute presentation = acute diseases only' reflects flawed reasoning and fixation on population-level statistics. This is a variation of the fallacy of 'you must always think of common diseases first'.

At a population level, patients who present with short-term suffering usually have short-term, acute illnesses. This does not mean patients who present with short-term suffering *always* have short-term, acute illnesses.

Chronic diseases must begin someday, and must be present long enough before they can be called 'chronic'. If a patient presents with the clinical features of a chronic disease and is suffering 'only for a few days', it is silly to think 'since you have only suffered a few days, I should not think of chronic diseases until you have suffered enough'.

Such thinking shows a lack of empathy and lack of reasoning. This fallacy is compounded by (flawed) diagnostic criteria, which insist on a minimum long duration of suffering before that disease can be diagnosed. Doctors often succumb to these fallacies even when there is no other likely diagnosis, and then refuse to accept and treat the clinically obvious diagnosis because 'the patient has not suffered long enough'. Thus, the patient suffers for much longer until the doctor decides to make the diagnosis.

I cannot agree with allowing patients to suffer because the doctor refuses to accept reality: the entirety of the patient's symptoms and signs.

The robust reasoner will avoid fallacies and promptly make the correct diagnosis.

GUIDELINES AND PROTOCOLS

Guidelines are documents that recommend steps in healthcare for particular symptoms, scenarios or diseases. Guidelines are derived from the interpretation of existing evidence, written with local infrastructure and population characteristics in mind, and influenced by the authors' experience and opinions.

Protocols are workplace-specific, shorter versions of guidelines.

There are 3 categories of guidelines and protocols:

- Defensive
- Neutral
- Best care

Defensive category

Intent and form of defensive documents

Defensive guidelines and protocols generally seem to assume that the intended audience cannot recognise and manage diseases, thereby increasing the chance of patient harm if the audience is not given appropriate help.

Unfortunately, the content of many defensive documents demonstrates and encourages poor reasoning, which *also* increases the chance of patient harm. Their hallmarks include:

- Encyclopaedic content and length
- Description of clinical information is unprioritised, such as focusing more on risk factors than clinical features for the diagnosis
- Focus on tests for ruling out an arbitrary list of dangerous diseases (ruling out OAF)
- Encourage early treatment for presumed, dangerous diseases without regard to probability or later consequences
- Primary outcomes are usually aimed at preventing disaster instead of ensuring optimal patient health. For example, if a chronic disease remains active but is not deemed life-threatening, this state is considered 'well-controlled'
- Evidence from the literature is interpreted defensively.

These hallmarks imply that the intended readers are any or all of the following:

- Cannot make the correct diagnosis
- Are ignorant
- Have poor or zero reasoning
- Clinical skills are questionable or nonexistent
- Cannot provide excellent care. Thus, the aim is to avert disaster instead.

Such documents may be useful for doctors who do not know what to do.

These documents often cannot recommend optimal decisions. Optimal decisions are based on the patient's diagnosis, which is in turn based on adequate clinical evaluation to understand the entirety of the patient.

Consideration of the entirety of the patient to make optimal decisions, is the responsibility of the doctor.

Consequences of following defensive documents, at the individual level

Though the intent of writing these documents was to help readers avoid missing and mishandling dangerous diseases, poor reasoners often misuse these documents. These documents are tools. Poor reasoners often misuse tools.

Readers of these documents will be tempted to rule out OAF. The doctor who rules out all the diseases on the checklist, still does not have the patient's actual diagnosis. It is sometimes implied (wrongly) that ruling out a fixed or arbitrary list of differentials means the doctor can then diagnose the single remaining disease the document is addressing, as if no other differentials are relevant to the unique patient.

Some patients will have part of their clinical picture fit the scenario described in the document, but have diseases that are not addressed in the document. Ignoring the rest of the patient's clinical picture to 'force the patient to fit the document', is to ignore reality. Following that document and doing nothing else, would mean automatically missing the correct diagnosis and mismanaging these patients.

I have heard poor reasoners argue that doctors should follow the defensive documents, and then tackle the most likely diagnosis afterwards. Such an argument ignores reality. Many doctors who rule out OAF, are trying to conceal their inability to make the most likely diagnosis. After ruling out OAF, they still have no idea what the most likely diagnosis is. How are they going to 'tackle the most likely diagnosis' afterwards? By wildly guessing a diagnosis, or hoping that the sole remaining diagnosis on their arbitrary list is the most likely diagnosis?

Even if the doctor could somehow rule out OAF and can subsequently tackle the most likely diagnosis, the initial defensive battery of tests and treatments can consume a significant amount of time, energy and money, and annoy the patient. Proposing yet more tests and treatments on top of the previous barrage of orders will further annoy some patients and creates mistrust: 'Doctor, what exactly are you doing? Can you make up your mind? You don't seem to know what is going on.' Some of these patients react by refusing the subsequent orders or filing complaints.

Decent reasoners do not follow defensive documents except as a final, desperate resort. Instead, they go for the most likely diagnosis. They know when to consider ruling out dangerous differentials, including differentials that were never mentioned in the document.

Wider consequences and proof of outcomes from defensive documents

Did these defensive documents improve the outcomes of healthcare in those countries where they originated, in the years and decades since their emergence? So far, I have not found any evidence to support this, which is unsurprising:

- If the intended audience did not learn to handle that symptom/scenario/disease in medical school despite being taught properly, why should they now read, memorise and follow a 100-page (or longer) document? (If the learners were not taught properly, the problem may not lie with the learners.)

- It is often impossible to memorise 100 pages or more for 1 symptom/scenario/disease alone, never mind multiplying this by the sheer number of symptoms/scenarios/diseases the doctor will encounter.

Even more harm is inflicted when these documents reach other parts of the world. When poor reasoners learn of the existence of a defensive guideline or protocol, the common reaction is: 'Great! There is a document and a process to follow! There is no need to think!'

The key questions of 'What is the healthcare outcome in countries where these documents originated?' and 'What is the healthcare outcome in countries where these documents were followed?' never seem to come up.

When these documents are followed in other parts of the world, the consequences of following these documents — ruling out OAF, failing to make the correct diagnosis, unnecessary tests and treatment in most patients, automatically missing every other dangerous disease, and more — spread across the world. This situation is tragic: the doctors who would have done better by *not* following these documents, now follow these documents and therefore have worse outcomes. Nationwide, more money is spent on tests and treatments. Despite this, the overall outcomes do not improve and might even worsen.

When defensive documents and the use of these documents encourage poor reasoning, healthcare outcomes are unlikely to improve. Instead, the reverse is more likely to occur: the outcomes worsen. These consequences are instantly obvious to a robust reasoner, which is why robust reasoners generally stay away from defensive documents.

The common and poorly reasoning reaction when the outcomes do not improve despite (and because of) the use of defensive documents, is to add even more defensiveness to such documents. Increased defensiveness can manifest in many ways, such as increasing the eligible pool of patients to undergo tests or suggesting more tests for every patient.

As a hypothetical example, if the previous recommendation was to perform a lumbar puncture in every child up to 12 months of age with suspected febrile seizures to rule out meningitis, increased defensiveness leads to the recommendation of including all children below 18 months of age. The use of a demographic (age) instead of the patient's clinical picture, to make a sweeping recommendation that ignores the patient's entire clinical picture, is typical of poor reasoning in a defensive document.

Insisting on the use of defensive documents instead of recognising that they are contributing to the problem, will not break the vicious cycle of discouraging reasoning, poor decisions, and poor outcomes.

Defensive guidelines and protocols **are not a part of the solution. Instead, they have become a part of the problem, and will worsen the problem.** Therefore, defensive documents and their widespread use, are products of flawed reasoning at multiple levels.

The path forward for defensive documents, and the problems underlying their origin

When diagnoses are missed, it is the 'dangerous' diseases that tend to cause major harm or death, which in turn captures attention when these are reported in the news. Other cases tend to arise when a dangerous disease, despite being known, is mismanaged.

A high prevalence of poor outcomes in a region or country points to systemic problems in training, practice and governance.

The vicious cycle of poor reasoning, poor decisions and poor outcomes cannot be broken without identifying and tackling the root cause of the poor outcomes: a lack of reasoning.

The answer is straightforward: fix the root cause. Clinical reasoning enables the training of the safest doctors: those who get it right, and know how to adapt when they are uncertain of the correct diagnosis. This requires a systematic and sustained effort from leaders and teachers. Medical schools should rework their teaching. Leaders of healthcare facilities and government officials need to pitch in too. (These teachers and leaders should buy this book.)

The solution to poor healthcare, is not a defensive document that perpetuates the disastrous chain of dominoes. In a sense, defensive documents have become excuses to avoid facing the truth and doing the hard work associated with this truth.

When someone (often a student or junior doctor) asks me if I would follow a defensive document, I laugh.

Seeing their mystified look, I say, 'If you do the same thing as other people, you get the same result they get. So, if you wanted to be successful and copy someone, do you follow the footsteps of the successful, or those who failed?'

The reply is always: 'The successful, obviously.'

I go on. 'Good. So, in healthcare, if you follow the footsteps of a country — their guidelines and protocols — should you look at their outcomes?'

The reply is always: 'Yes.'

I finish. 'Which countries have the worst healthcare outcomes? You can look this up online and in the literature. Chronic or acute disease, it does not matter. Then ask yourself which countries publish the most defensive documents.'

After a few seconds, the other person realises the countries with the worst outcomes are also the countries that publish the most defensive documents. Therefore, following in those footsteps (those documents) would predispose them to obtain the same outcomes.

Their expression of horror reflects the implications of themselves and their colleagues following defensive documents all this while.

Telling students what not to do, does not teach them what to do. Thus, this conversation often accompanies a short lesson on the basics of universal clinical reasoning. To be fair, I also tell the students the potential (but very limited) utility of these defensive documents.

Do these defensive documents have any utility? Yes, for a doctor who is just starting work in a new rotation, and has no idea how to recognise and handle the diseases in that rotation. Where this doctor might miss a dangerous disease, the defensive document can help to save a patient's life. However, this situation highlights the inappropriateness of throwing an unprepared doctor with inadequate or no supervision into the workplace, and then hoping a defensive document is a proper substitute for lack of preparation and supervision.

If the defensive document is used, the doctor must still try to make the correct diagnosis and make plans for the patient. The doctor must properly perform their fundamental jobs for the patient. Otherwise, the patient's care will be suboptimal.

Handling defensive documents

There are 3 ways to handle defensive documents properly:

1. Recognise and stay away from them
2. Rewrite them
3. Recycle them

The first way is automatic for any robust reasoner.

The second way means rewriting these documents to make them more useful, by accounting for human behaviour and incorporating robust clinical reasoning. However, such rewriting would be extensive. Even rewriting these documents may be insufficient because of their intended audience: poor reasoners. Poor reasoners readily misuse even the best-written documents. The time spent rewriting these documents may be better spent writing a neutral-category document instead.

The third way is to recycle them so that the paper can be reused for something more useful. If these documents are purely electronic, rendering recycling impossible, then the alternative is to scrap them entirely.

Neutral category

Documents in this category focus on standard care for diseases and scenarios. The target audience is very broad.

Unlike defensive documents, these documents assume the doctors are at least semi-competent in clinical evaluation and making diagnoses. Thus, their recommendations describe and are derived from, a proper clinical assessment. Even so, these documents may not be able to anticipate every situation for that topic.

Evidence from studies, if cited, tends to be interpreted objectively.

Best-care category

Being targeted at decent reasoners with the assumption of decent clinical skills and knowledge, these documents tend to be much shorter than the earlier categories' documents.

They aim to provide top-notch care.

These documents are rare, due to the expertise needed to write such documents. Expert reasoners in the speciality and evidence-based medicine must pool their efforts to impart the insights needed for top-notch care.

The role of reasoning in using all documents

These documents are tools and thus, have the same limitations as all tools. Doctors should be trained in the intent, form and proper use of all their tools.

Recall the carpenter analogy. If you were a carpenter who had dozens of tools for the many tasks you must accomplish (hammer, saw, chisel, screwdriver, tape measure, and so on):

- How good would you be if you did not know the exact purpose of each tool?

- How safe would you be if you did not know how to wield the tool properly?

- Would such a carpenter be a master who somehow did not bother to learn the basics? Or an amateur who thought that carpentry only involved copying what they saw other carpenters do, without learning the how and the why, and without checking the competence of the carpenters they were mimicking?

By extension, proper use of these documents is reliant on the clinical reasoning of the doctor. Any tool in the hands of the unskilled is often useless, and can be more dangerous than simply not having the tool at all. Would you give a saw to someone who did not know how to use it properly?

The provision of any guideline or protocol to a poor reasoner, often elicits complacency: 'I am safe because I have a guideline or protocol to follow.' Providing a neutral-category or best-care document to a poor reasoner will not solve the problem. Neutral and best-care documents assume the reader has some reasoning, knowledge and clinical attentiveness. The poor reasoner lacks these requirements. Being unable to follow the steps in these documents, the poor reasoner can either fumble through the steps when providing healthcare, or look for a defensive document that suits their preferences and situation.

Thus, should any of these documents (and other tools, such as tests) be made readily available to poor reasoners?

There is no adequate substitute for solid clinical reasoning.

Defensive documents seem to be targeted at poor reasoners, but their target audience lacks the reasoning to use these documents properly. If these tools are intended to avoid disaster in poor reasoners, they should account for their audience's limitations in reasoning. A tool that does not fully account for its intended audience, is flawed.

A decently reasoning junior doctor may face a tug-of-war internally between following defensive documents versus focusing on the patient's correct diagnosis and care. This tug-of-war comes from empathy for the patient, which is countered by seniors telling them to 'just follow the guidelines'.

A decent reasoner can use neutral and best-care documents well.

Robust reasoners recognise their fundamental duty to the patient and the absurdity of following defensive documents. They diagnose dangerous diseases that other doctors who followed the defensive documents, would have missed. They use the information in neutral and best-care documents perfectly.

Writing useful guidelines and protocols

A team of at least 2 people should write any guideline or protocol. These documents should either be neutral-category or best-care.

Many documents cite research. As many studies are flawed, expertise in reasoning and evidence-based medicine is required to accurately interpret research findings.

Mistakes can be unintentionally perpetuated through omission or vague wording. Poor reasoners are especially prone to misinterpreting documents to favour their personal preferences. A common example is the statement: 'This test is used for diagnosis'. One common (poorly reasoned) misinterpretation of that short sentence is: 'This test is 100% accurate. A proper history and examination are unnecessary; just perform the test and follow its results'. A counter to this potential misinterpretation would require stating the limitations of the test and its utility as a diagnostic aid.

Thus, the requirements for writing such documents include:

- Robust clinical reasoning
- Expertise in evidence-based medicine
- Awareness of the perspectives of poor reasoners
- Ability to explain recommendations to poor reasoners
- Willingness to admit and explicitly address uncertainty
- Clarity in grades of recommendation and documentation. For example: recommend; neutral (unclear whether to recommend for or against); recommend not performing
- Emphasis on patient-centred attention.

Capsule summary

- There are 3 categories of guidelines and protocols.
- Defensive documents have become part of the problem, not part of the solution.
- Writing accurate and practical guides for excellent healthcare, requires considerable expertise in reasoning.

Frequently asked questions

Q: What is your take on 'defensive medicine'?

A: Defensive medicine refers to the practice of ordering unnecessary tests or treatments, often out of self-interest and fear. The plethora of defensive documents worsens this problem because many poor reasoners (wrongly) assume that following these documents and thus, ordering unnecessary tests and treatments, will prevent mistakes and lawsuits.

Fear of being sued, without realising why lawsuits occur, is common.

The biggest irony of defensive medicine is that it does not prevent allegations of malpractice. If anything, the irrational behaviour of defensive medicine can increase the risk of such allegations. Look up the prevalence of defensive medicine within various countries, especially those with high rates. Then correlate that prevalence with the rate of medical malpractice allegations in those countries: the rates of complaints and lawsuits are either unchanged or rising over time.

What is likely to be the biggest factor contributing to the correlation?

One could argue that the prevalence of defensive medicine is due to high rates of complaints and lawsuits: doctors are responding in fear to these incidents. Though there can be an element of truth in this, the practice of defensive medicine is still a personal choice that boils down to the doctor's degree of competence, commitment to professionalism, wisdom, reasoning and courage.

One could argue that easy access to the Internet and media reports has increased everyone's awareness of lawsuits; maybe this increased awareness encourages unhappy patients to make similar allegations. This argument fails to address the key question, which is not whether unhappy patients are making allegations, but whether they are making such allegations *with a valid basis*.

Patients do not seek healthcare with the aim of becoming unhappy. If the doctor's patients are routinely becoming unhappy, the doctor should be questioning their own behaviour instead of blaming the Internet.

One could argue that the problem is increased patient knowledge and education, which may predispose to allegations of malpractice. After all, patients who have more knowledge may be more likely to know when the doctor is not thinking, communicating or making decisions properly. However, doctors are supposed to be thinking, communicating and making decisions properly! Furthermore, even an ignorant and uneducated patient can recognise when things are going badly for them.

Mistakes in medical practice do exist, and most do not end up in court.

Defensive medicine predisposes to making not one, or two, but multiple mistakes. Engaging in batteries of tests and polypharmacy, means patients suffer more and pay more. When there is no rational justification for the tests and treatment, counselling of the patient is often lacking and the doctor may try to conceal their ulterior motives. This is a lethal combination: a poor outcome, being made to suffer and pay more whilst achieving nothing useful, whilst the doctor seems unempathetic and deceitful. This combination predisposes to malpractice allegations.

I suspect that defensive medicine is the biggest factor driving the decades-long pessimistic trends in malpractice allegations in many countries. This trend reflects a vicious cycle of fear, insecurity and poor reasoning that keeps feeding itself.

Q: Do I have to memorise defensive guidelines? What if the defensive guidelines are tested in the clinical exams? (Often asked by medical students)

A: Consider this reply.

Me: 'First, you cannot remember everything in those documents. Second, if they must test you for content in these guidelines, you probably have failed the station.'

Student: 'Huh? Why?'

Me: 'Recall the usual clinical tutorial where you evaluate a patient, then present your conclusions. What happens if you get it wrong?'

Student: 'The tutor provides prompts about the patient's information. The tutor is trying to help.'

Me: 'Good. Notice that the tutor is using the patient's information, not the textbook or guideline, to help you. If you still do not get the answer, sometimes they ask you about the pathophysiology behind a symptom or sign, correct?'

Student: 'Hey, yeah.'

Me: 'That is because the tutor has realised you cannot put everything together, to suggest the most likely diagnosis and reasonable differentials. The tutor can fall back on the pathophysiology, trying to bring up previously learnt knowledge to help you.'

Student: 'Yes.'

Me: 'And even then, you may struggle to answer the question on pathophysiology. In desperation, the tutor then recalls the defensive guideline regarding this disease, and asks you if you remember what this guideline says. In some situations, the tutor does not use pathophysiology and directly asks you about the defensive guideline.'

Student: 'Oh dear. Yes.'

Me: 'An exam station must be fair; we cannot expect students to always get it right. Even so, there are minimum standards for competence. If you are in the exam station and failed all the other questions before the defensive guideline question, you are probably grossly inept. Thus, how many marks do you have? Even if you managed to answer the guideline-based question?'

Student: 'I see.'

Me: 'Let us look at it the other way around. If you got the correct clinical diagnosis and made appropriate plans for the patient, might the tutor ask you for higher-level information to see how much further you can go? An example would be a tumour of the thyroid, where you got the clinical diagnosis and plans right. The tutor could ask you about the staging of the tumour.'

Student: 'Yes. I have seen that happen before.'

Me: 'Is that higher-level information available in your textbooks?'

Student: 'Yes.'

Me: 'If you already got it right, would any tutor or examiner ever ask you about the content of a defensive guideline as if you were wrong?'

Student: 'No.'

Me: 'So why would you need to memorise a defensive guideline for the exams? Assuming you wanted to pass the exams, which I am sure you do. Assuming you do not have infinite time to learn everything, which I am sure you do not. The only situation you might use the guideline is if you have already flunked every single question before the final, desperate question about defensive guidelines. At that point, answering the defensive question might get you an "E" grade instead of an "F" grade. You can spend the hours preparing for the exam in a better way, such as learning to do better, so that you do not face that final, desperate question about the defensive guideline.'

SCHOOL

Medical schools train the doctors of the future.

As good doctors must possess considerable knowledge, reasoning ability and positive qualities such as compassion, the selection and training of doctors should be a rigorous process.

The sheer amount of knowledge is vast, encompassing the basic sciences relevant to the human body, pathophysiology, and diseases across multiple specialities. Thus, much of the years-long curriculum time is focused on imparting knowledge.

Ethics, compassion, communication skills, and information technology proficiency (given the rise of medical cybercrimes) are other important areas.

Clinical reasoning is often neglected. Given the importance of reasoning in clinical performance, the literature on doctors' often-poor diagnostic and management skills is unsurprising.

Medical school is the best time to teach clinical reasoning. The longer clinical reasoning is omitted from training, the less receptive students and doctors become towards learning this reasoning. The drop in receptiveness is particularly marked once the final year of medical school has begun. As described in the 'Tiers of performance' chapter, the window of maximum receptiveness probably closes soon after the completion of training. Graduates who must cope with the burdens of work, family life and greater financial responsibility, have less free time and energy to devote to honing clinical reasoning.

Aside from receptiveness, opportunity cost is the other compelling reason to teach clinical reasoning as early as possible. Students learn something from each patient encounter. If they have not learnt reasoning to deliver excellent healthcare and avoid mistakes, they are more likely to be learning mistaken approaches and behaviours. If this erroneous learning goes on long enough, the mistakes become habits.

Old habits die hard: many humans do not willingly 'unlearn' their bad habits. To adopt the behaviours of robust clinical reasoning, students and doctors with bad clinical habits would have to 'unlearn' their bad habits whilst practising clinical reasoning.

To make matters worse, humans often take the easy way out. Even when medical students and doctors are taught clinical reasoning, it is tempting to order unnecessary tests and polypharmacy instead of putting in the effort to reason. Witnessing one's teachers and seniors indulge in these poorly reasoned behaviours, increases this temptation.

Let us examine some of the areas where clinical reasoning should be incorporated into medical school.

Selection of medical students

Many medical schools use interviews, pre-medical school grades, non-academic achievements, and additional selection tests for selecting medical students.

Clinical reasoning is difficult to incorporate into these interviews and selection tests. However, *overall* reasoning can and should be incorporated into these. After all, clinical reasoning is the medical application of overall reasoning. A terrible overall reasoner, even if taught clinical reasoning, is unlikely to become skilled at clinical reasoning.

The association between poor overall reasoning and poor clinical reasoning is due to more than just ineptitude. Even when taught clinical reasoning soon after the start of medical school, some students will flat-out refuse to accept clinical reasoning. Further questioning often reveals a lack of robust overall reasoning too, which implies they have not learnt or seen the need to reason properly since childhood. When poor reasoning has become a habit, it may be too much to expect receptiveness to lessons on robust reasoning, clinical or otherwise.

Given the limited vacancies to enter medical school, it makes no sense to choose a poor overall reasoner over a robust overall reasoner. Even if all the teachers in the medical school are the best in the world (which is unlikely), most of the outcome is decided by the student's effort and openness to learning, not the quality of the teachers.

Since clinical reasoning directly affects healthcare, selecting poor overall reasoners over robust reasoners is likely to cause indirect harm to patients in future.

The crucial and tricky bit is to ensure that the selection process will deliberately check for overall reasoning instead of the other areas that are often mistaken for reasoning. Intelligence, 'street smarts', 'exam smartness' and knowledge, are not reasoning.

This distinction between each area would help to accurately select the better reasoners out of the crowd of applicants. These robust reasoners are the future doctors who are likely to learn and wield clinical reasoning effectively, thus contributing to excellent outcomes for future patients and the country.

Humility, adaptability, courage and empathy are important qualities for future doctors. Doctors must be willing to understand their patients and learn from their mistakes. Selection for such qualities requires more effort and interviewer training, than asking untrained faculty to conduct interviews and assessments of the resume.

It is ideal to select for and embed these qualities in medical students. Embedding requires far more effort than selection for these qualities; I will not cover such embedding in this book.

Selecting medical students without checking for overall reasoning and qualities

How are medical students usually selected?

Sometimes this selection is purely based on academic grades. Grades do matter somewhat; doctors must be able to study and demonstrate knowledge. However, grades often do not correlate with professional performance. Knowledge without reasoning is unlikely to produce consistent and excellent healthcare.

Sometimes there are selection tests, such as writing essays and providing answers to theoretical scenarios. If selection tests are to accurately assess the quality of the applicants, the topics must be unpredictable. Having predictable topics that allow applicants to easily 'spot' the test topic beforehand, defeats the purpose of the test.

The test creators must differentiate between knowledge, reasoning, qualities and 'exam-smartness' as separate domains. Each domain is different in value. Without these safeguards, selection tests are limited by:

- Testing knowledge instead of reasoning. Educators and faculty often conflate knowledge with reasoning.

- Failure to recognise that selecting for qualities is difficult. It is much easier to superficially sound empathic than to truly be empathic.

Sometimes there are interviews to evaluate applicants for medical school. At the interviews, the appearance, manners, resume, connections, and other 'risk factors' for potentially capable doctors can play to the biases of the interviewers. Robust interviewer training is required to minimise biases. Interviewers who have potential conflicts of interest, such as being friends with the parents of an applicant, should not participate in the interview or selection process of such applicants.

When either interviewer training or selection is lacking, biased comments are often heard during the discussion of the candidate's suitability for medical school. Examples include:

- 'This candidate speaks so well.'

- 'This candidate has top grades.'

- 'I know this candidate's parents.'
- 'This candidate is very intelligent.'
- 'This candidate won an academic prize.'

Interviewers often use these statements to recommend certain candidates after the interview. Biased interviewers tend to decide that their preference overrules everything else.

Even after interviewer training, many interviewers are unaware that they are psychologically 'projecting': a factor they deem valuable in themselves, becomes a valued factor for selecting candidates. When this interviewer meets a candidate who shows the same factor, they favour this candidate because they are projecting themselves into the shoes of the candidate: 'This factor is important for a doctor. I am a doctor. This candidate is like me.' The interviewer is essentially validating *themselves* when they favour this candidate. This projection is particularly obvious when the valued factor clashes with the objective selection criteria.

For example, the interviewer is eloquent because he or she has always valued eloquence. When selecting candidates, the interviewer is biased towards eloquent candidates. The interviewer then insists on selecting a favoured candidate because: 'this candidate is so eloquent'. If the eloquent candidate flunked the selection criteria, this interviewer often argues that the objective criteria should be ignored because the eloquent candidate flunked the criteria.

Intelligence, manners, fashion sense, eloquence, family background, resume, awards, grades and other advantages (all of these can be considered 'risk factors' for being capable doctors) do have some importance. However, just as direct manifestations of the underlying current diagnosis are the core requirement for getting the correct diagnosis, direct manifestations of excellent doctors derive from the core requirements: qualities and reasoning.

Just as risk factors are less important than the core requirements (clinical features) for the patient's diagnosis, risk factors are less important than the core requirements for excellent doctors:

- Though it is tempting to believe that having a family member in the same profession means the candidate will be an excellent doctor, history shows that competence is often not dynastic. A candidate who cannot outperform other candidates despite having this advantage (such as one or more of their parents being doctors), is often less suitable than their relatively disadvantaged peers. They lack the reasoning to use their advantage properly. Recall the story of the tortoise and the hare.

- Many intelligent doctors reason poorly and struggle to make patient-centred decisions.

- Do top grades correlate with professional performance? Often, no.

- Can candidates buff up a resume to appear to have good qualities, instead of really possessing those qualities? Yes. Thus, interviewers should be trained to recognise the differences between an impressive-looking resume without substance, and an impressive-looking resume with substance.

- Polishing the appearance of a less-impressive-looking candidate with outstanding qualities and reasoning, is easier than inculcating qualities and reasoning in a superficially impressive candidate who lacks these core requirements.

I have heard it argued that reasoning is unimportant for selecting potential medical researchers or leaders in healthcare. The argument goes along the lines of 'candidates who are intelligent with good grades can make good researchers, whilst candidates with connections and polished appearances can make good leaders. It does not matter if they cannot reason'. This argument ignores reality and reasoning (and is disturbing, since it is used by interviewers):

- Clinical reasoning is the medical application of overall reasoning. I have yet to meet a poor overall reasoner who could learn or apply clinical reasoning with any competence. Likewise, poor clinical reasoners often struggle with overall reasoning. Conversely, every superb clinical reasoner I encountered, was strong in overall reasoning too.

- Overall reasoning to make good decisions for formulating studies, making design choices, paying attention to research results and adapting correctly to surprises, is more important to a researcher than raw intelligence and school grades. The description of stellar researchers in human history, some of whom did not have excellent school grades and were not as intelligent as many of their peers, is consistent in this regard.

- Overall reasoning to pay attention to the facts on the ground and make excellent decisions that affect many others, is necessary for excellent leaders. If a candidate is predisposed to poor reasoning and thus, more likely to harm patients who trusted and paid them, how can you expect such a candidate to be a good leader and do the right thing for others who are *not* directly incentivising them?

- History has shown that selecting leaders based on appearances (height, speaks well, dresses well, and so on) often results in a mediocre or terrible leader.

If a candidate lacks reasoning and genuine empathy, that candidate is predisposed to causing harm to patients. The selection committee has indirect responsibility to those future patients. Thus, the committee that selects such a candidate over another candidate superior in reasoning and empathy, is inadvertently demonstrating a lack of reasoning and empathy too.

If a candidate has outstanding qualities and reasoning, with at least a street-level decent intelligence and dress sense, I would pick such a candidate over any other candidate who lacks those qualities or reasoning. A candidate without the core requirements for excellence is less deserving, no matter how knowledgeable, connected, intelligent, charming and impressive-looking they are.

These core requirements are even more important when selecting specialist trainees. By the time a patient needs to see a specialist, the illness is more likely to be complex and therefore requires more robust reasoning, empathy and courage to handle optimally, than a simpler illness.

Teaching reasoning

Explicit instruction in universal clinical reasoning should be required.

Every student and trainee should buy this book.

Every learner should participate in interactive teaching and case discussions, where the 'language of reasoning' is woven into their clinical diagnosis, justifications and decisions. This weaving of reasoning into the teaching, requires the teachers to be proficient in the technique and language of clinical reasoning. (The teachers should also buy this book.)

The school should select or appoint faculty in charge of clinical reasoning. Training faculty in this technique can be as simple as getting 4 to 6 doctors, each in different specialities, to participate in a case discussion. Each participant presents 1 recent patient they have seen, with the clinical diagnosis, justifications and decisions explained aloud using the principles of universal clinical reasoning. This exercise shows the would-be tutors, the universality of this method and language.

When the tutors use the same language of reasoning across the many lessons that students will receive, the students will rapidly grasp the universally applicable concepts of robust reasoning and extrapolate the lessons to other topics, maximising the learning impact.

Assessment

'Assessment drives learning', as Professor Dujeepa often says.

Clinical reasoning must be woven into assessments to replicate the patient-centred, real-world context.

The domains of knowledge and reasoning should be explicitly separated and scored, with a significant proportion of the marks assessing patient-centred reasoning.

When commonplace assessments do not check the underlying reasoning of would-be doctors, there are 3 predictable and unhappy consequences:

1. Students who are 'exam smart' can exploit the system to graduate despite lacking genuine reasoning and critical qualities, to the detriment of the profession and their patients. These students obtain and use 'tips' to score in knowledge-based assessments.

2. Some teachers can take advantage of the students' desire to pass exams by giving exam tips, which in turn incentivises students to give these teachers high teaching scores. These tips may help the students to pass exams, but do not help them to be competent doctors. Knowledge-based tips are much easier to give than reasoning- or quality-based tips. Thus, knowledge-based exams are easier to subvert in this manner than exams that test reasoning and qualities.

3. The lack of correlation between academic scores and real-world clinical competence worldwide is unsurprising. Many 'top medical students and trainees' who perform well in regular assessments and exams, do not go on to excel professionally.

The necessary modifications to incorporate clinical reasoning into assessments, require a fundamental shift across all assessments in medical schools and specialist training.

Since clinical reasoning and patient-centred care are reliant on the qualities outlined earlier in this chapter, assessment for these qualities may also be important before graduating as a doctor. If a medical student is found to be grossly deficient in the necessary qualities, remediation of this deficiency is likely to be a long and arduous process.

Avoiding methods that ignore reasoning

Teaching cannot ignore the real-world context and patient-centred clinical reasoning. Unfortunately, ignoring reasoning and real-world context to focus on knowledge, is common worldwide.

For example, when teaching students about laboratory or radiological test results, the clinical context and relevant differential diagnoses should be presented comprehensively and clearly, before showing or discussing any test results. This format matches and reinforces the optimal chain of dominoes: the patient receives a proper clinical evaluation, a clinical diagnosis is then made, and then excellent decisions about tests are made.

The alternative, which is to present lab or radiological results alone without clinical context, sends the wrong messages:

1. Decisions about tests are not based on the clinical context or relevant differentials.

2. Test results do not need interpretation within the patient's clinical context.

3. Tests are more important than the clinical evaluation and clinical context.

Encouraging, or even condoning, any of these 3 messages is a recipe for disaster.

Students should be taught how to react appropriately to surprises.

Defensive documents should not be used for teaching, as the use of these documents discourages reasoning and patient-centred care. The only page(s) in those documents that might add value, is the page that states the contraindications: 'the tests and/or treatment you must never use'. However, since these contraindications should have been taught in routine training, this redundancy further highlights the unimportance of these documents. Given the proliferation of defensive documents, students may be better served by educating them on the intent, identification, and dangers of following such documents.

Capsule summary

- Optimal selection for medical students and trainees, requires a focus on reasoning and qualities instead of superficial 'risk factors'.

- Schools should systematically incorporate clinical reasoning into their teaching and assessment, explicitly and implicitly.

HOSPITAL

Teaching clinical reasoning alone, is insufficient to encourage its continued use. Clinical reasoning can be subsequently encouraged or suppressed by the doctors' working environment.

Doctors tend to copy other doctors. Thus, robust clinical reasoning must be enshrined in medical training and practice.

I will briefly discuss 8 areas (this list is not exhaustive):

1. Documentation
2. Handover
3. Feedback on actions
4. 'Just follow the guideline/protocol'
5. Radiology rounds
6. Morbidity and Mortality rounds
7. Electronic healthcare systems
8. Performance

Documentation

Format

The documentation often reflects the reasoning of the healthcare team. Robust reasoners are comprehensive, concise and clear.

The common S-O-A-P format is adequate for the daily medical documentation of most hospitalised patients. It has 4 sections: Subjective (symptoms), Objective (signs), Assessment (diagnosis) and Plan (decisions). The most important information in each section must be described first, followed by less-important information:

<u>S</u>ubjective — Presenting a complaint with relevant details, followed by other symptoms and new symptoms. Relevant risk factors are mentioned at the end of this subsection.

<u>O</u>bjective — Vital signs and physical signs, including relevant negatives for the diagnosis and its differentials.

<u>A</u>ssessment — Assessment must be a diagnosis that tries to fulfil the 3 criteria for the correct diagnosis, with explicit justification. Results of diagnostic tests and response to treatment, may be cited to support or refute the diagnosis. Unexplainable clinical features and test results must be highlighted separately, and their significance understood as rapidly as possible (through getting help, if necessary).

If you have more than 1 active diagnosis, be careful. The more active diagnoses you have beyond the first, the greater the chance that you are missing a single, potentially lethal unifying diagnosis. All background diseases such as chronic co-morbidities are summarised after the active diagnoses.

<u>P</u>lan — Plans must be prioritised for the active diagnosis. All other plans, such as plans for opportunistic care, should be stated after the top priorities. The aims of care should be explicit, such as citing the time to expected recovery or the 'balance' point if 100% cure/control is not viable. Explicitly stating the aims of care helps to facilitate precisely targeted plans, realistic expectations, accurate handovers and clear communications.

EXAMPLE OF FOCUSED ASSESSMENT
(Middle-aged man admitted to the hospital general ward)

Active diagnoses:

1. Moderate exacerbation of chronic obstructive pulmonary disease (COPD), controlled after initial treatment at the Accident and Emergency (A&E)

2. Uncontrolled COPD, likely moderate severity, due to non-compliance with preventers (forgets). Has stopped smoking

Background/inactive diagnoses:

1. Alcoholic fatty liver disease, likely mild severity, mostly controlled as evidenced by no clinical features, function intact, mild transaminitis 2 months ago. Trigger: still taking 1 can of beer a month

2. Prolapsed intervertebral disc (L4–L5), pain-free, conservatively managed

EXAMPLE OF MATCHING, PRIORITISED PLAN
(in order of descending priority)

1. Continue Salbutamol and oxygen therapy from A&E; next review at 1100 hours today. Consider weaning thereafter if no breathlessness, no signs of increased work of breathing, and SaO_2 >90%

2. Address understanding and lifestyle regarding preventer therapy, to aid compliance

3. Inform the primary physician (cite physician's name) of the patient's admission and discuss this plan

4. Review history and alcohol intake. Explore potential motivators for cessation of alcohol

5. Review records of recent follow-ups with the orthopaedic surgeon

6. (Insert ongoing monitoring plan whilst in the general ward)

7. (Insert expected discharge date)

Clinical reasoning should be applied to all new and existing information before writing the next SOAP note.

If dealing with a diagnostic puzzle, fall back on the style of the clinical vignettes in Section 1. Summarise the patient's clinical entirety, and demonstrate the basic diagnostic reasoning requirement in your documentation. See Case #29.

CASE #29: Jerrald

Jerrald is a 65-year-old man who comes to the Emergency Department at lunchtime. He was brought by his wife. He complains of tiredness for a week, followed by smelling a strange scent of lavender whilst at home the night before. He is adamant there is no lavender in his home, and his wife agrees. The tiredness is a general feeling; he has been performing his usual activities at home. He is now complaining of a headache all over his head, pain score 6/10, for the past 2 hours. He cannot remember anything else he was doing that morning.

There are no other symptoms.

There is no history of chronic disease. He denies using any recreational drugs. He is retired. He did not perform any strenuous activity in the week prior to the onset of tiredness.

His vital signs are normal. He seems lucid and oriented to time, person and place. The physical examination, including a complete neurological examination, is normal.

--

You are unable to fit all the bizarre symptoms into 1 diagnosis. You do your best, documenting your top differentials whilst stating all the bits that do not fulfil the basic diagnostic reasoning requirement for each differential.

(Continued)

DOCUMENTATION:

Assessment: 65-year-old man with acute generalised headache now; strange smell the night before; feeling tired for 1 week. Differentials:

1. Acute hallucinogen ingestion (does not explain tiredness; lacks risk factor of known hallucinogen ingestion)

2. Viral encephalitis (does not explain current headache; physical examination of mental state is oddly normal)

Poor documentation and its implications

Poor documentation showcases the manifestations of poor reasoning. Given the varied manifestations of poor reasoning, this documentation is likewise varied in length, vagueness, omission of crucial information, and so on. Every mistake in this book that is ascribed to poor reasoning, can be deduced from the documentation.

Three of the most common manifestations of poor documentation are:

1. Failure to document crucial clinical information

2. No proper diagnosis in the Assessment, or no Assessment at all

3. Dissociation between the subsections

1. *Failure to document crucial clinical information*

Being comprehensive, prioritised and relevant showcases robust reasoning. By extension, an absence of comprehensiveness, prioritisation, or relevance, is often due to poor reasoning.

Poor reasoners are unable to prioritise information properly and often skimp on the proper clinical evaluation. Thus, the clinical information can be scant or nonexistent. The entry can be very short.

Sometimes, with the inability to prioritise information properly, the poor reasoner wants to appear comprehensive and documents everything: encyclopaedic walls of unprioritised text, long lists of significant negatives, and copying and pasting every line of every test result into the entry. Though these entries are very long, they lack depth in the crucial clinical information. Despite putting so much information in, the poor reasoner often skimps on the most crucial parts of the clinical evaluation, and thus puts a tiny fraction of the most important clinical information somewhere in the long entry.

Unthinking copying is often seen when doctors perform an electronic copy-and-paste with no alterations or thought. When a poor reasoner does not know what is going on, they can copy another doctor's entry instead. Sometimes, when they are caught for copying an outdated or inadequate entry, a poor reasoner pushes the blame on the previous doctor's documentation instead of admitting their own responsibility to evaluate and document properly.

The difference in documentation between poor and robust reasoning becomes rapidly obvious when a robust reasoner intervenes for that patient: trimming a lengthy-and-mostly-irrelevant entry to become concise yet comprehensive, identifying the correct clinical diagnosis, interpreting the results of tests correctly, and providing an effective management plan.

Ironically, poor reasoners often distrust the shortened, relevant and prioritised entries of robust reasoners. Subsequent documentation by poor reasoners often reverts to the original encyclopaedic and unprioritised mess, demonstrating that poor reasoners often do not want to learn from their better-performing colleagues.

2. No proper diagnosis in the Assessment, or no Assessment at all

A poor reasoner is often tempted to avoid making a diagnosis or think of differentials. Thus, there is either an Assessment without a proper diagnosis, or no Assessment at all.

This Assessment can list individual problems/issues instead of diagnoses. Each problem/issue is an individual symptom, sign, or test result, which is described in isolation. The subsequent plans superficially and illogically treat each problem/issue in isolation. The following example is the Assessment listing issues for one patient:

- Issue #1: Fever for 5 days for investigation, to rule out sepsis. Plan: Full septic workup. Start antibiotics if cultures are positive.
- Issue #2: Dysuria for investigation. Plan: Refer to Renal.
- Issue #3: Right lumbar pain. Plan: Analgesia.
- Issue #4: Right lumbar tenderness for investigation. Plan: Refer to Orthopaedic Surgery to rule out musculoskeletal disease.

This patient had acute pyelonephritis of the right kidney. Is the multitude of plans targeting individual 'issues' as if they are unrelated, including the delay in starting antibiotics, optimal?

When doctors work in a team, poor reasoners may wait for their colleagues to make the diagnoses and plans. The poorly reasoning junior doctor waits for everyone else. The poorly reasoning senior doctors can also wait for everyone else to do their job for them. Everyone in the team waits for everyone else to do the job. Referring to a specialist in hopes that they make the diagnosis may not help either; the specialist may also be a poor reasoner. This is especially true in places where poor reasoning and refusal to commit to diagnoses, is the norm.

3. Dissociation between the subsections

Dissociation refers to recording information in 1 subsection of documentation, and then ignoring that information later in the same entry when making diagnoses or plans. Dissociation is a manifestation of deliberately ignoring inconvenient information about the patient.

An example would be mentioning in the Subjective portion that the patient is distressed by the pain whilst on analgesia, and then ignoring the pain entirely in the Assessment and Plan subsections. A variation could state in the Plan: 'keep the same (inadequate) analgesia'.

Presentation of patient information

In hospital rounds, 1 doctor often presents the patient's information to the rest of the team.

Poor reasoners present patients in a manner that mirrors their reasoning, and thus often mirrors their documentation. Common styles include:

1. Spending several minutes at the start to talk about everything else except the patient's primary concerns, clinical features and most likely diagnosis. This predisposes to long ward rounds and weariness all around.

2. Skipping the clinical context, to rush straight to tests, test results and treatments.

3. Virtually all specific information is omitted. The presentation is a one-line 'the patient is fine', which is not necessarily true. The documentation in this situation is often slightly longer than the one-line-statement, or a copy-and-paste of the previous day's entry.

Senior doctors and documentation

It is the senior doctor's job to supervise and check on the documentation of juniors. This job ensures the documentation serves its purpose, and simultaneously teaches juniors the standards of proper documentation.

When a senior doctor does not check the documentation or does not challenge poor documentation, junior doctors readily realise they are not being held accountable for proper clinical evaluation and documentation.

Lack of accountability predisposes to sloppiness. Incoherent, outdated documentation confuses anyone else reading that documentation, such as the doctors on the next shift attending to the patient. Even more damage is done when junior doctors follow their seniors' example in later years: 'Since my boss does not care enough about the patient and the rest of the healthcare team to ensure proper evaluation, decision-making and documentation, why should I?'

I have never seen sloppy documentation and inattentiveness to juniors, in excellent doctors. Sloppy documentation and other behaviours of poor reasoning, including inattentiveness to juniors and patients, often coexist.

Robust reasoners are attentive to everyone, write excellent and concise entries, and will insist on the same standards in their junior colleagues. These doctors recognise that everyone in the healthcare team, including juniors and the patient's subsequent doctors, is important for patient care.

The robust reasoner who is a junior doctor, and surrounded by poor reasoners

At times, the robust reasoner may be the most junior member of the healthcare team. This position often frustrates them, because their poorly reasoning seniors often dismiss the opinions of juniors. These seniors:

- Do not know the correct diagnosis
- Cannot accept the truth of their inadequacies
- Refuse to accept help because this might mean having to admit their inadequacies
- Are willing to allow the patient to suffer rather than accept the truth.

Some of these seniors do not just dismiss their juniors' opinions; they totally ignore their juniors and do not deign to talk to them. It is not always clear if this aloofness is out of arrogance, or fear of being asked questions that require reasoning (or both).

If these seniors do respond to their juniors' opinions (and still dismiss the opinions), the grossly illogical statements the seniors use, include:

- 'I will not listen to you because you are my junior.' (Seniority has nothing to do with accuracy, as this senior is inadvertently revealing.)
- 'If you decide on a diagnosis, you are being narrow-minded.' (Being narrow-minded implies you are doing *some* thinking. Not

deciding on the diagnosis often means zero thinking. The senior is inadvertently admitting that they are not thinking at all.)

- 'If you never decide on a diagnosis, you can never be wrong. So do not try.' (If you never try, you automatically fail. The senior is inadvertently admitting they do not want to try.)

When the seniors are poor reasoners, it takes courage for the junior to speak up. Many junior doctors fear being 'marked down' for challenging the senior colleagues grading them. They realise they may be marked down for being right, because being right means disagreeing with their seniors' mistakes. Thus, many junior doctors silently follow along despite realising that clinical reasoning and good patient care have been abandoned.

Case #30 illustrates this situation.

CASE #30: Leon

Leon is a 50-year-old man who presents to the Accident and Emergency Department at 5 p.m. He complains of 2 days of vomiting (1 episode per day), 2 days of diarrhoea (1 episode per day, large amount), and dizziness starting on the day of presentation. Oral intake was unchanged. There are no other symptoms. His blood pressure is 80/50 mmHg and heart rate is 80 beats per minute. The other vital signs are normal. The physical examination shows a capillary refill time of 3 seconds and cool peripheries, but is otherwise unremarkable. His mucous membranes are moist and skin turgor is good.

He is labelled as 'gastroenteritis with severe dehydration and hypovolemic shock'. An intravenous (IV) fluid bolus of 2 litres is administered, without any change in the vital signs. A battery of tests is sent off, which shows elevated troponins. The electrocardiogram is unremarkable.

He is admitted to the general ward that same night. An intravenous dopamine infusion is administered, which brings the blood pressure up to 85/55 mmHg, and heart rate to 85 beats per minute. He is placed on a 2-litre normal saline drip for the next 24 hours.

(Continued)

The next morning, the ward consultant dictates the assessment and plans.

DOCUMENTATION OF ASSESSMENT AND PLANS:

1. Gastroenteritis with severe dehydration. Plan: continue IV rehydration.
2. Shock unresponsive to IV fluids. Plan: rule out septic shock. Perform cultures. Cover with IV Ceftriaxone. Refer to Infectious Disease.
3. Raised cardiac enzymes. Plan: refer to Cardiology to rule out myocardial infarction.
4. Dizziness for investigation. Plan: refer to Neurology to rule out central nervous system causes of dizziness.

Doctor W, a 2nd-year doctor, has just joined the team that same morning. She asks: 'Isn't this classic viral myocarditis with vomiting, diarrhoea, symptomatic hypotension and an inappropriately normal heart rate? The history and examination do not fit hypovolemic or septic shock. There is no response to IV fluids. The patient may die if we continue with this. The IV fluids being administered may result in pulmonary oedema, and the patient may end up being intubated in the Intensive Care Unit!'

None of the doctors in the team who rank between Doctor W and the consultant, say anything.

The consultant says: 'How dare you question your seniors! Do as I say. You cannot be narrow-minded. Anything is possible.'

Doctor W: 'Instead of putting all the clues together to make the diagnosis? Doesn't saving the patient, matter?'

(Continued)

(Continued)

Consultant: 'Even if the patient dies, no one can say whose fault it is. We would not get checked, so do not worry. The other consultants would do the same thing. Do not waste time thinking. Let us round on the other patients.'

Doctor W was correct about the diagnosis and her predictions.

This case simultaneously illustrates the apathetic tier of performance at multiple levels:

- Tunnel vision
- Refusing to obey Rule #1 of clinical reasoning
- Cherry-picking 1 problem/issue for each symptom, sign or test result
- Pretending that probability and pathophysiology do not exist
- Refusing to consider the consequences of one's decisions
- Refusing to admit mistakes
- Referring to everyone else instead of doing their job
- Attacking challengers whilst using excuses to dismiss different opinions
- Flimsy rationalisation of behaviour, such as 'others are doing the same thing, therefore I can'. This is similar to insisting 'others are hurting people, therefore I can'.

The other doctors in the team may think: 'I should do whatever I want. After all, the consultant is getting away with doing whatever they want.' They may mimic the same behaviour, with the same or worse consequences for future patients.

Insights into the preceding doctor's accuracy

If taking over the care of a patient, be sure of the diagnosis and proper management. The last thing you want is a patient collapsing under your care.

Thus, when you review the previous doctor's documentation, focus on the clinical evaluation and the basic diagnostic reasoning requirement.

A useful clue is the proportion of assessment devoted to the presenting complaint and details of symptoms, versus significant negatives in the Clinical Features, and the 2 categories of information. Recall the table on illness scripts in Section 1 of this book. I have replicated the relevant rows here:

	Novice, freshly graduated from medical school, and did not obey Rule #1	Novice, spent 5 years working and trying to memorise defensive guidelines, and did not obey Rule #1	Expert-to-be, spent 2 years asking patients in detail about clinical features and building expert-level illness scripts to obey Rule #1
Pattern of questioning on Clinical Features	Asks about presenting symptoms and other symptoms, then launches into a list of significant negatives and less-important information	May ask about presenting symptoms and other symptoms briefly, then rapidly launches into questions to rule out dangerous diagnoses. Goes through a long list of significant negatives	Focuses on presenting complaint, exploring details and using targeted questions that check for details in detailed illness scripts. Asks about other symptoms broadly and in a targeted manner without pause
The usual proportion of enquiry on risk factors	10–40%	20–50%	5–20%

The most dangerous of the 3 doctors, is the doctor who is obsessed with ruling out OAF (middle column). Their note will have scant information on the patient's symptoms. This is often followed by 10 to 30 lines of significant negatives. The beginning of the note may list all the patient's co-morbid diseases without any summarisation, prioritisation or apparent relevance to the current diagnosis.

Thus, if the preceding doctor's documentation suggests defensive obsession, you must clinically evaluate the patient yourself.

Templates for documentation

Some hospitals have 'templates' for clerking patients.

Beware templates that prioritise less-important information over the most important information. Ironically, some templates encourage poor documentation and poor reasoning. One example is the insistence on listing all chronic co-morbid diseases up front without prioritisation or summarisation, before paying attention to the patient's clinical features.

The most important priorities must come first. Doctors tend to put in more effort to fill in or read the earliest areas, and then get more tired as they go down the template. By reversing the optimal sequence of information, the risk-factors-first template wears down the doctors who fill it, and the doctors who read the filled template, and gives the wrong impression of the priorities of healthcare. A template that encourages doctors to focus on risk factors and skimp on the assessment of the clinical features, invites disaster.

Handover

'Handover' refers to the process of conveying information to the next team of doctors taking over the care of the patients.

Doctors will take over the care of patients when they rotate to new locations, as well as during the day (shift work, or going on-call).

The clarity and conciseness of the handover often mirror the original doctor's documentation, and thus mirror the doctor's clinical reasoning.

A useful handover is accurate and concise. When the initial team's reasoning is robust, the diagnosis is usually correct and optimal management has been instituted. Predictions about the patient's subsequent progress and anticipated problems will likewise be accurate. Providing the clinical context of each patient is crucial to understanding and anticipating subsequent changes in the patient's status and test results. Describing the reasoning of the initial team provides insight into the basis of the diagnosis and the suggestions. The new team taking over is tasked with continuing the excellent care that the previous team had begun.

Conversely, if the initial team was reasoning poorly, the handover is often filled with inaccurate predictions of the patient's progress, and irrelevant suggestions for healthcare. Inadequate handovers are dangerous for the patient and tiresome for decently reasoning recipients, who realise that nothing they were told can be trusted. Instead of continuing with the diagnosis and care plan of the previous team, the new team may suddenly discover they have to make the correct diagnosis themselves and institute the appropriate management for the patients, because the previous team got everything wrong. Sometimes, the new team's first warning that the handover was totally wrong, is the emergency code informing them that the 'stable patient at the handover' has unexpectedly collapsed.

The chapter 'Interpreting test results' in Section 2, described inadequate handovers in greater detail.

Feedback on actions

Senior colleagues may give feedback to junior doctors after a ward round, duty shift or rotation.

The accuracy of this feedback correlates with the seniors' reasoning. Extra problems arise when poor reasoners give feedback. They tend to give illogical feedback, sometimes scolding their juniors for doing the right thing!

Poor reasoners can illogically find fault even though they do not know what is going on. Instead of admitting they do not know the right thing to do, they randomly choose a quick fix like 'do an electrocardiogram in all patients with tachycardia', and then criticise the junior doctor for failing to use the quick fix. The senior can illogically reprimand the junior even when the robustly reasoning junior doctor fixed the mess the poorly reasoning senior created. The senior doctor's behaviour gives the strong impression that they resent the junior doctor, and cannot accept that this junior doctor did a better job than them.

Illogical scoldings are confusing and demoralising to many junior doctors. Robustly reasoning junior doctors are horrified that the seniors they are supposed to obey and learn from, show no reasoning, gratitude, remorse or sense of responsibility.

Illogical feedback has different effects on different juniors:

- Poor reasoners tend to obey suggestions of quick fixes, because these quick fixes imply there is no need to think. When they become seniors, they recommend these mistakes to their juniors.

- Semi-decent reasoners may be tempted to become just like their seniors: 'Why should I bother to think? My seniors are getting away with their behaviour.'

- Robust reasoners become annoyed and ignore the poor reasoner. They will not copy the senior because they realise that their future is decided by their priorities. The senior has amply demonstrated that they do not care if the junior is harmed by poor advice.

'Just follow the guideline/protocol'

Hospitals often have many protocols for various situations. The protocols usually aim to provide a minimum level of safety and adherence to the rules. Guidelines and protocols can be useful in fixed situations where the user does not know what to do. However, these documents cannot handle every situation.

Optimal decisions are based on the patient's diagnosis, which is in turn based on recognising the entirety of the patient. Getting this diagnosis is the duty of the doctor, not the document.

Instead of explaining the limited utility and the caveats of using these documents, a 'hospital orientation' often emphasises following the documents, full stop. Senior doctors often reinforce this by telling others: 'Just follow the protocol.'

'Just follow the protocol', stated as it is, is often interpreted as: just follow the protocol regardless of the patient's presentation.

However, the full and accurate statement is different: just follow the protocol *unless the patient's presentation suggests another course of action.*

Many junior doctors have this misinterpretation because their senior never stated the exact role and limitations of the protocol. The seniors may never have thought about the role and limitations of the protocol.

Some seniors ignore the patient's entire clinical context, demonstrate unthinking obedience to a protocol, and then blame the protocol when mishaps occur.

Juniors can assume that since seniors are getting away with ignoring the patient's entirety, and there was no mention of paying attention to the entirety of the patient, such attention is unimportant. This assumption discourages clinical reasoning and patient-centredness, with predictably tragic results. When these doctors become senior doctors, they can encourage their juniors to make the same mistake.

Radiology rounds

During Radiology teaching rounds, the patient's clinical context, relevant differentials and basis for ordering the radiological investigation, must be presented before any discussion of the radiological findings. The folly of doing otherwise has been discussed earlier in this book.

Morbidity and Mortality rounds

Reporting of major events, such as patient demise and catastrophic deteriorations, can be used for teaching and accountability. These patients are presented in group sessions; the sessions have names such as 'Morbidity and Mortality rounds'.

If these sessions aim to help doctors improve to prevent such recurrences, robust reasoning must be demonstrated. The language of clinical reasoning is required. All decisions must be linked to a diagnosis. By fully laying out the mental process, fallacies and weaknesses are identified in the doctors who were managing the patient. This exercise increases useful learning for everyone, because the doctors in the audience who did not manage that patient, often have the same fallacies and weaknesses as the doctors who did manage that patient.

Electronic healthcare systems

Electronic healthcare systems are used to record patient information. These systems must capture enough information for various healthcare functions.

Since the anchor point for good decision-making is the correct diagnosis, the assessment must focus on proper diagnoses, as described in this book.

Distinguish between these 2 categories: Diagnoses versus Problems. The Problems are unexplained clinical features and results. The system programmers cannot rely solely on existing international classification codes as of the end of 2022, which do not differentiate between these 2 categories.

Performance

It is easy to assess performance based on quantity alone, such as the 'number of patients seen' by each doctor. Seeing many patients to earn money, is useful.

However, the qualitative component is at least as important as the quantity. Minimising waste, dramatically reducing unnecessary hospitalisations, reducing the length of stay, saving patients' lives, and impressing patients with superlative care to the point they spread the word so that other patients would choose that hospital for healthcare,

are crucial. Lowering wastage and thus, lowering expenses, also increases overall profits.

Quantity matters, but it is more important to deliver excellent care to 1,000 patients than deliver rushed, half-erroneous care (or worse) to 2,000 patients. This is like choosing between baking 100 tasty cakes versus 200 mediocre-to-awful cakes, or choosing between training 100 competent doctors versus 200 half-baked doctors. The issue here is not whether the hospital refuses patients unnecessarily; the issue is whether the hospital encourages rushing through patients in the clinics and wards for various reasons, such as to earn more money.

If rushing through patients to make money is preferable to delivering excellent care, the clinic or hospital is not truly an institution focused on helping the sick. Instead, this hospital or clinic is a profit-driven business, first and foremost.

If 2,000 patients must be cared for, the quantity of patients is not an excuse to deliver poor care. Though it may not be possible to deliver ideal care to all 2,000 patients, there is a difference between genuinely trying, and not bothering to try at all.

Clinical reasoning allows superior care and the evaluation of such care.

Without measuring this qualitative component and factoring it into the performance rating, it is difficult to:

- Incentivise excellent care.
- Hold doctors accountable. Lack of accountability opens the door to flimsy rationalisation such as 'since no one is checking the outcomes, I can just follow the process or do what I want, and ignore the outcome'.
- Properly acknowledge skilled clinicians whose other responsibilities (be it in administration, education or research) greatly reduce the number of patients they can see in a given year.

If the performance evaluation only counts the 'number of patients seen each year', skilled clinicians may not be recognised (or promoted) for the high-quality care they provide despite seeing half the number of patients a poorly reasoning doctor sees (or operates on).

The absence of attention to qualitative aspects of care, leads to ongoing and tragic consequences in healthcare facilities.

Capsule summary

- Hospitals have a major role to play in encouraging and incentivising clinical reasoning, thereby improving patient outcomes, avoiding wastage, and increasing the hospital's overall profit.

- Robust clinical reasoning is evident through the quality and accuracy of documentation and handover, which will match the excellent outcomes of care. Conversely, poor reasoning leads to inaccurate diagnoses, terrible care, shoddy documentation and inaccurate handovers.

Frequently asked questions

Q: You emphasise the importance of Assessment being diagnoses as far as possible. How about non-disease problems, such as personal circumstances?

A: Even for non-disease problems, you should try to 'diagnose' the root cause of those problems. Such diagnosis enables targeted, effective intervention. The benefits of targeted and effective intervention are considerable, regardless of whether the problem is a disease or a non-disease.

Identifying and addressing the root cause of a problem is based on robust overall reasoning.

Consider this common example of 'problems':

1. High risk of nutritional deficiencies due to diet

2. Struggling to wake up on time to get to work, because of sleeping late

3. Non-compliance with chronic therapy

The interventions that doctors can reflexively (but unthinkingly) list, include: Advice on proper diet, Refer to a dietitian, Advise on sleep hygiene and the need to sleep on time, Educate the patient on the importance of compliance with chronic treatment, and Check the patient's understanding of the chronic disease.

When I was told of one such patient with these 3 'problems', I gently asked the team of doctors: 'What is the root cause of all these problems?'

I was told that the patient was juggling family care, studying and work.

My next question was: 'Has anyone enquired about the patient's daily schedule, ascertained the exact degree of her (tremendous) strain, and demonstrated empathy and understanding of her perspective?'

Everyone looked puzzled. Someone said: 'No.'

I continued. 'If you want to effectively treat the disease, you must understand the patient. Especially if the patient has difficulties coping with the treatment plan. Does anyone in the team understand *the patient?*'

To recap what was written in the chapter 'Getting additional information to manage patients': Understanding the patient to treat *the patient and the disease* as a whole, separates the best (doctors) from the rest (of the doctors).

There was silence. Eventually, someone mumbled, 'No.'

The patient had been hospitalised for a few days. The healthcare team was about to discharge the patient that day. These 'problems' had been documented daily and in previous admissions over several months, with the same interventions proposed each time and the same failure to resolve these problems at each admission.

No one had thought about understanding the patient to discover *why* the previous attempts at these interventions did not work. There had been ample opportunity in the past to execute the tasks I suggested. The notion of truly understanding the patient did not seem to have occurred to anyone during this admission, or in the previous admissions.

I said: 'We can lecture and educate patients and perform other superficial actions, but please accept reality. If you do the same thing as your predecessors, you can expect the same result your predecessors got: *you would not fix these problems.* The most effective solution begins with understanding the patient, regardless of whether you are the first team or the fifth team of doctors that she has encountered.'

'Obtain all the information I requested. Once you know her schedule and burden, you can support her adequately. Without solving the root cause of her difficulties, she is unlikely to be able to follow your advice and comply with interventions. When the patient's burdens have been cushioned and supported, thereby proving to her that you genuinely care about her, she is more likely to trust you and comply with your suggestions.'

A junior doctor protested, 'We have referred to the Medical Social Work service previously. The social worker would have assessed and tried to help the patient...'

She trailed off as she saw my eyes hardening with each word she uttered.

I replied, 'Ah. So now it is *someone else's* job to understand the patient and help them comply with the treatment plan? Are we doctors, or not? Are we supposed to understand the patient as a whole, no matter who else we rope in to help? Who knows our plans best and can work with the patient to make these plans feasible, ourselves or our colleagues? Are we supposed to push the job of understanding the patient to someone else, and expect them to also do our job for us?'

She replied quietly, 'I see. It is our job.'

I nodded. 'Doctors can get help from others, like the Medical Social Work services, to assist the patient. However, getting additional help is different from abandoning our job to others. This is the same debate in social media about whether parents should push the job of teaching children to the schoolteachers, and blame the schoolteachers if the children behave or do poorly in anything. Good parents know that the ultimate responsibility lies with the parent, not the teacher. Teachers are supposed to teach and help, but the parents must do the work of understanding the child and work alongside the teacher, not abandon their duty to the child and treat the teacher as a scapegoat.'

'Our profession is like the position of the child's parents. In that analogy, the "child" is the patient before us. Doctors work together with others. Teamwork is not the same as an abandonment of our job to others.'

A junior doctor asked: 'What should we document in the Assessment?'

I said, 'How about "Heavy burdens in personal and work life"? Then state the diet, non-compliance and work lateness as manifestations and consequences of this "diagnosis". That "diagnosis" focuses you on the proper, target-the-root-cause intervention that will finally make solving the difficulties, a reality.'

SECTION 6

Wrapping Up

This section summarises the steps of the clinical approach, diagnosis and management. It also covers miscellaneous information: answers to the quizzes, closing thoughts, additional resources, and so on.

SUMMARY OF THE CLINICAL APPROACH, DIAGNOSIS AND MANAGEMENT

This chapter summarises the action steps and their principles for a diagnostic encounter, across Sections 1 to 4.

Omit any step at your peril.

1. The presenting complaint

Listen carefully. Explore the details of the presenting complaint.

Then ask for other accompanying symptoms.

2. Generate early differentials

Generate the most likely differentials for this patient by the 3rd minute of the consultation (this can overlap with Step 1). Begin by trying to explain all the clinical features and their known details, first.

The most likely disease is the disease that Clinically Fits the patient. The mental Venn diagram helps.

Epidemiology/Risk Factors are then considered, the main purpose being to re-rank differentials of equal Clinical Fit. Occasionally, new differentials may arise from this category of information.

3. Target the clinical evaluation

This evaluation includes history and physical examination.

The highest yield steps always go for the most likely diagnosis. The highest yield answers will lie in the Clinical Features.

Thus, start with the most likely diagnosis. There are 2 ways to approach the evaluation of clinical features:

1. Only familiar with Rule #1: recall your illness script for that disease. Evaluate for other clinical features of this disease. Repeat for each subsequent differential.

2. Proficient in all 3 rules of clinical reasoning: recall your illness scripts for all the relevant differentials. Evaluate for Universal and Secondary Specific Clinical Features of the most likely diagnosis, and then repeat for subsequent differentials if necessary.

Risk Factors for each disease, starting with the most likely disease, are then checked.

Sometimes, doctors complete the history for clinical features and risk factors, before performing the physical examination.

Sometimes, doctors complete the evaluation for clinical features (history and examination), then return to the history for risk factors.

4. Put it all together

Rule #1 of clinical reasoning (explain all clinical features and their details) decides the most likely diagnosis. The less a differential explains all the clinical features, the less likely that differential is.

Decide the most likely diagnosis and top 1 or 2 other differentials, the certainty of each possibility, and the severity of the disease.

Since severity is not always the same as activity, ask about recent treatment that addresses your most likely diagnosis and differentials. Mentally 'add' that treatment intensity to the apparent disease activity to get the true disease severity.

The most likely disease decides the potentially relevant management options.

Disease severity decides overall management urgency and intensity.

5. Are diagnostic tests needed?

Diagnostic tests are indicated when:

- The certainty of the most likely diagnosis does not reach the treatment threshold for that disease, or
- A less-likely differential fulfils all 3 criteria for ruling out, and is in the testing window.

If performing diagnostic tests, prioritise the most likely diagnosis. Ruling this in with at least 97% certainty automatically 'excludes' the less-likely differentials.

Under rare circumstances, rule-out tests for the dangerous differentials are performed instead of the rule-in test for the most likely diagnosis.

Choose the appropriate tests. Rule-in tests have strong positive likelihood ratios. Rule-out tests have strong negative likelihood ratios.

Factor in the clinical context and pre-test probability when interpreting the test results.

6. Are tests needed to adjust treatment?

Tests for adjusting treatment can:

1. Assess disease activity/severity

2. Detect treatment-related risks, due to the patient's co-morbid diseases or status conditions

3. Assess disease presence and activity, in diseases that can be present but clinically occult

7. Decide and implement other decisions for management

Overall management must match disease severity.

Treatment intensity must at least match disease severity.

8. Follow-up

Follow-up of the patient depends on the setting.

In a patient who is sick enough or the diagnosis uncertain enough to be hospitalised, the certainty and severity of the correct diagnosis, speed of progression and duration of symptoms before admission, decide the closeness of follow-up.

In an outpatient setting, the danger level of the diagnosis, the estimated ability of the patient to cooperate with care, and the timing of the next decision point decide the interval of follow-up.

Follow-up accomplishes multiple goals, including:

- Ascertain if the patient is recovering as expected
- Obtain new information, which may change your diagnosis
- Rescue the situation, if surprises arise
- Learn when you were right, thereby reinforcing your correct thought processes
- Learn when you were wrong, thereby giving you an opportunity to recheck and correct your erroneous thought processes
- Learn the final diagnosis, so that you can accurately add information to your illness script for that disease
- Add more information to your illness script for that disease.

Surprises

If a patient ever surprises you, be it in a test result, new clinical feature or failure to respond as expected during follow-up, recheck your clinical assumptions.

Restart from square one of the clinical evaluation.

ANSWERS TO QUIZZES

Quiz (Clinical Approach)

Q1a: The basic diagnostic requirement is the application of

- The priorities of diagnostic information — Clinical Features take priority over Risk Factors — in acquiring and analysing patient information, and

- Rule #1 of clinical reasoning: explain all clinical features.

Q1b: The priorities drive efficient, effective evaluation and diagnostic thinking. These priorities help you to avoid fixating on risk factors, and help 'de-conflict' your differential diagnoses.

Rule #1 of clinical reasoning recognises that symptoms and signs are manifestations of the current, correct diagnosis (or diagnoses). The diagnosis that explains the patient's clinical features better than the other differentials, will usually be the most likely diagnosis.

Q2a: The top differentials are:

- Parasitic diseases classified as visceral larva migrans, especially *Strongyloides stercoralis* and *Toxocara*

- Gut vasculitis caused by diseases such as systemic lupus erythematosus
- Eosinophilic gastroenteritis
- Idiopathic Hypereosinophilic Syndrome.

Patients with these diseases may have multiple other symptoms and signs.

Q2b: Check for clinical features of the differentials, and risk factors for the abovementioned parasites. The risk factors include eating raw vegetables, raw meat or liver from potential parasitic hosts such as chickens, lambs or calves.

A full complete count can be useful, as eosinophilia is present in most of the differentials except the usual inflammatory diseases that cause gut vasculitis. Some patients with systemic lupus erythematosus have lymphopenia, anaemia or thrombocytopenia.

Thereafter, definitive testing and decision-making would depend on the most likely diagnosis. Specialist referral may involve Infectious Diseases (parasites), Rheumatology (gut vasculitis), Gastroenterology and Allergy (eosinophilic gastroenteritis) or Haematology (Idiopathic Hypereosinophilic Syndrome).

Q3a: The top differentials are:

- Intermittent ovarian torsion
- Early acute appendicitis

The clinical vignette describes a patient whose disease is rapidly progressing, with initial intermittent activation of visceral pain fibres. The distribution of pain suggests the structures involved are innervated by the nerve plexuses in the abdomen and pelvis.

Q3b: Check for symptoms and signs pointing to sacral dermatomal involvement. Check for prior history of such episodes. If there are such prior episodes (which may have resolved spontaneously) or the sacral dermatomes appear to be involved, then the most likely diagnosis is intermittent ovarian torsion.

Imaging to discern between the 2 differentials may help. An ultrasound of the abdomen and pelvis is often preferable to a CT scan because CT scans slightly increase the chance of future cancers. As both differentials are potential emergencies, testing and referral to the appropriate specialist(s) are urgent.

If intermittent ovarian torsion is suspected in a young child, the rarity of this diagnosis in this age group should prompt suspicion of a predisposing, previously undetected concomitant disease such as an ovarian dysgerminoma.

A common mistake in the approach is to assume 'common things happen commonly', instead of obeying Rule #1 of clinical reasoning. This assumption is often followed by diagnosing these patients with viral vomiting or gastroenteritis, even though the rapidly progressive pain and abdominal tenderness cannot be explained by most infections. Appropriate care is delayed.

Q4: The amount of consultation time left over for anticipatory care depends on the accuracy and speed used to handle the patient's primary concern in that consultation. The 'leftover time' afterwards can be split between the patient's other chronic diseases (if any) and anticipatory care.

Quiz (Tests)

Q1: Diagnostic tests are usually necessary when the probability of your most likely clinical diagnosis falls within the testing window. Sometimes, differential diagnoses that fulfil the 3 criteria to rule out, will also fall into this window. This window lies between the test threshold and the treatment threshold. Usually, the first step should be to attempt to rule in the most likely diagnosis.

Q2: A single most accurate diagnostic and invasive test has the advantage of accuracy, but is usually more expensive and has greater risks than several non-invasive, less-accurate diagnostic tests.

Several noninvasive tests are often preferred. However, if these tests' results disagree with the clinical context, the doctor must recheck their clinical assumptions. If the clinical diagnosis remains unchanged after this recheck, that single most accurate test becomes necessary.

Q3: The 3 categories of information that tests help with for adjusting treatment, are:

- Assess disease activity/severity
- Detect treatment-related risks, due to the patient's co-morbid diseases or status conditions
- Assess disease presence and activity, in diseases that can be present but clinically occult.

--

Quiz (Treatment)

Q1: As treatment intensity must at least match disease severity, an appendectomy is a more 'intense' treatment and thus, is more likely to cure the patient than intravenous antibiotics.

Q2: This patient seems very anxious. Thus, the 3 extra elements to cover are:

- Rarest and worst side effects
- Contingency plans if the patient becomes unwell on the operating table
- The scenario if general anaesthesia was not administered. Without general anaesthesia, the surgeon may be unwilling to operate on the patient, with the attendant consequences. Sometimes, an alternative method of treatment and/or anaesthesia may be viable.

CLOSING

I have defined and explained the method of universally applicable clinical reasoning, its components, its manifestations, and its benefits. It is difficult to overstate the necessity of robust clinical reasoning for excellent healthcare and training.

Becoming skilled in this method requires sustained effort. My strongest students know this well.

There is much to be gained from this method in the long term. For a lazy person (like me), there are added benefits because:

- I dislike re-reading textbooks. If I did not have a way to cement my knowledge for the long term, I would either have to re-read textbooks, or fail my exams and my patients. Therefore, I came up with the pathophysiology-based idea of cementing of knowledge.

- If I made mistakes, I would have to fix them. This means extra work. I dislike extra work. If I minimise mistakes, I have less extra work.

- If I ensure I catch virtually all mistakes (through follow-up) early, preventing disasters means less extra work.

- If I fix the weaknesses that led to mistakes, thereby preventing recurrences of mistakes, I do not have to keep fixing the same mistakes.

- Handling complaints from patients which allege inappropriate care, is potentially stressful. If mistakes are not made in patient care and communication, valid complaints become almost impossible.

'Wise' laziness involves putting in more work initially to perpetually reap rewards and avoid even more (painful) work later on. Its opposite, unwise laziness, means going with whims and ignoring mistakes to stumble through life.

I mention my laziness because I could not come up with a 'lazier' way or journey to get these outcomes. If I could, I would have described it. If you can think of a way, please let me know.

Will everyone believe the content of this book? Of course not.

Human reactions to a novel concept differ:

- Some will jump in right away, recognising the benefits are worth the effort. The sooner you begin in earnest, the sooner you begin reaping the benefits personally.

- Others will adopt a wait-and-see approach for years before joining in.

- A fair proportion of humans tend to oppose anything different, instantly and irrationally, purely because it is different and thus, threatens their 'comfort zone' of beliefs and habitual behaviour.

I will not insist that you believe me. However, do not expect the commonplace methods that have failed to fix (and sometimes, created) the problems of healthcare for decades, to fix those problems. If you do the same thing as everyone else, you can expect to get the same result as them.

Inattention and poor reasoning: the relationship

Inattention is often accompanied by poor reasoning. I have described their coexistence throughout this book. Their coexistence is not a coincidence.

The question arises: does inattention cause poor reasoning, or does poor reasoning cause inattention, or do both feed each other in a vicious cycle?

My answer: Both feed each other in a vicious cycle.

Attentiveness is a choice. Most people have 5 senses. Whether they choose to use their senses and believe their senses, is a choice. The saying 'to see but not to notice; to hear but not to listen' aptly describes this choice.

Inattention and poor reasoning often feed each other in a vicious cycle. Throughout the book, I have explained how poor reasoning encourages inattentiveness towards anything. This inattention can be global, or targeted only to the inconvenient information the doctor dislikes accepting. Inattention, deliberate or not, likewise drives poor reasoning because this inattention deprives you of the knowledge you need, to practise reasoning. Without knowledge, you cannot employ reasoning. I have never seen a robust reasoner who was ignorant. To argue that someone is skilled without having the knowledge necessary to use the skill, is like arguing that a tennis player is skilled despite never having used a tennis racket or hit a tennis ball in their life.

Can a poor reasoner seem to be attentive? Yes, if you cannot recognise the difference between attentiveness and confusion. I have explained how outward manifestations, such as encyclopaedic entries, are not truly manifestations of focused attention but rather, an inability to reason and prioritise properly. Even if the poor reasoner was truly attentive for brief moments, their poor reasoning leaves them struggling to understand any information they acquired.

Robust reasoning, either clinical or overall, derives from attentiveness to the patient and the world we operate in.

Some of the conversations are hard to believe.

Some of the statements in the conversations are outrageous. You may want to believe that they are exaggerations or fabrications. When I first heard those statements, I could barely believe my ears too. I did not want to believe what I was hearing, because the implications were horrifying. However, robust reasoning is about accepting reality, not about blind obedience to your personal beliefs.

The full truth is sometimes worse than the content of those conversations. If you had difficulty believing some of those encounters and conversations, then I am glad I did not further upset you by describing even more of what you do not want to believe. I have been as diplomatic as I could, without concealing the essence of the truth. If you struggle with believing the descriptions in this book, ask yourself if you are truly open-minded and attentive to what has been going on around you.

To quote: 'Evil flourishes when good men and women stand by and do nothing.' Neither intelligence nor reasoning is required to do evil; ignorance of reality and outcomes, often combined with disrespect to others, is enough. The unthinking schoolyard or workplace bully who repeatedly harms others, regardless of motivation or intent, is doing evil even if they never bother to find out if their victims are hurt. This is true for all of humankind; healthcare is no exception. A more diplomatic translation can be 'Harm flourishes when doctors stand by and ignore mistakes'.

Excellent doctors are being called 'strange' and 'crazy' by some of their peers because they bother to put in the extra effort to excel and deliver excellent patient care. How wide has the rot in our profession spread? How far have some in our 'lofty' profession fallen?

Consider other professions. Would you expect athletes to call the opponents who outperformed them, 'strange' or 'crazy'? Would you expect engineers to denigrate the best engineers? If you are someone who relies on professionals to provide you with a safe car or aeroplane or house or food, would you want the poor performers in that profession discouraging their properly performing peers from giving you what you want or need?

This book has illuminated the unthinking behaviours and deceptions that often go unchallenged. If you are a leader, teacher or researcher, you have more power than many doctors to change these situations.

I challenge you: will you accept the truth and act? Will you actively encourage your peers, students, and subordinates to do the right thing? Will you hold them accountable for their actions? Or will you remain silent and inactive, thereby being part of the problem by appearing to condone the behaviours and deceptions?

The outcomes, and the standards needed to reach those outcomes, are considerable.

Some have told me that my standards are very high.

To call my standards high, implies that there are other standards to compare them with.

Given the outcomes of healthcare worldwide, the real question is: are the conventional standards of training and healthcare worldwide, too low?

When the real-world outcomes that matter to patients are not tracked and tackled by institutions and doctors themselves, do we even *have* standards for the outcomes?

If a medical school either:

- Focuses on getting high pass rates for final exams instead of tracking the real-world outcomes of the graduates, or

- Tracks the real-world outcomes of the graduates but will not make the necessary changes to the training to improve the outcomes of these graduates,

does the school really have standards for the outcome that matters: the real-world competence of its graduates?

Are we conflating the process with the outcome?

Are we assuming a standard process automatically leads to an excellent outcome?

The standards and learning journey I describe are the minimum standards for excellent training and healthcare.

Talking about standards without taking effective action to meet those standards, is just that: talk. Actions and outcomes speak louder than words.

I hope I have taken enough action in describing this learning journey, to help others meet the minimum standards of care that patients should be getting.

This journey does not require genius, great wealth, photographic memory, vast experience, or most other advantages. Most students and doctors can undertake this journey, provided they are willing. The journey requires effort in a different direction from much of conventional training, and a genuine openness to learning.

By seeking and facing the truth about yourself, and then acting upon this truth, this journey will make you a better *person* as well as a better doctor.

Even if you undertake the journey and then give up at some point (which you should not), merely striving to become better in this way will make you a much better doctor than you otherwise would have become. What you get, is what you put into it.

There is more. This book is just the tip of the iceberg.

The genesis of this method and the (wearying) years-long journey to refine it, are described in the later section 'How this came about'.

The Additional Resources section provides other suggestions for enhancing your clinical reasoning. My electronic mail address is there too.

Is there more to clinical reasoning than the content of this book? Yes.

This book focused on the basics. Mastery of the basics opens the door to the even-more-powerful, advanced-level reasoning methods. A glimpse of the potency of 1 aspect of advanced-level reasoning — timelines — was provided in the chapter 'Theoretical disease approaches'. Beyond their clinical diagnostic potency, time-based illness scripts also enable the accurate interpretation of test results based on the exact day of disease when the test was performed. As of end-2022, no literature or textbook has described this time-based interpretation across many tests.

Given the intended audience for this book, I have withheld mention of all other aspects of advanced-level reasoning, including cases that require advanced-level reasoning. Such cases are virtually impossible for most doctors to handle optimally, would pose a challenge to a master of the basics, and are relatively clear to a master of advanced-level reasoning.

Undertaking the learning journey described in this book will yield some of those advanced-level insights after years of dedicated pursuit.

The world needs better healthcare. I have done my part.

Now it is your turn.

ADDITIONAL RESOURCES

A small team from the National University of Singapore (NUS) and I partnered Med2Lab, an innovative education technology company based in the United States of America. Our mutual aim: to create the world's first universal clinical reasoning-based assessment and reinforcement, virtual patient platform. The framework provides users with automated insight and feedback on separate components of their mental reasoning process and decision-making process.

By separating cases into tiers of reasoning complexity, the assessment and teaching of reasoning can be built into learners in a manner akin to the construction of a tall and sturdy building. The foundations must be laid down and properly organised to provide maximum strength for the layers that follow. Otherwise, embedding an accurate and clear reasoning process is less certain in users.

With this method, users are expected to benefit greatly in all-around clinical reasoning just by completing a handful of cases, with increasing benefit as more cases of greater variety and complexity are undertaken. The benefits of superior, universally applicable clinical reasoning carry over to other diseases the user encounters, not just for the diseases in those cases alone.

This approach is novel compared to other existing platforms at the end of 2022, which rely on users completing dozens and hundreds of cases, each case providing knowledge-based lessons specific to that case alone.

Faculty may find this platform useful for their medical schools and postgraduate training programs, as these insights reveal both individual-level as well as cohort-level weaknesses. Awareness of your learners' weaknesses can enable effective remediation, be it personally or as a curriculum-level change.

As the exact mental process of students and doctors has never been described before, the insights also open new areas for research: how the mind seeks and analyses information, the correlation between reasoning and performance, and so on.

The NUS-Med2Lab link is: https://www.med2lab.com/

--

Two of my former students undertook a systematic review of diagnostic reasoning in undergraduate teaching. I was honoured to provide my input. The summary of the evidence, and the insights they shared at the end, is available at: https://pubmed.ncbi.nlm.nih.gov/34159542/

--

For feedback, further questions, discussions on clinical reasoning and collaborations, I can be reached at paesjy@nus.edu.sg.

If I do not reply in 3 days, I have probably missed your email. If so, I apologise in advance; I get a lot of emails. =(Just drop me another! Or contact me directly in another way.

GLOSSARY (AND SIGNIFICANCE IN CLINICAL REASONING)

Anticipatory care — provision of health education and interventions to maintain health and detect the disease as early as possible. Performed at the end of consultations.

Basic diagnostic reasoning requirement — application of the priorities of diagnostic information (Clinical features versus Epidemiology/Risk Factors), together with Rule #1 of Clinical Reasoning: explain all clinical features. Maximises the chance the doctor will get the correct clinical diagnosis and think of relevant differential diagnoses.

Clinical Features — symptoms and signs of the disease. This category also includes the absence of symptoms and signs (e.g. normal vital signs), as many diseases should not cause abnormalities in unrelated systems.

Cognitive load — the amount of mental energy diverted towards comprehending the form and format of any knowledge or skill being taught. This mental energy is 'wasted' because it was not directly used to embed or organise the knowledge/skill in the learner. Reducing cognitive load maximises learning effectiveness and efficiency.

Complication — another disease that often requires management separate from the original disease. Complications tend to occur when the original disease has been inadequately treated or uncontrolled for a sufficiently long period. Complications can occur after the onset of acute as well as chronic diseases.

Correct diagnosis — fulfilled by 3 elements: Rule #1 of Clinical Reasoning, explained with a specific disease, and an estimated severity level.

Diagnosis of Exclusion — a common, benign disease that requires you to think of relevant differentials, which are mimickers of that unique patient's clinical features.

Differential diagnoses — all the relevant diseases the doctor must consider for the patient. Generating these differentials helps you to avoid target fixation.

Disease activity — the degree of clinical, biochemical and other evidence of disease still being present in the patient. This decreases in proportion to the treatment intensity. Effective care usually aims to reduce disease activity to zero.

Disease severity — dictates the current harm, and risk of future harm to the patient. In turn, disease severity decides the overall management, including the degree of testing, the intensity of treatment choices, disposition, monitoring and counselling. Disease severity is the sum total of treatment intensity and disease activity.

Disposition — decisions regarding where the patient goes, whom they see, and when. Mostly dictated by the disease and its level of severity.

Epidemiology — the patient's demographics, applied to the commonality of the disease in their demographic groups. Also includes the commonality of the disease in the general population.

Presenting Complaint — the symptom(s) the patient volunteers, usually in the first 30 seconds of consultation.

Risk Factors — all patient-unique information other than the clinical features, that may increase or decrease the likelihood of that disease in the patient.

Rule In — the process of becoming certain that a disease is the most likely diagnosis. This is mostly a clinical process, assisted by the Rules of Clinical

Reasoning. When the reasoning is robust, the most likely diagnosis is almost always the correct diagnosis.

Rule Out — the process of deciding that less-relevant differential diagnoses, are truly absent in the patient. This should be undertaken if the 3 criteria for ruling out are fulfilled, and ruling in the most likely diagnosis to the point of near-100% certainty is not feasible. A synonym for 'rule out', is 'exclude'.

Ruling out OAF — the process of ruling out a disease Only, Always or First. Is the basis of defensive obsession and many adverse outcomes in healthcare.

Treatment Intensity — the sum total of all treatment measures' effectiveness. This should always match or exceed the severity of the disease.

Velocity of improvement — the speed at which clinical features and test-based indicators of disease activity resolve, and the patient's functional impairment (if any) improves. This velocity is a reflection of the degree by which the treatment intensity exceeds disease severity.

HOW THIS CAME ABOUT

In 2006, at the suggestion of Professor Yap Hui Kim, I joined the Department of Paediatrics at the National University Hospital of Singapore. I had graduated from medical school 18 months before.

Acceptance into this Department was considered an honour, given the number of former top students and prize-winners among the faculty.

My initial observations, and reasoning

Within a few months, I noticed an invisible 'glass ceiling' in the diagnostic accuracy and decision-making of my colleagues and teachers. They were far more experienced than I; many were far more intelligent and knowledgeable; some were more meticulous.

However, none of these advantages got these brilliant, knowledgeable and experienced doctors above the conventional ceiling of performance.

Therefore, I concluded that the limiting factor was not inherent to the faculty as individuals, but had to be a systemic factor. The systemic factor was obvious: the conventional, mixed bag of different approaches and teaching and work that everyone went through.

As the saying goes: if you do the same thing as everyone else, you get the same result as them.

Therefore, if I hoped to get past that ceiling, I would have to do something different and better. Specifically, I had to train myself to think differently and learn from my patients differently. 'Different' can be better or worse than everyone else. Thus, my 'different' had to be better.

Such thinking might be seen as ludicrous or even blasphemous: 'This department has many of the smartest doctors in the country. How dare you challenge traditional teaching here? Do you really think you can come up with a technique superior to our standard training?'

I could not announce what I intended. That would offend a lot of seniors, who would perceive such thoughts as arrogance. Human history is replete with automatically hostile, irrational reactions towards people who challenge commonplace thinking and behaviour. The scientific studies echo human history: look up the 'anti-creativity bias'.

I decided the best way to get above the ceiling of conventional performance was to develop a new, 'best' method of approaching all patients, no matter what their diagnosis was. This method had to figure out their diagnosis as soon as possible, thereby enabling optimal decisions as early as possible.

Since the best patient-centred care could only come from patient-centred clinical diagnosis, I realised that my first step had to be the careful observation of the patterns of information-gathering. The next step would be to analyse this information for every patient, trying different ways to find the optimal analytical process that would maximise the chance of being correct.

Creating a new method could be dangerous. History shows that inventors often experienced many mishaps before they succeeded. If I was to do this as a doctor, patients might die unnecessarily if no one could counter-check me. I could not attempt this after I completed my specialist training. As a consultant, I could not expect anyone to check on or question my plans.

Thus, I had to undertake this creation as a junior doctor. I could always present my conclusions about the patient, to the supervising senior. If they disagreed, the patient would still receive conventional care. If they agreed, the patient would get conventional-or-better care.

If I failed, the worst that could happen would be getting kicked out of speciality training for being a 'difficult trainee'. Not so high a price to pay if the potential reward was a new method that would consistently produce superior outcomes.

Creating and testing the Universal Clinical Reasoning method/technique

I began that same year. The standard specialist training in the Department was intensive. I had to care for patients in different subspecialties. This broad exposure gave me many patients across specialities to observe, question, and analyse in terms of the approach, the diagnosis, the decisions made for them, and their outcomes.

I tried different approaches and analyses for each patient's information.

The extra effort devoted to creating and testing this universally applicable method, took a tremendous amount of time and energy.

I struggled to simultaneously juggle the punishing training, work, and my efforts at creation. Something had to be sacrificed.

I cut back on my studying of textbooks, relying on my grasp of pathophysiology (which had been cemented during medical school) to help me answer any questions posed to me.

(I had not stopped studying entirely, and I do not encourage trainees to cut back on their studying.)

At the end of my first 6 months as a Paediatrics trainee, my first supervisor, Professor Low Poh Sim, summoned me to her office. I sat down facing her.

She asked, 'You are not studying, are you?'

I was taken aback. 'Er…yeah. How did you know?'

I was puzzled. Most of the questions assessing us were posed at various teaching sessions. I had been answering the questions correctly and consistently, even the most-feared questions at the weekly Intensive Care Unit grand rounds. There should have been no outward clue that I was not studying much.

She replied, 'I have seen you answer the questions at the grand rounds. You always pause for a few seconds, then state the answer. That means you do not have the answer at your fingertips. You are deriving the answer from first principles.'

Back then, 'first principles' was the synonym for 'pathophysiology'.

Professor Low was half-right. She was right about my not spending much time studying the standard Paediatrics references. However, her deduction about the reason behind my pauses was not entirely correct.

Recall the analogy of the house of bricks and cement in the chapter 'Pathophysiology in reasoning'. Most of the time, I did have the answer at my fingertips. I did not blurt out that answer right away because I would use my pathophysiological understanding to double-check the answer before I said it. At other times, I would derive the answer from the pathophysiological understanding I had built up since medical school.

Calling upon the pathophysiology inevitably took a few seconds, regardless of whether I was using it to double-check or derive. This was the 'few seconds' pause that she was alluding to.

There was no point explaining the bit about the double-checking. She clearly wanted me to study more, which was a fair suggestion. And she had been partly right about the 'not studying' bit.

I said, 'Yes, that's right. Sorry, Professor. I will study more.'

She continued thoughtfully, 'Having said that, you always get it right. That means you are very powerful at first principles.'

I continued to struggle with the juggling. The extra time taken to think through each patient — the conventional ways and my experiments with different mental approaches — meant that I could take a long time to make decisions. This was most prominent in the first year of my efforts.

That did not sit well with many of the nurses, who wanted rapid decisions from the doctors.

Back then, we trained ourselves to know all our patients mentally; no patient lists or other handheld assistants.

Limited mental space meant we had to prioritise information. Since clinical features mattered much more than risk factors and demographics, I would prioritise demographics last. My exhaustion from juggling my training and my 'creation' efforts, meant that the patient demographics often received the least attention. Thus, I sometimes got the demographics of one patient mixed up with another patient. That left more than one professor perplexed when I mixed up the gender of the patient whilst presenting, such as saying the patient was a girl, when the patient was actually a boy.

I also disagreed a lot with my seniors. Some of those times, I was wrong. At other times, I was not wrong. Following up on the patients over the subsequent days to weeks, taught me whether I was right or wrong. This following up further affirmed my perception of the performance ceiling; even senior consultants could not get above that ceiling with their standard approach and conventional practice.

I annoyed many seniors, who were surprised that a junior doctor had the gall to question them. Whispers went around that I was a 'difficult trainee'. I was not deaf. I ignored them.

They did not know why I was doing all this, so how could I expect them to think otherwise?

Near the end of the second year after I joined the Department, Professor Yap — the same professor who had suggested I apply to the Department — took me aside and scolded me roundly. She told me about the negative feedback she had received. She told me she was disappointed that I was not performing as she had expected. Given the tremendous respect I had for her, I was in tears.

However, my universal reasoning technique was nearly complete. Having defined the information categories and the rules of clinical reasoning, I no longer needed a long time to make the right decisions. I was also armed with prioritised and detailed illness scripts from 2 years of scrutinising patients thoroughly. I was beginning to incorporate the dimension of time into those scripts, transforming them into advanced time-based illness scripts.

I could not be certain of her response if I told her what I had been doing all this while. Would she agree that I should finish my endeavour? Or order me to abandon my efforts?

I gritted my teeth, apologised, decided not to tell her, and decided not to abandon my efforts. After all, if I was right, all would eventually become clear to her.

Before that scolding, the half-formed method was already yielding benefits. I was demonstrating 'moments of diagnostic brilliance' for patients. For example, within the first year of joining the Department, I saw a young boy in the middle of the night who complained of crushing, left-sided chest pain. I noticed the whiteness of the boy's face, checked his vital signs, and became alarmed. I grabbed the electrocardiogram (ECG) machine to perform an ECG, and then called the cardiologist on duty.

The cardiologist scoffed at my description of the clinical picture and diagnosis. To quote him: 'Myocardial infarction?! You must be kidding! Do you know how rare that is in kids?'

I then told him what the ECG showed: changes consistent with a myocardial infarction, and the likely location of the infarct. I insisted that the myocardial infarction had just set in, and thus immediate treatment would make a difference to the long-term outcome.

The cardiologist shook off his disbelief (specialists are unused to having junior doctors tell them what to do), and the child was moved to the Intensive Care Unit immediately for monitoring and treatment. The child did have a myocardial infarction, and the appropriate treatment was commenced immediately.

Several months after that discussion with Professor Yap, I took and passed my MRCPCH exam. Now I was a registrar, responsible for making most of the major decisions for patient care, both on-call and during the working day.

It was time to demonstrate the technique.

Within the first few months, the results silenced all my critics. I was pleased. The preceding, punishing 3 years had been worth the results. Professor Yap did not hear any more complaints about my clinical performance. To everyone back then, it was a mystery how the 'difficult trainee' had suddenly transformed into a consistently accurate registrar with regular 'moments of clinical diagnostic and management brilliance'.

I had broken through the ceiling.

I met various role models along the way. I observed their behaviour and studied their thought processes. The best doctors followed a consistent and systematic thought pattern, one that was virtually identical to my universal technique. There were minor differences in style, but the key principles and steps were similar.

For example, just before I took the MRCPCH exam, I was assigned to the Department of Neonatology at the National University Hospital, and ran into Professor Lee Jiun once more. When I first met him in the Department of Neonatology in another hospital, I had been impressed with his apparent clinical prescience.

In that first hospital where I had met him, the consultants reviewed all the babies once a week by walking together as a group, through the wards. Dozens of babies lay in rows of cots, all swaddled head to toe. The only visible part of each baby was their face.

Despite being the most junior consultant and walking at the back of the group, Lee Jiun would point to 1 baby amidst the rows of swaddled babies and say, 'That baby is sick.' This would mystify junior doctors like me, especially if we had just reviewed the baby a mere hour ago. Whenever he said those words, we would hurry over and recheck the baby.

He did this twice. One was a baby who had a bacterial infection upon re-examination. The other had no apparent symptoms or signs, but then developed a fever (also due to a bacterial infection) within the next 2 hours.

Identification of these sick, fully swaddled neonates with a single glance when no other doctor could tell, was incredible. Early identification of these neonates allowed us to intervene earlier and commence the correct antibiotics earlier, thereby maximising their chance of cure, minimising their suffering, and shortening the length of hospitalisation.

When he demonstrated this skill for the third time (and was right, again!) in the National University Hospital, my curiosity finally got the better of me. I sought him out in his office and described what I had seen, and then asked: 'How do you do that?'

He told me that as a junior doctor, given the dozens of healthy babies he had to see every day, he would study their faces, noting the colour and breathing pattern of these 'normal' babies. This observation of hundreds of normal babies gave him the ability to recognise subtle abnormalities in the faces of babies, instantly.

I understood what he was describing: mastery of Normal. I had been doing the same observation of 'Normals', albeit with older children in the Department of Paediatrics.

Since I was a paediatrician, most of my patients were children. The question arose: was the technique as useful in adult patients?

Over the years, I had opportunities to test the universal reasoning technique on adult patients through referrals, direct care, and advising colleagues in other specialities. It became clear that the technique was equally useful in adult patients too.

As I taught others, I noticed medical students and postgraduate specialist trainees, locally or internationally trained, were making the same pattern of mental mistakes at the same time points in doctor–patient scenarios and simulations, regardless of the final diagnosis and setting.

I found that I was using the same phrases and same language to teach, regardless of the seniority of the learners, patient diagnosis and setting. Those phrases and language came from the universal technique I had created and honed.

Along the way, I met Professor Amdekar, an internationally renowned paediatrician and teacher. I was also entrusted with the care of the works of the founder of the Department of Paediatrics, the late (and legendary) Professor Wong Hock Boon. Professor Wong's works contain insights into a wide spectrum of diseases.

Making the technique widely accessible

In February 2018, Professor Lau Tang Ching, the Vice-Dean of the Yong Loo Lin School of Medicine, National University of Singapore (NUS), put out a call for teaching clinical reasoning to medical students. I mentioned this technique to him and was tasked with teaching it to the students.

I converted the rudimentary basics of the technique into video recordings.

In 2019, Professor Chen Zhi Xiong told Bao Truong, the founder of Med2Lab, an American-based health education technology company, that 'a guy in Singapore has created something you should see'.

Bao flew to Singapore with the company's plans for a virtual patient platform. I listened to his pitch, and then told him that his plan shared the same weaknesses as existing commercial platforms. I then asked him 2 questions, letting his answers show him his thought process when he was going to get the diagnosis right.

The NUS-Med2Lab partnership was born.

As awareness and interest in this technique grew, I began teaching in the Masters of Nursing program at NUS, which has students across the hospitals, polyclinics, and nursing homes in Singapore. I also became responsible for teaching all incoming first-year doctors (house officers) across all the speciality rotations in the National University Hospital too.

I created a case presentation template using Powerpoint slides, based on the principles described in the first few chapters of this book. To fill up this template properly, learners were compelled to obey the basic diagnostic reasoning requirement. Each slide instructed them on the exact steps to fill that slide.

They picked a real patient of theirs. They had to fill out the template as instructed. The template required them to decide the most likely clinical diagnosis, and then make decisions for tests and treatment based on that diagnosis. Their diagnosis and decisions would then be compared side-by-side with the diagnosis and decisions of the team of experienced doctors who took care of the real patient.

Following the template invariably pointed these lone house officers and nursing students to the correct clinical diagnosis (or diagnoses. The template also allowed discernment of two or more simultaneous diagnoses) and relevant differentials. The correct diagnosis in turn suggested the appropriate tests and treatment.

In contrast, the teams of experienced doctors often performed inappropriate tests, had a higher tendency to misinterpret the results of those tests, and sometimes did not treat the patient appropriately.

Thus, these first-year doctors and nursing students were consistently outperforming experienced doctors in clinical diagnostic accuracy and optimal decision-making. The template was drastically (albeit temporarily) boosting the performance of these inexperienced healthcare workers who were generally unaware of the Universal Clinical Reasoning method.

In 2022, the first cohort of medical students from NUS who had been exposed to the reasoning videos, graduated. I received word from those employing this technique. They credited it with enabling them to make clinical diagnoses accurately and then make optimal decisions. Some helped their seniors (if those seniors were humble enough to accept suggestions) make the correct diagnosis and decisions. The wiser seniors realised that if they did not want to be consistently proven wrong and wanted their patients to get better as soon as possible, they should defer to these junior doctors. Which is exactly what these seniors did.

These former students also described how many of their peers and seniors followed the disastrous chain of dominoes consistently: 'They do not care about a proper clinical evaluation, they ignore whatever they want, they ignore all other opinions except their own, their plans are often irrelevant, and they do not learn from the poor outcomes of their patients.' They described how their peers kept shushing them and called them 'strange', 'difficult' and 'crazy' because they dared to question the seniors' (mistaken) diagnoses and plans.

Following up on the patient inevitably revealed the final correct diagnosis and by extension, the appropriate management. When they disagreed with their seniors, these former students were often, but not always correct.

In following up, these former students learnt from their mistakes. Their colleagues did not. Furthermore, the opinions, working style, and lack of patient-centredness of their colleagues rarely changed even when these colleagues were consistently proven wrong *and knew the outcome was poor*.

Those who deny being wrong, deny the need to learn and improve. Without improvement, the mistakes continue, and the denial continues. This is a self-created vicious cycle common to humankind.

Do you own your fears and accept reality, or do you let your fears own you and thus run away from reality?

The answer to this question is the essence of courage versus cowardice. The answer also decides your outcomes.

Over the years, my students have taken turns to independently suggest I write this book. One of the best was so persuasive that I finally agreed.

I thought, 'Okay. Besides, this could help the world.'

On 7 July 2022, I began writing. The first draft of 102,000-odd words took 3 weeks. Work continued until its final form of over 170,000 words in August 2023. At its completion, I felt a sense of contentment: this is my life's work, my journey, part of my legacy, and my hope for a better world. My best students were particularly helpful; one of them brilliantly suggested the cover picture of this book, which shows a slightly oversized brain and a heart. The brain symbolises reasoning, and the heart symbolises positive qualities. Both are needed for excellent healthcare.

At the time of this writing, over 16 years have passed since I embarked on this journey of discovery. Why did I wait so long to write this book?

- **Clarity.** Mental clarity leads to verbal clarity and clarity in decision-making.
- **Completeness.** How can one expect to consistently train a fully competent professional, with an incomplete process?

- **Simplicity.** Simplicity means less cognitive load and a wider audience that can understand the book.
- **Replicability.** Others had to be able to learn and replicate the results of this method of clinical reasoning.
- **History.** History has repeatedly demonstrated that half-formed or ineffective 'innovations' have mixed or negative receptions.

It took me this long to render the entire process into a complete, coherent step-by-step method simple enough for an educated teenager to understand. Simplicity and clarity are essential for training others to break through the 'glass ceiling' of conventional performance.

Some of my students pointed out that even with clarity, completeness, simplicity and replicability, there would be automatic naysayers to clinical reasoning. There are 4 groups of naysayers:

1. The first group comprises those who do not know what reasoning is. They decide that reasoning cannot be important because they do not know what it is. If I do not know how to sanitise and prepare water for human consumption, does that make the preparation of safe water unimportant for me or humankind?

2. The second group comprises those who instantly oppose anything different purely because it is unfamiliar to them. Human history is consistent in this regard. Something new is often met with immediate irrational hostility and outright rejection purely because it is new and unfamiliar: the anti-creativity bias.

3. The third group comprises those who recognise the need to change themselves if circumstances change, but refuse to change anyway: 'I do not want to change what I am doing.' If a huge boulder comes tumbling down the hill and would crush me if I remained stationary, I will change my position by getting out of the way. Refusing to change when it is necessary, is akin to remaining in the boulder's path and yelling at the oncoming boulder: 'Fly back up the hill! I refuse to change my position! The world must obey me!'

4. The fourth group comprises those who fear admitting the hidden shame in our profession. Since reasoning requires patient-centredness

and respecting the patient, all other behaviour that is inattentive to patients, ignores reality, is self-serving, exploitative, or worse, is revealed for what it truly is. Without reasoning, it is easier to claim that 'there is no best approach' to the patient, and then claim that anything the doctor does is therefore justified.

I agree with my students, as I have run into members of all 4 groups. These members include faculty, doctors and medical students. Some even ran away when I offered to share or demonstrate the technique, as if they were afraid of the truth. When I encounter the naysayers, I am unsurprised and not offended: this is not about me. Each person is entitled to their opinions, and gets the results they deserve.

I hope you are not in any of these groups. If so, the choice to remain in the group is yours.

Think this over, try it, and decide for yourself.

What more is there?

More can be written to complement this book, such as:

1. An encyclopaedia of detailed illness scripts that identify universal and secondary specific clinical features for multiple diseases
2. A workbook of anonymised clinical vignettes and diagnoses across multiple specialities and settings
3. A book that describes the important, reasoning-centred changes across multiple aspects of healthcare
4. A book on the simultaneous wielding of ownership and reasoning
5. A book that analyses, modifies and simplifies external descriptors of reasoning, to make them practical and useful
6. A book on advanced-level reasoning, filled with advanced illness scripts and reasoning techniques

The value of the first 2 suggestions is self-explanatory. I will elaborate on the other suggestions.

Reasoning-centred changes in aspects of healthcare

Major changes to many aspects of healthcare can be made, to encourage clinical reasoning and excellent outcomes. Glimpses of these changes were provided in this book. The full extent and practical steps to embed reasoning into all aspects of healthcare would require another book.

The aspects include:

- Selection of trainees
- Textbooks
- Curricula
- Teaching methodology
- Exams
- Healthcare teamwork and dynamics
- Healthcare records
- Research design, audits and approvals
- Standards of accountability and transparency
- Health and medicolegal insurance
- Governmental oversight

Simultaneous wielding of ownership and reasoning

Clinical reasoning is an offshoot of overall reasoning. This relationship was illustrated through general examples such as primary-school mathematics, identifying specific travellers at airports, recognising that moving a street bus requires adequate force, and proper usage of tools through the acquisition of skill. All of these analogies apply to healthcare.

Overall reasoning goes hand-in-hand with ownership.

Reasoning without ownership of your choices is often useless; if you never take the right actions despite knowing what they are, there is no practical difference between you and a poor reasoner. In a world where hyperbole and words are freely used to deceive oneself and others, it is easy to forget that actions and outcomes, sustained over time, speak louder than words alone.

When both reasoning and ownership are exercised simultaneously, other elements of effectiveness such as altruism, humility, courage, open-mindedness, objectiveness, self-regulation, adaptability, emotional intelligence, resilience, and impactful creativity, emerge. Many effective people are living examples of this synergy. I have woven in these elements throughout the book.

However, I have not explicitly described how ownership and reasoning synergise outside of the work scope of the healthcare professional. This is important to healthcare workers (and all other humans too), because the aspects of our non-working lives do affect ourselves and our work.

Analysis, modification and simplification of external descriptors of reasoning

In the Introduction of this book, I listed the many descriptors of clinical reasoning along with an overview of their limitations. If properly understood and simplified, some descriptors can be useful.

For example, dual-process theory refers to the theory of 2 types of thinking processes, 1 type known as 'fast' thinking and 1 type known as 'slow' thinking. The mass-market description of these processes explicitly separated the 2 types, so that the concept was easier for the readers to understand. If you tried to teach this theory to medical students as it is, they might understand that there can be 2 types of thinking processes, but you would still have failed to teach them what reasoning itself, truly is.

Suggesting these types of thinking should be wielded as separate processes just because they were described separately, is a mistake. Robust clinical reasoning uses a *simultaneous fusion* of the 2 processes, the relative proportion of each process varying with the degree of uncertainty in each patient.

An expert-tier doctor who sees a 'straightforward' patient will not mentally go 100% 'Type 1 thinking'. Instead, the expert is likely to go 98% or 99% 'Type 1 thinking' (the patient seems to fit their illness script) with the remaining 2% or 1% being 'Type 2 thinking' (double-check: does this patient fulfil Rule #1 of clinical reasoning?). I showed these proportions and the fusion of the 2 types, in the templates in the chapter 'Putting it all together: the most likely diagnosis'.

By extension, other descriptors of clinical reasoning may be modifiable for teaching purposes.

Advanced-level reasoning

The first 2 milestones of the learning journey (discussed in the FAQ section of the chapter 'Tiers of performance'), proficiency in the basics and mastery of the basics, come into play. To wield advanced-level reasoning to a limited degree, requires proficiency in the basics of the universal clinical reasoning method. To wield advanced-level reasoning with some proficiency, requires mastery of the basics. The third milestone of the learning journey for this method, focuses on the mastery of advanced-level reasoning. If there is a milestone beyond the third, at the time of this writing (August 2023), I cannot conceive of it.

Advanced illness scripts contain extra details of clinical features and thus, confer superior diagnostic speed and accuracy over basic illness scripts. The extra details include the aspects of clustering and time. For example, the different types of lung infections in children can be diagnosed clinically, using a simple time-based flowchart of my own devising. The time-based checks are for clinical 'phases of illness' and 'speed of progression'. This flowchart has a clinical accuracy of at least 98%. In addition, the flowchart accurately predicts the results of tests that are often ordered for these patients, such as blood tests and chest X-rays, thereby rendering these tests unnecessary.

Advanced decision-making includes higher-level applications of healthcare decision-making. One example is the use of patient decision thresholds to make decisions with and for the patient. Basic decision threshold theory focuses on the doctor's model of disease for the average patient, balancing factors such as costs, risks and benefits. However, patients do not use the same models in the doctor's head; they care about what happens to themselves, not the general balance of costs, risks and benefits for the average patient. The literature has shown significant discrepancies between the decision thresholds of doctors compared to patients. Additional information such as the patient's perspective will help with patient-centred decision-making, but such decision-making is not as optimal as using the patient's decision thresholds.

Patient decision thresholds are particularly important for high-stakes decisions. For example, as a junior consultant, I had a patient with Omenn syndrome where the option to perform an expensive bone marrow transplant was extremely risky. This led to a deadlock in the discussion and decision-making. I intervened by ascertaining the decision thresholds of the baby's parents. The subsequent discussion using their decision thresholds helped to break the deadlock. They then made the right decision, saving their child's life.

To ascertain the patient's decision thresholds, the doctor combines 3 factors:

1. Their knowledge of the usual costs, risks and benefits of each decision,

2. Their estimates of the probability of the costs, risks and benefits for those same decisions for that unique patient, and

3. That unique patient's perspective.

To be consistently accurate in the 2nd factor, requires a minimum of proficiency in the basics of universal clinical reasoning. Without this accuracy, the doctor can easily be wrong in ascertaining the patient's decision thresholds and then mislead the patient during the decision-making. This is 1 example of the necessity of great skill in the basics if a doctor wishes to use advanced-level reasoning.

If and when basic universal clinical reasoning becomes widespread, a book on advanced-level reasoning may be worth writing.

REFERENCES

These are the most relevant references for this book.

Introduction

1. Yazdani S, Hosseinzadeh M, Hosseini F. Models of clinical reasoning with a focus on general practice: A critical review. *J Adv Med Educ Prof.* 2017 Oct; 5(4):177–84. PMID: 28979912; PMCID: PMC5611427.

2. Tikkanen R, Abrams MK. U.S. health care spending from a global perspective, 2019: higher spending, worse outcomes? https://www.commonwealthfund.org/publications/issue-briefs/2020/jan/us-health-care-global-perspective-2019

3. Hertwig R, Meier N, Nickel C, Zimmermann PC, Ackermann S, Woike JK, Bingisser R. Correlates of diagnostic accuracy in patients with nonspecific complaints. *Med Decis Making.* 2013 May; 33(4):533–43. doi: 10.1177/0272989X12470975. PMID: 23295544.

4. Meyer AN, Payne VL, Meeks DW, Rao R, Singh H. Physicians' diagnostic accuracy, confidence, and resource requests: a vignette study. *JAMA Intern Med.* 2013 Nov 25; 173(21):1952–8. doi: 10.1001/jamainternmed.2013.10081. PMID: 23979070.

5. Schewe JC, Kappler J, Dovermann K, Graeff I, Ehrentraut SF, Heister U, Hoeft A, Weber SU, Muenster S. Diagnostic accuracy of physician-staffed emergency medical teams: a retrospective observational cohort study of prehospital versus hospital diagnosis in a 10-year interval. *Scand J Trauma Resusc Emerg Med*. 2019 Apr 2; 27(1):36. doi: 10.1186/s13049-019-0617-3. PMID: 30940205; PMCID: PMC6446382.

6. Pauker SG, Kassirer JP. The threshold approach to clinical decision making. *N Engl J Med*. 1980 May 15; 302(20):1109–17. doi: 10.1056/NEJM198005153022003. PMID: 7366635.

7. Morgan DJ, Pineles L, Owczarzak J, Magder L, Scherer L, Brown JP, Pfeiffer C, Terndrup C, Leykum L, Feldstein D, Foy A, Stevens D, Koch C, Masnick M, Weisenberg S, Korenstein D. Accuracy of practitioner estimates of probability of diagnosis before and after testing. *JAMA Intern Med*. 2021 Jun 1; 181(6):747–55. doi: 10.1001/jamainternmed.2021.0269. PMID: 33818595; PMCID: PMC8022260.

8. Cooper N, Bartlett M, Gay S, Hammond A, Lillicrap M, Matthan J, Singh M; UK Clinical Reasoning in Medical Education (CReME) consensus statement group. Consensus statement on the content of clinical reasoning curricula in undergraduate medical education. *Med Teach*. 2021 Feb; 43(2):152–59. doi: 10.1080/0142159X.2020.1842343. PMID: 33205693.

The initial information, categories of diagnostic information, and illness scripts

9. Ericsson, KA, Krampe, RT, Tesch-Römer C. The role of deliberate practice in the acquisition of expert performance. *Psychol Rev*. 1993; 100(3):363–406.

10. Ericsson, KA. The danger of delegating education to journalists. https://radicalscholarship.com/2014/11/03/guest-post-the-danger-of-delegating-education-to-journalists-k-anders-ericsson/

Pathophysiology in reasoning

11. Höck M, Zelger B, Schweigmann G, Brunner B, Zelger B, Kropshofer G, Kiechl-Kohlendorfer U. The various clinical spectra of juvenile xanthogranuloma:

imaging for two case reports and review of the literature. *BMC Pediatr.* 2019 Apr 24; 19(1):128. doi: 10.1186/s12887-019-1490-y. PMID: 31018833; PMCID: PMC6482499.

Anticipatory care

12. Lennerz BS, Mey JT, Henn OH, Ludwig DS. Behavioral characteristics and self-reported health status among 2029 adults consuming a "carnivore diet". *Curr Dev Nutr.* 2021 Nov 2; 5(12):nzab133. doi: 10.1093/cdn/nzab133. PMID: 34934897; PMCID: PMC8684475.

13. The carnivore diet: a beefy leap of faith. https://www.mcgill.ca/oss/article/health-nutrition/carnivore-diet-beefy-leap-faith.

14. Ham OK, Lee BG. Screen time and cardiovascular risks among middle-aged women. *J Cardiovasc Nurs.* 2019 Nov/Dec; 34(6):474–82. doi: 10.1097/JCN.0000000000000598. PMID: 31373954.

15. Lissak G. Adverse physiological and psychological effects of screen time on children and adolescents: literature review and case study. *Environ Res.* 2018 Jul; 164:149–57. doi: 10.1016/j.envres.2018.01.015. PMID: 29499467.

16. Madigan S, Browne D, Racine N, Mori C, Tough S. Association between screen time and children's performance on a developmental screening test. *JAMA Pediatr.* 2019 Mar 1; 173(3):244–50. doi: 10.1001/jamapediatrics.2018.5056. Erratum in: *JAMA Pediatr.* 2019 May 1; 173(5):501–2. PMID: 30688984; PMCID: PMC6439882.

17. Violence in the media: psychologists study potential harmful effects. https://www.apa.org/topics/video-games/violence-harmful-effects.

18. Hensch TK, Bilimoria PM. Re-opening windows: manipulating critical periods for brain development. *Cerebrum.* 2012 Jul; 2012:11. PMID: 23447797; PMCID: PMC3574806.

19. Santos RMS, Mendes CG, Marques Miranda D, Romano-Silva MA. The association between screen time and attention in children: a systematic review. *Dev Neuropsychol.* 2022 Jul; 47(4):175–92. doi: 10.1080/87565641.2022.2064863. PMID: 35430923.

20. Kushima M, Kojima R, Shinohara R, Horiuchi S, Otawa S, Ooka T, Akiyama Y, Miyake K, Yokomichi H, Yamagata Z; Japan Environment and Children's

Study Group. Association between screen time exposure in children at 1 year of age and autism spectrum disorder at 3 years of age: the Japan Environment and Children's Study. *JAMA Pediatr.* 2022 Apr 1; 176(4):384–91. doi: 10.1001/jamapediatrics.2021.5778. PMID: 35099540; PMCID: PMC8804971.

Quiz: clinical approach

21. Jariwala S, Langman Y, Benson AA, Wolf E, Moss J, Zhu CC, Brandt L. Strongyloidiasis presenting as eosinophilic ascites. *Ann Trop Med Parasitol.* 2011 Jun; 105(4):335–8. doi: 10.1179/136485911X12987676649863. PMID: 21871171; PMCID: PMC4090796.

Interpreting test results

22. Helweg-Larsen J, Astradsson A, Richhall H, Erdal J, Laursen A, Brennum J. Pyogenic brain abscess, a 15 year survey. *BMC Infect Dis.* 2012 Nov 30; 12:332. doi: 10.1186/1471-2334-12-332. PMID: 23193986; PMCID: PMC3536615.

Diagnosis: disease, severity and treatment

23. DREAM (Diabetes REduction Assessment with ramipril and rosiglitazone Medication) Trial Investigators, Gerstein HC, Yusuf S, Bosch J, Pogue J, Sheridan P, Dinccag N, Hanefeld M, Hoogwerf B, Laakso M, Mohan V, Shaw J, Zinman B, Holman RR. Effect of rosiglitazone on the frequency of diabetes in patients with impaired glucose tolerance or impaired fasting glucose: a randomised controlled trial. *Lancet.* 2006 Sep 23; 368(9541): 1096–105. doi: 10.1016/S0140-6736(06)69420-8. Erratum in: Lancet. 2006 Nov 18;368(9549):1770. PMID: 16997664.

24. DREAM Trial Investigators. Incidence of diabetes following ramipril or rosiglitazone withdrawal. *Diabetes Care.* 2011 Jun; 34(6):1265–9. doi: 10.2337/dc10-1567. Epub 2011 Apr 22. PMID: 21515846; PMCID: PMC3114353.

25. Horimukai K, Morita K, Narita M, Kondo M, Kitazawa H, Nozaki M, Shigematsu Y, Yoshida K, Niizeki H, Motomura K, Sago H, Takimoto T, Inoue E, Kamemura N, Kido H, Hisatsune J, Sugai M, Murota H, Katayama I, Sasaki T, Amagai M, Morita H, Matsuda A, Matsumoto K, Saito H, Ohya Y. Application of moisturiser to neonates prevents development of atopic

dermatitis. *J Allergy Clin Immunol.* 2014 Oct; 134(4):824–30.e6. doi: 10.1016/j.jaci.2014.07.060. PMID: 25282564.

26. Simpson EL, Chalmers JR, Hanifin JM, Thomas KS, Cork MJ, McLean WH, Brown SJ, Chen Z, Chen Y, Williams HC. Emollient enhancement of the skin barrier from birth offers effective atopic dermatitis prevention. *J Allergy Clin Immunol.* 2014 Oct; 134(4):818–23. doi: 10.1016/j.jaci.2014.08.005. PMID: 25282563; PMCID: PMC4180007.

27. Chalmers JR, Haines RH, Bradshaw LE, Montgomery AA, Thomas KS, Brown SJ, Ridd MJ, Lawton S, Simpson EL, Cork MJ, Sach TH, Flohr C, Mitchell EJ, Swinden R, Tarr S, Davies-Jones S, Jay N, Kelleher MM, Perkin MR, Boyle RJ, Williams HC; BEEP study team. Daily emollient during infancy for prevention of eczema: the BEEP randomised controlled trial. *Lancet.* 2020 Mar 21; 395(10228):962–72. doi: 10.1016/S0140-6736(19)32984-8. Epub 2020 Feb 19. PMID: 32087126; PMCID: PMC7086156.

28. Ng PSM, Wee LWY, Ho VPY, Tan WC, Bishnoi P, Alagappan U, Wong SMY, Gan EY, Quek BH, Shen L, Su B, Common JE, Koh MJA. Moisturisers from birth in at-risk infants of atopic dermatitis — a pragmatic randomised controlled trial. *Australas J Dermatol.* 2021 Nov; 62(4):e539–e545. doi: 10.1111/ajd.13703. Epub 2021 Aug 23. PMID: 34424533; PMCID: PMC9291182.

29. Pendharkar S, Mehta S. The clinical significance of exhaled nitric oxide in asthma. *Can Respir J.* 2008 Mar; 15(2):99–106. doi: 10.1155/2008/463762. PMID: 18354750; PMCID: PMC2677842.

30. Song WJ, Kim HJ, Shim JS, Won HK, Kang SY, Sohn KH, Kim BK, Jo EJ, Kim MH, Kim SH, Park HW, Kim SS, Chang YS, Morice AH, Lee BJ, Cho SH. Diagnostic accuracy of fractional exhaled nitric oxide measurement in predicting cough-variant asthma and eosinophilic bronchitis in adults with chronic cough: a systematic review and meta-analysis. *J Allergy Clin Immunol.* 2017 Sep; 140(3):701–9. doi: 10.1016/j.jaci.2016.11.037. PMID: 28088474.

Applied clinical reasoning for improved healthcare

31. Payares-Salamanca L, Contreras-Arrieta S, Florez-García V, Barrios-Sanjuanelo A, Stand-Niño I, Rodriguez-Martinez CE. Metered-dose inhalers versus nebulization for the delivery of albuterol for acute exacerbations of

wheezing or asthma in children: a systematic review with meta-analysis. *Pediatr Pulmonol.* 2020 Dec; 55(12):3268–78. doi: 10.1002/ppul.25077. PMID: 32940961.

32. Iramain R, Castro-Rodriguez JA, Jara A, Cardozo L, Bogado N, Morinigo R, De Jesús R. Salbutamol and ipratropium by inhaler is superior to nebulizer in children with severe acute asthma exacerbation: randomized clinical trial. *Pediatr Pulmonol.* 2019 Apr; 54(4):372–77. doi: 10.1002/ppul.24244. PMID: 30672140.

33. Lin HL, Restrepo RD, Gardenhire DS, Rau JL. Effect of face mask design on inhaled mass of nebulized albuterol, using a pediatric breathing model. *Respir Care.* 2007 Aug; 52(8):1021–6. PMID: 17650358.

34. Lavorini F. The challenge of delivering therapeutic aerosols to asthma patients. *ISRN Allergy.* 2013 Aug 5; 2013:102418. doi: 10.1155/2013/102418. PMID: 23984095; PMCID: PMC3747606.

35. Burger C, Vendiola DF, Arnold DH. Nebulized albuterol delivery is associated with decreased skeletal muscle strength in comparison with metered-dose inhaler delivery among children with acute asthma exacerbations. *J Am Coll Emerg Physicians Open.* 2021 Apr 8; 2(2):e12422. doi: 10.1002/emp2.12422. PMID: 33855311; PMCID: PMC8032924.

36. Cates CJ, Welsh EJ, Rowe BH. Holding chambers (spacers) versus nebulisers for beta-agonist treatment of acute asthma. *Cochrane Database Syst Rev.* 2013 Sep 13; 2013(9):CD000052. doi: 10.1002/14651858.CD000052.pub3. PMID: 24037768; PMCID: PMC7032675.

37. Fidler L, Green S, Wintemute K. Pressurized metered-dose inhalers and their impact on climate change. *Can Med Assoc J.* 2022 Mar 28; 194(12):E460. doi: 10.1503/cmaj.211747. PMID: 35347049; PMCID: PMC8967439.

Tiers of performance

38. Carley B. The surprising benefits of being an introvert. *Time.* 2018 Aug 27. https://time.com/5373403/surprising-benefits-introvert/

39. Cain S. Quiet: the power of introverts in a world that can't stop talking. *Crown.* 2013 Jan 29.

Theoretical disease approaches

40. Tse SM, Silverman ED, McCrindle BW, Yeung RS. Early treatment with intravenous immunoglobulin in patients with Kawasaki disease. *J Pediatr.* 2002 Apr; 140(4):450–5. doi: 10.1067/mpd.2002.122469. PMID: 12006960.

41. van Stijn D, Korbee JM, Netea SA, de Winter VC, Zwinderman KAH, Kuipers IM, Kuijpers TW. Treatment and coronary artery aneurysm formation in Kawasaki disease: a per-day risk analysis. *J Pediatr.* 2022 Apr; 243:167–72. e1. doi: 10.1016/j.jpeds.2021.12.054. Epub 2021 Dec 27. PMID: 34968497.

42. Bar-Meir M, Kalisky I, Schwartz A, Somekh E, Tasher D; Israeli Kawasaki Group. Prediction of resistance to intravenous immunoglobulin in children with Kawasaki disease. *J Pediatric Infect Dis Soc.* 2018 Feb 19; 7(1):25–9. doi: 10.1093/jpids/piw075. PMID: 28062554.

43. Li X, Chen Y, Tang Y, Ding Y, Xu Q, Sun L, Qian W, Qian G, Qin L, Lv H. Predictors of intravenous immunoglobulin-resistant Kawasaki disease in children: a meta-analysis of 4442 cases. *Eur J Pediatr.* 2018 Aug; 177(8):1279–92. doi: 10.1007/s00431-018-3182-2. PMID: 29948255; PMCID: PMC6061038.

Guidelines and protocols

44. Baungaard N, Skovvang PL, Hvidt EA, Gerbild H, Andersen MK, Lykkegaard J. How defensive medicine is defined in European medical literature: a systematic review. *BMJ Open.* 2022 Jan 20; 12(1):e057169. doi: 10.1136/bmjopen-2021-057169. PMID: 35058268; PMCID: PMC8783809.

45. Ng SL, Thirumoorthy T. The current medico-legal climate and defensive medicine. https://www.sma.org.sg/UploadedImg/1631082437_2019Nov SMA%20CMEP.pdf

Additional resources

46. Xu H, Ang BWG, Soh JY, Ponnamperuma GG. Methods to improve diagnostic reasoning in undergraduate medical education in the clinical setting: a systematic review. *J Gen Intern Med.* 2021 Sep; 36(9):2745–54. doi: 10.1007/s11606-021-06916-0. PMID: 34159542; PMCID: PMC8390726.

How this came about

47. Mueller JS, Melwani S, Goncalo JA. The bias against creativity: why people desire but reject creative ideas. *Psychol Sci.* 2012 Jan 1; 23(1):13–7. doi: 10.1177/0956797611421018. PMID: 22127366.

48. Devereaux PJ, Anderson DR, Gardner MJ, Putnam W, Flowerdew GJ, Brownell BF, Nagpal S, Cox JL. Differences between perspectives of physicians and patients on anticoagulation in patients with atrial fibrillation: observational study. *BMJ.* 2001 Nov 24; 323(7323):1218–22. doi: 10.1136/bmj.323.7323.1218. PMID: 11719412; PMCID: PMC59994.

ACKNOWLEDGEMENTS

I thank my patients. This book would not have been possible without them.

I thank my trainees, who made me a better teacher. Special thanks go to Doctors Xu Hongyun, Benson Ang, Valencia Long, Cheryl Chong, Annushkha Sinnathamby and Nicholas Ng for their passion for excellent healthcare. They were instrumental in refining this model and encouraging me to write this book.

Thanks to Professor Lau Tang Ching, the Vice-Dean of the Yong Loo Lin School of Medicine, National University of Singapore. In February 2018, it was he who put out the call for teaching reasoning and has since supported my efforts to promulgate clinical reasoning.

Thanks to the National University of Singapore's Edutech team, especially Nyssa Ho and Esther Tan, who patiently worked and reworked the initial video courses over the years. Feedback on those videos further refined the content of this book.

Thanks to Professor Chen Zhi Xiong, Assistant Dean of the Yong Loo Lin School of Medicine, National University of Singapore. He has passionately advocated for pathophysiology in clinical reasoning, and has been supportive of teaching clinical reasoning too. It was he who linked me up with Bao Truong and Med2Lab.

Thanks to Bao Truong, founder of Med2Lab. He is a passionate and foresighted co-worker and leader, on the cases in the virtual patient platform. Many fruitful discussions on the presentation of the cases sharpened my awareness for this book.

Thanks to my excellent senior colleagues and role models in patient care. Special mention goes to Professors Abu Rauff, Low Cheng Hock, Raja C Rajasoorya, Zubair Amin, Lee Jiun, Lee Bee Wah and Yap Hui Kim.

Two of the generalists deserve special thanks. Professor Yeshwant Amdekar is highly skilled in teaching pathophysiology in clinical medicine. I regret never having met Professor Wong Hock Boon, but had the opportunity to peruse the many volumes he typed about diseases.

I thank the National University Hospital of Singapore, where I gained much experience and insight while caring for patients.

I thank Mr Lam Nam Soon from Raffles Institution, for his crucial advice long before I entered medical school. Rest in peace.

Thanks to my family for supporting me in many ways while I wrote this book.

Thanks to the World Scientific Publishing team for working with me to publish this book. They promptly responded to my requests; in my experience, it is rare to meet a team that consistently replies within 24 hours. They patiently put up with my many queries (I am new to writing books). Joy Quek and Gregory Lee deserve special mention in this regard.

Lastly, I thank everyone else who supported my endeavours to refine and teach clinical reasoning over the years.

ABOUT THE AUTHOR

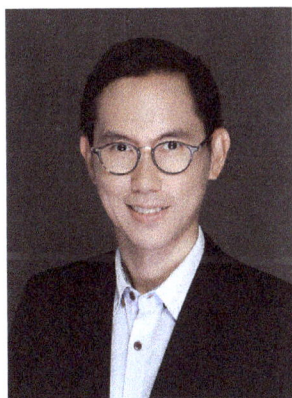

Born in 1980, Soh Jian Yi passed through Raffles Institution and Raffles Junior College. He graduated from medical school at the National University of Singapore in 2004.

In 2006, at the behest of Professor Yap Hui Kim, he joined the Department of Paediatrics, National University Hospital of Singapore.

He juggled his official paediatrics training with his creation and refining of the technique of universal clinical reasoning. He completed his basic specialist training in 2012 and has been working in the Division of Allergy and Immunology in the Department ever since. He sees patients with atopic diseases, allergies and immunodeficiency disorders, as well as children in the hospital wards who have a broad range of illnesses.

He founded the first clinical service providing oral immunotherapy for food allergies in Singapore in 2015. This service has been recognised by the global non-profit OIT101 network.

As Core Faculty of his department's residency program, he holds the portfolios of clinical reasoning and evidence-based medicine.

He created the Universal Clinical Reasoning videos in 2019. These were incorporated into the curriculum of the Masters of Nursing program at the Alice Lee School of Nursing in the university and the postgraduate year-1 program for all doctors joining the National University Hospital. He is the lead teacher for clinical reasoning in these programs.

He was a regular contributor to *The Straits Times* of Singapore on health issues and a volunteer with TOUCH Community Services. His physical fitness regime includes working out in the gym, twice a week.

INDEX

www.ingramcontent.com/pod-product-compliance
Lightning Source LLC
Chambersburg PA
CBHW070709220326
41598CB00026B/3676